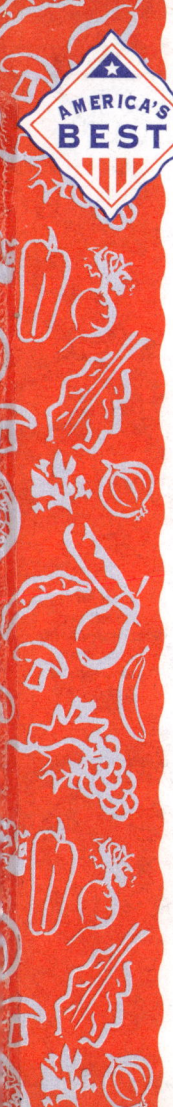

Contents

- ▶ **WEIGHT CONTROL GUIDE** 2-19
- ▶ **CALORIE & FAT COUNTER**
  - Milk, Soy, Yogurt 20-22
  - Icecream & Ice Confections 23-28
  - Fats, Oils, Cream, Cheese, Eggs 29-36
  - Meats, Poultry, Fish 37-48
  - Frozen & Packaged Meals 49-62
  - Soups, Sauces, Dressings 63-76
  - Breakfast Cereals, Rice, Pasta 77-82
  - Bread, Crackers, Cookies 83-89
  - Cakes, Pastries, Pies, Baking 90-95
  - Pancakes, Puddings, Desserts 96-97
  - Sugar, Syrups 98-99
  - Candy, Chocolate, Snacks 100-107
  - Nuts, Fruits, Vegetables 108-122
  - Beverages: Coffee, Tea, Sports, Soda ...123-132
  - Alcohol: Beer, Wine, Spirits, Cocktails ...123-132
  - Restaurant & Ethnic Foods 133-138
- ▶ **FAST-FOOD CHAINS & RESTAURANT SECTION** 139-218
- ▶ **DIET GUIDES & COUNTERS**
  - Alcohol Guide & Counter 128-132
  - Caffeine Guide & Counter 224-225
  - Diabetes & Weight Control 17-18
  - Fats & Cholesterol Guide 219-223
  - Fiber Guide & Counter 232-237
  - Osteoporosis Guide & Calcium Counter ..226-227
  - Protein & Iron Guide & Counter 238-243
  - Salt, Hypertension & Sodium Counter ...244-249
- ▶ **INDEX** 250-255

BODY FAT DISTRIBUTION & HEALTH

BODY FAT DISTRIBUTION & HEALTH

Fat above the hips carries a far greater health risk than fat on or below the hips - better to be a '**pear-shape**' than an '**apple-shape**'.

Abdominal obesity greatly increases the risk of developing diabetes, coronary heart disease, high blood fats, hypertension, stroke and some cancers.

Visceral Fat Versus Subcutaneous Fat

Specifically, it is an excess of **visceral fat** (which surrounds organs in the abdomen) that is a potential health danger. Visceral fat is more metabolically active; and is much easier to shed than fat on the hips and buttocks.

By contrast, **subcutaneous fat** (just beneath the skin and including fat on the hips, thighs and buttocks), carries a relatively minor health risk, if any. So-called '**cellulite**' carries no extra health risk.

The relative amount of visceral and subcutaneous fat varies greatly between individuals and is genetically determined - and while not distinguishable by eye, waist circumference still best indicates health risk.

WAIST MEASUREMENTS
~ HIGH HEALTH RISK ~
- Men - Waist above 39 inches
- Women - Waist above 34 inches

Abdominal obesity greatly increases the risk of ill-health and earlier death.

INCREASED RISK

Diabetes (x30), Heart Attack (x5)
Stroke (x11), Endometrial Cancer (x15).
Breast Cancer (x2), Gall Stones (x2)
High Blood Pressure (x3) Arthritis (x4)

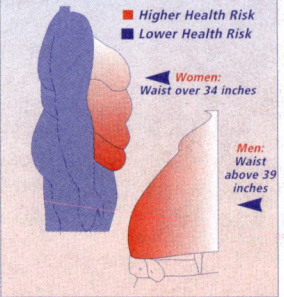

- Higher Health Risk
- Lower Health Risk

◄ Women: Waist over 34 inches

Men: Waist above 39 inches ◄

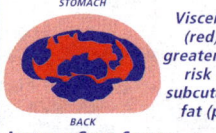

STOMACH

BACK

ABDOMEN: CROSS-SECTION

Visceral fat (red) is a greater health risk than subcutaneous fat (pink).

WOMEN'S HIPS & THIGHS

The fat in women's thighs serves the biological function of an energy storehouse were a famine to occur during pregnancy or lactation.

Women who become obsessed with dieting away their thighs and buttocks on an otherwise lean body, are fighting mother nature and may well be inviting health problems.

If you are within a healthy weight range, it is better to exercise regularly to maintain body shape, rather than to be constantly dieting and lacking in energy. Accept your body shape and focus on other pursuits and enjoying life!

Fat in women's hips and thighs is not a health risk.

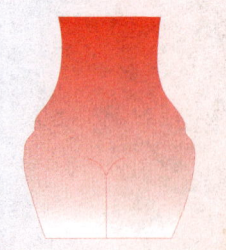

WEIGHT CONTROL TIPS

✓ EAT SENSIBLY

- Avoid fad diets. Eat 3 sensible meals daily.
- Limit fats and fatty foods
- Limit alcohol

(Sample Diet Plans, Page 11)

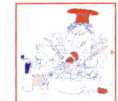

✓ EXERCISE DAILY

Exercise religiously every day!

Regular exercisers lose more fat and keep it off. You'll feel and look better, and can eat a little more food. *(See Page 13)*

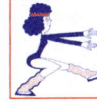

✓ RESHAPING EATING BEHAVIORS

Especially those behaviors that lead you to over-eat and compulsively snack. *(Extra Notes - Page 14)*

✓ KEEP A FOOD & EXERCISE DIARY

- A diary helps you see exactly what you eat and drink, and your exercise habits.
- An excellent motivator
- Keeps you honest! *(Page 15)*

✓ ARRANGE MORAL SUPPORT

Gain the support of family and friends. Get extra professional help if required, from your doctor, dietitian, psychologist, exercise trainer, or slimming group. Beware of family saboteurs!

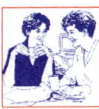

DOCTOR CHECK-UP

Ask your doctor to check you for high blood pressure, diabetes, and high blood cholesterol.

HEALTHY WEIGHTS FOR MEN AND WOMEN
(Over 18 Years)

- Based on weights with least risk of disease or death from heart disease, diabetes, stroke and cancer.
- Based on Body Mass Index - range 20-25.

BMI calculated as: $\frac{Weight\ (kg)}{Height\ (m)^2}$

HEIGHT (No Shoes)	HEALTHY WEIGHT RANGE
Ft Ins	Pounds
4'7"	86-108
4'8"	88-110
4'9"	92-114
4'10"	97-121
4'11"	99-123
5'0"	101-127
5'1"	105-132
5'2"	110-136
5'3"	112-140
5'4"	114-145
5'5"	199-149
5'6"	123-156
5'7"	127-158
5'8"	129-162
5'9"	134-167
5'10"	138-173
5'11"	143-178
6'0"	145-182
6'1"	149-187
6"2"	156-193
6'3"	158-198
6'4"	162-202
6'5'	170-211
6'6"	172-215
6'7"	175-220

RECOMMENDED FAT INTAKE

FAT IN THE DIET

- Fats in the diet are essential for good health. However, too much fat can contribute to obesity, and a higher risk of heart disease, high blood pressure, diabetes, gall stones and certain cancers.

- Dietary fats/oils have over double the calories of carbohydrates and protein:

CALORIE VALUES PER GRAM		
Carbohydrate	~	4 Calories
Protein	~	4 Calories
Fat/Oil	~	9 Calories
Alcohol	~	7 Calories

- **Dietary fat** is more readily converted to and stored as body fat compared to carbohydrates and protein.

- **Excess carbohydrates** over body needs may also be converted and stored as body fat - especially in women in their fertile years when extra fat pads are more readily laid down in the thighs and buttocks.

- **Excess alcohol** lessens the body's ability to burn fat. Fat storage is promoted, particularly in the belly - a danger zone.

RECOMMENDED FAT INTAKE

Americans consume too much fat with many having over 40% of total calories from fat - either as fat or oil, or as fat in foods and drinks A range of 20-30% is considered healthier.

FAT INTAKE - HEALTHY RANGES		
Children	~	30-60g
Teenagers (Active)	~	40-80g
Women	~	30-60g
Men: Active	~	40-80g
Heavy Activity/Athlete	~	80-120g

The chart below shows the recommended maximum fat intake for different calorie levels.

INFANTS FAT INTAKE

Infants and toddlers under 3 years should not be restricted in their fat intake because much larger volumes of food would be required to guarantee adequate calorie intake and growth. Whole milk should be used rather than light milk (1%) or nonfat milk.

Similarly, a high fiber diet is also not suitable for infants.

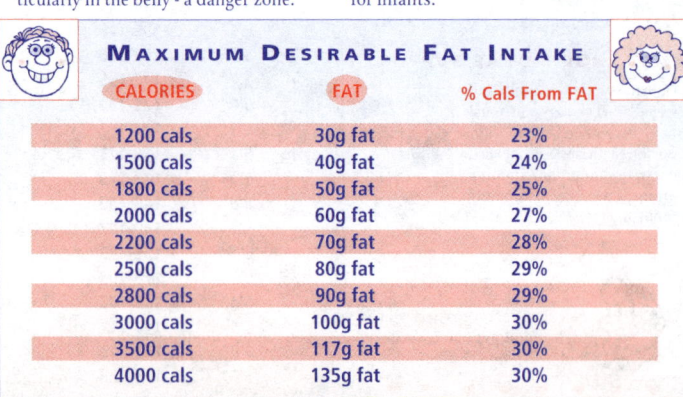

MAXIMUM DESIRABLE FAT INTAKE

CALORIES	FAT	% Cals From FAT
1200 cals	30g fat	23%
1500 cals	40g fat	24%
1800 cals	50g fat	25%
2000 cals	60g fat	27%
2200 cals	70g fat	28%
2500 cals	80g fat	29%
2800 cals	90g fat	29%
3000 cals	100g fat	30%
3500 cals	117g fat	30%
4000 cals	135g fat	30%

FAT PERCENTAGES

PERCENTAGE OF CALORIES FROM FAT

While health authorities recommend that not more than 30% of our total food calories should come from fat, it is not implied nor even recommended that you eat only those foods with less than 30% calories from fat.

Our normal diet is made up of foods that are either well above or below 30%. Only on average should the total diet be less than 30% calories from fat.

Some higher fat foods such as avocados, nuts and seeds, are highly nutritious and favor lower blood cholesterol levels. **Moderation is the aim . . . not elimination.**

Nevertheless, knowing the percentage of calories from fat can be useful in spotting high-fat foods and drinks.

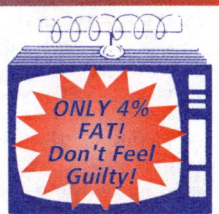

PERCENT FAT CONTENT IN FOODS

Don't be fooled by promotion of foods claiming to have a low percentage of fat. It's serving size and total grams of fat that count.

For example, whole milk with 3.5% fat sounds low (3.5g fat/100ml) but an 8fl.oz cup contains 8g fat (and 2 cups contain 16g fat).

Icecream with 10% fat seems high, yet a medium scoop (3fl.oz) has only 5g fat. (Low-fat icecream has less than 2g fat/serve.)

❖   ❖   ❖

Also note that the percentage of fat in a food is not the same as the percentage of calories derived from fat.

Foods with a low percentage of fat can still have a high percentage of calories derived from fat - as shown below.

For example, almost 50% of total calories in whole milk comes from fat - yet whole milk has less than 4% fat. Lowfat/light milk with less than 1% fat has only 18% of total calories from fat - a much better choice.

FORMULA FOR CALCULATING PERCENTAGE CALORIES FROM FAT

$$\frac{\text{Grams of Fat/Serve} \times 9}{\text{Total Calories/Serve}} \times \frac{100}{1}$$

EXAMPLE:
Mars Bar (11g fat, 240 cals)

Percentage Calories from Fat

$$= \frac{11 \times 9}{240} \times \frac{100}{1}$$

$$= 41\%$$

FAT CONTENT & PERCENTAGES OF MILK

	WHOLE MILK	REDUCED FAT	LOW-FAT (LIGHT)	NON-FAT (SKIM)
Percent Fat	3.5%	2%	1%	0%
Fat (Grams) in 8fl.oz. Cup	8g	5g	2g	0g
Calories	150	120	100	95
Percent Calories From Fat	48%	38%	18%	0%

HINTS TO REDUCE FAT

MEATS & POULTRY

- **Choose lean cuts** of meat with little marbling. Choose the white meat of chicken and turkey, and extra lean ground beef. Avoid organ meats.
- **Trim all visible fat** from met and remove the skin from poultry.
- **Eat modest portions** (3-4 oz cooked weight) of meat, poultry or fish. **Add extra** beans, lentils, tofu, tempeh, vegetables, potatoes, rice, pasta, bread, bagels, plain tortillas.
- **Avoid high-fat meat products;** e.g. salami, bacon, sausage, frankfurters. Choose lean luncheon meats (90% or more fat-free).
- **Broil or bake. Avoid frying.** Allow casseroles to cool and skim off any surface fat.

FISH & SEAFOODS

- **Choose fresh or frozen fillets,** canned fish (in water pack).
- **Avoid fried fish,** frozen fish in batter, canned fish in oil.

FATS & OILS

- **Use minimal amounts** of all types of fat and oil. All are high in calories.
- **Avoid** butter, lard, dripping, ghee, margarine (other than polyunsaturated).
- **Avoid** coconut oil and hydrogenated palm oil products. (Regular palm oil does not raise blood cholesterol).
- **Choose** fat-reduced polyunsaturated or canola margarines. Use polyunsaturated oils or monounsaturated oils (e.g. canola, olive) in moderation.
- Use minimal amounts of oil when stir-frying with a wok.

SALAD DRESSINGS & SAUCES

- **Limit mayonnaise and oil dressings.** Choose low-oil or fat-free dressings (e.g. *Hidden Valley Ranch, Kraft Free, Pritikin*).
- **Choose** lowfat or fat-free sauces.

MILK, DAIRY, SOY DRINKS

- **Choose** lowfat or skim milks and yogurts. **Avoid** full-cream milk, cream, *Half & Half* coffee creamers.
- **Soy Drinks:** Choose lowfat brands.
- **Choose:** Choose lowfat and fat-reduced (e.g. cottage, part-skim ricotta). Cheese substitutes can still be high in fat.
- **Icecream:** Choose lowfat milks, frozen yogurt, sorbet, sherbet and ices. Limit regular ice-cream to a small serving. Avoid rich high-fat icecreams.

FROZEN ENTREES & MEALS

- **Choose low fat varieties** such as *Lean Cuisine, Healthy Choice* and *Weight Watchers*.

FRYING ADDS FAT!

The greater the surface area of potato exposed to fat or oil, the higher the fat content.

Whole Potato (3oz))
Nil fat, 65 Cals/

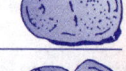

Roast Potato (3oz))
8g fat, 155 Cals

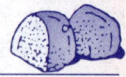

**French Fries
Large Cut (3 oz)**
12g fat, 220 Cals

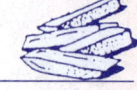

**French Fries
Small Cut (3oz)**
15g fat, 275 Cals

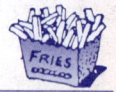

Potato Chips (3oz)
36g fat, 540 Cals

HINTS TO REDUCE FAT

BREADS, BAGELS, CRACKERS

- **All breads are suitable** as well as pita, bagels, English muffins and rice cakes. Avoid croissants, sweet rolls, danish pastry and doughnuts. **Avoid** fat-soaked toast and garlic bread.
- **Choose lowfat crackers** such as graham, saltines, matzo, bread sticks, crispbreads. **Avoid** regular cheese or butter crackers.

CEREALS, PASTA, RICE

- Most cold and hot cereals are low in fat and nil in cholesterol. Avoid granola made with hydrogenated oils.
- **Choose** plain pasta or rice. Avoid dishes made with cream, buitter or cheese sauces. **Avoid** high-fat ramen noodle blocks/soups.

FRUITS & VEGETABLES

- **Choose all types.** (Note: Avocados contain no cholesterol. Their fat and fiber can help lower blood cholesterol.) Use mashed avocado on bread in place of fat.
- **Choose** dried beans, lentils, chick peas, baked beans.
- **Avoid** french-fried potatoes and regular potato salad. Avoid vegetables made in butter, cream or sauce.
- **Avoid** deli-style salads made with high fat dressings. Use low-calorie salad dressings.

SNACKS, COOKIES & CANDY

- **Avoid** high-fat snacks such as potato chips, corn/tortilla chips, *Chee-Tos*, *Cheez Balls*, buttered popcorn, chocolate and carob bars.
- **Choose** plain popcorn, lowfat cookies and muffins, hard candy, jelly beans, fruit rolls and frozen fruit bars/popsicles.
- **Avoid** french-fried potatoes and regular potato salad. Avoid vegetables made in butter, cream or sauce.
- **Choose** fresh and dried fruits, vegetables. Limit nuts and seeds if overweight.

SNACKS, COOKIES (CONT)

- **Choose** low fat vegetable or noodle soups. Most *Cup-A-Soup* varieties are suitable.

DESSERTS/SWEETS

- **Avoid high-fat desserts**, e.g. fruit pies, pastries, cheesecake, cheese board.
- **Choose** fresh fruits, fresh fruit salad, low fat custard, yogurt, frozen yogurt, sorbet. Use yogurt in place of cream or ice cream.

FAST-FOODS & TAKE-OUT

(Check the Fast Foods Section of this book for actual fat counts and wise selections.)

- **Delis:** Choose sandwiches/bread rolls, pitas with low fat fillings and plain salad. Limit meat/cheese to small portions.

  Avoid high-fat diet salads. Choose plain salads and add your own low fat dressing. Eat more fruit.

- **Chicken & Fish:** Avoid deep-fried chicken or fish, BBQ chicken with fat or skin, chicken nuggets. Choose broiled or baked chicken breast without fat or skin.

- **Hamburgers:** Choose medium size, lower fat burgers. Avoid bacon. Have a side salad (without dressing).

- **Pizzas:** Avoid sausage/pepperoni. Choose vegetarian topping and modest quantity of cheese. Eat a moderate serving. Eat extra salad and fruit.

- **Desserts & Drinks:** Avoid apple pie, danish, choc chip cokies. Choose low fat muffins (e.g. *McDonald's*).

  Avoid regular shakes, sundaes. Choose lowfat milk, lower fat shakes (such as *McDonald's*), frozen yogurt, fruit salad and orange juice.

Hints To Reduce Sugar

- While reducing the amount of fat is an important dietary focus for weight control, sugar intake also needs to be watched.

- Many overweight, inactive persons consume over 500 calories of refined sugars per day (equivalent to over 30 level teaspoons) - a significant amount in weight control terms. Halving this amount would be reasonable and worthwhile.

Note: Naturally occurring sugars in fruits, vegetables and milk are fine when consumed in normal recommended amounts.

- Most sugar in our diet is 'hidden' in processed foods such as soft drinks, fruit drinks, candy, cookies, cake, jam, sauces, ice-cream, desserts, canned foods, and breakfast cereals.

Certainly enjoy moderate quantities of these foods, but for serious weight control, look for 'low calorie', 'diet' or sugar-free alternatives. Be careful not to substitute sugar-rich foods with high-fat foods which might boost calories even more!

- Sweeteners such as *Equal, NutraSweet,* and *Sweet'n Low* make it easy to greatly cut back on sugar we add to drinks and in recipes. (Most recipes can be adapted to contain less sugar with little effect on taste or quality.)

Reduced-calorie sweeteners (such as *Isomalt*) used by the food industry also expand our food choices and help limit sugar intake.

- The body can obtain sufficient sugar for its needs from carbohydrate-rich foods such as bread, rice, spaghetti and other pasta, potatoes, corn, fruit, vegetables, beans, nuts, seeds and lactose in milk.

These foods are also rich in other nutrients. Refined sugar is referred to as 'empty calorie' because it supplies calories but negligible nutrients and no fiber.

DIFFERENT FORMS OF SUGAR
*Be aware that sugar comes in different forms. Check the label.

- Sugar
- Brown Sugar
- Dextrose
- Fructose
- Corn Syrup
- Honey
- Maple Syrup
- Sucrose
- Confectioners' Sugar
- Glucose
- Malt, Maltose
- High-Fructose Corn Syrup
- Molasses
- Turbinado Sugar

SUGAR CONTENT OF SOME COMMON FOODS:

Food	Teaspoons of Sugar
Coca Cola; Pepsi, 12 oz	10
20 oz size	17
Iced tea, sweetened, 12 oz	8
Choc malted Milk, 12 oz	4.5
Honey Smacks Cereal, 1 oz	4
Popcorn, caramel, 1 cup	3.5
Chocolate Bar, 1.5 oz	6
M&M's, 1.7 oz pkg	7
Cake, sponge, jam-filled	8
Choc Chip Cookie, 1 oz	2
Donut, iced	6
Apple Pie, 1 piece	7
Jell-O, 1/2 cup	4.5
Jam, 1 Tbsp, 20g	2.5
Syrup, maple, 1 Tbsp	3

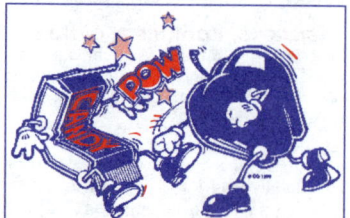

Reach for fresh fruit when you want to snack instead of candy or snack products rich in sugar and fat.

TEN DIETING HINTS

1. Avoid fad diets. They don't re-educate your eating habits. Eat 3 moderate-sized meals daily that are nutritionally balanced. (Sample Eating Plan ~ Next Page)

2. Carefully plan each meal rather than just grabbing haphazardly whatever comes into your line of vision. Keep a food diary. (See Page 15)

3. Don't skip meals. You are more likely to snack on high calorie, high-fat foods.

4. Use minimal amounts of fat and oil. Trim fat from meat, and skin from poultry. Use lowfat dairy products and low calorie salad dressings. Use fat-free cooking methods. Avoid fried foods, high-fat snacks and high-fat fast foods, cookies, cakes and icecream. Limit nuts.

Note: Changing to lower fat foods is not a licence to eat larger quantities. Ultimately, it is the total calories that count. (Remember, cows get fat on grass!)

5. Avoid sugar and foods high in sugar such as soft drinks, fruit drinks, jams, chocolate, cookies, cakes, icecream and ice confections. Use sugar substitutes and sugar-free diet products.

6. Eat adequate fresh fruits, vegetables and wholegrain cereal products. They are healthy, filling and their fiber helps to prevent constipation.

7. There is no food that cannot occasionally be eaten; e.g. chocolate, cake, dessert, wine. It is the quantity that is critical. Total deprivation can lead to bingeing. (Also see 'Reshaping Eating Behavior' ~ P. 14)

8. Avoid alcohol when dieting. Alcohol may lessen the body's ability to burn fat and promote fat strorage. (See Alcohol Guide ~ Page ??).

9. When dining out, avoid fried and sauce-laden dishes as well as pastries, regular salad dressings and desserts. Eat moderately. Quench your thirst on water, mineral water or low calorie diet drinks.

10. Take a multi-vitamin and mineral supplement when dieting particularly if tired and irritable.

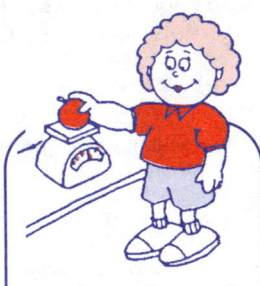

Weigh your food until you can accurately estimate food portion sizes. Better control of calories will result.

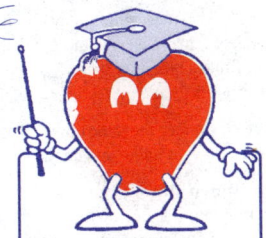

Eating a high fiber breakfast gives you a good start to the day ...and helps prevent high calorie snacking.

Desirable lower calorie snacks include apples, oranges, carrot sticks and plain popcorn.

BODY WEIGHT VARIATIONS

BODY WEIGHT VARIATIONS

- Misinterpretation of weight changes is a constant source of frustration amongst dieters. Weight changes are rarely the result of changes only in fatty tissue.

- **Day to day weight fluctuations result** mainly from changes in body fluid/water levels - which, for example, can be affected by the amount of salt, carbohydrate or water in the diet, by hormonal changes (e.g. monthly period), or the amount of exercise.

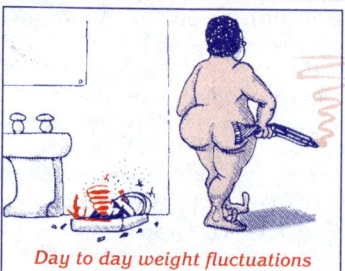

Day to day weight fluctuations are due to body fluid variations

- **Weight change over several weeks** is more likely to reflect changes in body levels of fat and muscle - rather than fluid. Unfortunately, the scales do not distinguish between weight changes due to water, fat or muscle.

While weekly weighing may eliminate this dilemma, many people find the daily weighing ritual a reminder that weight control is a daily event that requires daily attention.

Weigh at much the same time of day, in similar clothing or nude - and on the same scales.

- **When dining out,** be aware that the extra pound or two that might show on the scales the next morning, is not necessarily the result of a **small** dietary indiscretion. It is more likely to be due to **fluid retention** resulting from the more highly seasoned and salted food - or a large dietary indiscretion!

Of course, it is important to drink adequate water when thirsty.

When dining out, a glass of wine is fine but quench your thirst on water, mineral water or diet soda drinks.

PLATEAUS... THE DIETER'S BANE!

- The 'plateau' is possibly an example of how the body adapts to a famine situation. Weight may be static for several weeks after initial weight losses.

  The body's metabolism slows down to preserve as much body mass as possible - a welcome situation in a famine, but not appreciated by the dieter!

  So, treat plateaus as a rest period for the body to adjust to the weight loss.

- **Self-discipline and perseverance** are the keys to success. The longer the plateau, the closer you are to getting to the next phase of weight loss. Now, that's positive thinking!

- **Regular exercise is important.** If you have not been exercising, now is an excellent time to start. It could make all the difference (especially if you add in strength training.)

Note: Weight on the scales does not tell the complete story, particularly as you approach your ideal weight. Fatty tissue losses from increased exercise may be cancelled on the scales by muscle gains - a healthy situation. Weight can be static even though you are still losing inches and reshaping your body. Body fat determinations will give more insight.

SAMPLE EATING PLAN - 1200 CALORIES

(FOR OVERWEIGHT, INACTIVE PERSONS. CHECK WITH YOUR DOCTOR)
(Contains approximately 30 - 35 Grams Fat)

BREAKFAST (Approx. 250 cal)
1 small Fruit or ½oz Dried Fruit
Plus Cereal: 1½oz Dry (high fiber)
or 1 cup cooked, e.g. Oatmeal
Plus Milk (from daily allowance)

BREAKFAST - CHOICE 2
1 small Fruit
Plus 1 Egg (no added fat)
or 20g Cheese
or 60g Cottage Cheese
or 75g, ¼ c., Baked Beans
Plus 1 Toast or ½ EnglishMuffin

MILK ALLOWANCE (160 Calories)
2 cups Skim Milk or 1½ cups Low Fat Milk
or equivalent Soy Milk, Yogurt, Cheese, Tofu

FAT ALLOWANCE (140 Calories; 15g Fat)
4 tsp Fat or 6-8 tsp Diet Margarine or 3 tsp Oil
or 1½ Tbsp Mayonnaise or ½ medium Avocado
or 1½ Tbsp Peanut Butter or 30g Nuts/Seeds

LUNCH (Approx. 440 Calories)
2 slices Bread (2 oz) or 1 medium Roll or 1 Bagel
or 4 Crispbreads/Crackers 6" Pita
Plus 2 oz lean Meat, Chicken or Turkey
or 3½oz Tuna (in water) or 70g Salmon
or 1oz Cheese or 3 oz Cottage Cheese
or 2½oz Ricotta Cheese
or ½ cup, 120g Fruit Yoghurt (lowfat)
or ½ cup (4 oz) Baked Beans or Bean Salad
Plus Large Salad (oil-free dressing)
Plus 1 small Fruit or ½oz Dried Fruit

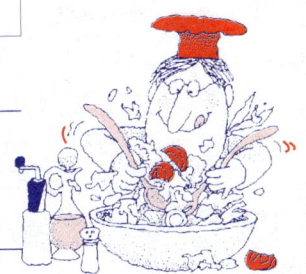

DINNER (Approx. 360 Calories)
Soup (fat-free)
Plus 3 oz lean Meat (cooked weight)
or 4 oz Chicken Breast (no skin)
or 3 oz Chicken Thigh/Leg (no skin)
or 5 oz Fish (grilled, no fat)
or ¾ cup Beans (Soy, Baked, Haricot etc)/Lentils or Vegetarian Entree (lowfat)
or Low Fat Recipe Dish (e.g. Lean Cuisine)
Plus 1 small Potato or ½ cup Rice/Pasta or 1 slice Bread
Plus 2-3 servings Vegetables/Salad
Plus 1 small Fruit + Diet Gelatin Dessert

BETWEEN MEALS: Water, Coffee, Tea, Diet drinks
Fruit from main meals; Raw vegetable pieces, Milk from Allowance
Note: Take a multivitamin/mineral supplement daily while dieting.

EXERCISE AND WEIGHT CONTROL

- Persons who exercise regularly **lose more weight** and keep it off longer than non-exercisers.
- Exercise also improves general health and well-being. **Confidence and self-esteem** are enhanced by a sense of control and accomplishment.
- **Exercise increases the metabolic rate** of the body even for hours after exercise - a good way to 'wake up' a sluggish metabolism.

  Exercise compensates for any decrease in metabolic rate with increasing age and also in some heavy smokers who stop smoking.
- **Strength training** further builds muscle and aids body reshaping. You can also eat more food!

  Note: When fat is lost and muscle gained, there may be little change in weight. Yet fatness has been reduced as evidenced by a smaller size of clothing fitting the reproportioned body. Weight from exercised muscles is okay. It is surplus fat that is potentially harmful.

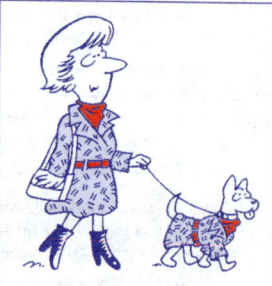

Brisk walking each day is a safe and effective way to keep trim and fit. Try it - you'll like it!"

Strength-training with light weights helps to retain or rebuild muscle tissue and enhances weight control.

- **Avoid injury** by beginning with walking, low impact aerobics, or weight-supported exercise (e.g. swimming, cycling). Avoid competitive sports.
- **How Much?** Start with 10 - 20 minutes/day and progress to 30-45minutes/day - even if broken into 5-10 minute lots. It all adds up! Aim to achieve 250-500 calories of exercise daily.

  Also walk up stairs instead of using lifts. Take a brisk walk at lunch. Use an exercise bike, treadmill or stepper while watching TV.
- **How Often?** While aerobic fitness requires only 3 - 4 sessions weekly, **weight control is a daily event which requires daily exercise.**

TV CAN BE FATTENING!

Many adults and children watch over 20 hours of television per week and indulge in high-fat snacks at the same time - potent contributors to obesity.

Are you a TV couch potato? Limit your TV hours and plan healthy physical activities. At least use an exercise bike or treadmill while watching TV!

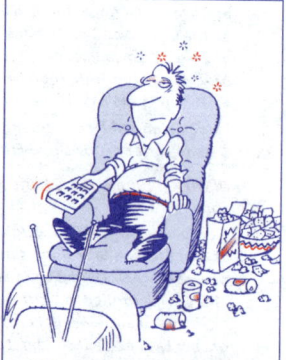

Middle-age spread has little to do with getting older. Too little exercise is the main culprit.

Daily exercise and sensible eating can prevent middle-age spread.

Are you a couch potato?

AVERAGE CALORIES USED IN EXERCISE

LIGHT
4 Calories Minute

Walking, slow
Cycling, light
Gardening light
Golf, social
Tennis, doubles
Housework, light
Callisthenics
Ten Pin Bowls
Table Tennis, social
Horse-riding
Ice Skating
Aquarobics
Skate Boarding

MODERATE
7 Calories Minute

Walking, brisk
Cycling, moderate
Swimming, crawl
Weight-training, light
Tennis, singles
Squash, beginners
Aerobics, light
Football, Grid Iron
Basketball, Baseball
Walking Downstairs
Snow Skiing (downhill)
Line/Square Dancing
Dancing, Jazzercise

HEAVY
10 Calories Minute

Walking (power), Jogging
Cycling, strenuous
Swimming, strenuous
Weight-training, heavy
Wrestling/Judo, advanced
Squash, advanced
Skipping
Football, training
Basketball (Pro)
Climbing Stairs
Skiing (cross country)
Aquarobics, advanced
Dancing, strenuous

Note: Only those sports or activities that are sustained over a period of time (e.g running) qualify for heavy exercise. Stop-start sports such as tennis are considered 'moderate' or average.

WALKING PROGRAM

Weeks	Distance To Walk	Time Taken	Calories Used (140lb Person)
Weeks 1-2	1 mile	20 mins	140 calories
Weeks 3-5	1.5 miles	28 mins	200 calories
Weeks 6-8	2 miles	35 mins	250 calories
Weeks 9-10	2.5 miles	45 mins	310 calories
Weeks 11+	3.5 miles	60 mins	420 calories

MINIMAL EXERCISES FOR LAZY SLIMMERS

 After finishing a set meal, place both hands on edge of table and P-U-S-H back hard!

 Shake your head vigorously from side to side, every time you are offered a second helping of rich food.

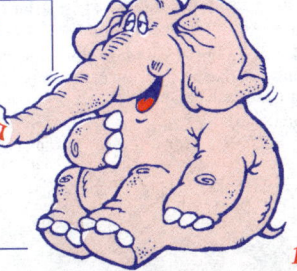

Reshaping Eating Behavior

- Eating is a behavior that is largely controlled by people with whom we live or socialize, places in which we carry out our lives, and our emotions. Become aware of those situations that commonly lead to extra food being eaten.

- We may also be unaware of 'bad' eating habits that can lead to excess calorie intake; e.g. eating quickly, large mouthsful, eating when tense or bored, finishing a large serving of food when not hungry.

Hints to help uncover and correct those 'bad' eating habits include:

- **Don't eat while engaged in other activities;** e.g. watching TV, reading. Eat only at the table, not at the fridge or while standing.

- **Don't eat quickly.** Chewing slowly allows time to register a feeling of fullness. Don't use fingers, only utensils. Cut food into smaller pieces. Don't load your fork until the previous mouthful is finished.

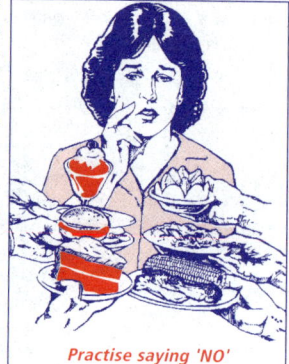

Practise saying 'NO' politely but assertively.

- **Don't purchase problem high calorie foods.** Shop from a set list to prevent impulse buying. Avoid shopping with children. Plan meals in advance. Stick to a set menu.

- **Plan a strategy to avoid uncontrolled eating** and drinking at social events, or when your emotions urge you to binge.

  Rehearse repeatedly in your mind exactly what you will do in such situations. Remind yourself several times each day that you are in charge of your actions and that you can be strongwilled. Seek counselling or coaching on various strategies.

- **Promise yourself** that when you feel the urge to snack, you will engage in some activity that will distract you away from food (e.g. go for a walk, brush your teeth, phone a friend.)

  If you eat out of boredom, find some new lobby or interest that gets you out of the house; even enrol in an adult education class.

Notes:
- Obese persons who can't stop snacking may benefit from counselling and a doctor-prescribed weight reducing agent
- Persons with deep-seated emotional problems and eating disorders require counselling.

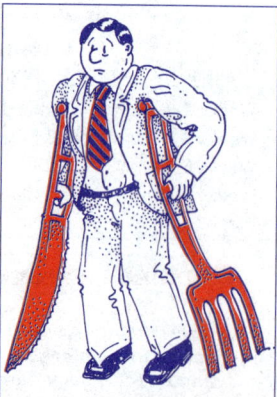

Do you use food as an emotional crutch? If so, professional counselling may be helpful.

THE VALUE OF A FOOD DIARY

The food diary is the most powerful proven aid for dieters. Persons who keep a food and exercise diary not only lose more weight they also keep it off. Here are some of the reasons:

- Recording your eating and exercise habits jolts you into realizing just what you do eat and drink each day; and also whether you exercise sufficiently.
- **Helps you identify problem foods** and drinks with excessive calories and fat.
- **Helps identify moods**, situations and events that lead to excessive eating of unwanted calories. You can then plan to overcome or avoid them.
- **Prevents 'calorie amnesia'**, the forgetfulness that leads to rebound weight gain after successful weight loss. Recording puts you back on the right track.
- **Helps you develop greater self-discipline.** You will think twice about over indulging if you have to record it - especially if someone checks your diary regularly. It certainly keeps you honest!
- **Motivates you** to carefully plan your meals and to exercise each day.
- **Serves as a check system** for your doctor, dietitian or counsellor to assess your progress and make recommendations.

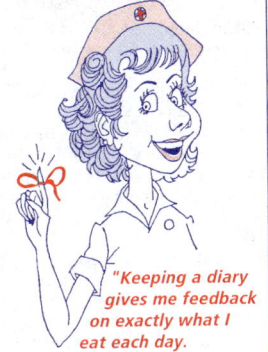

"Keeping a diary gives me feedback on exactly what I eat each day.

It helps prevent 'calorie amnesia' and reminds me to exercise each day.

It's a must for successful weight control!"

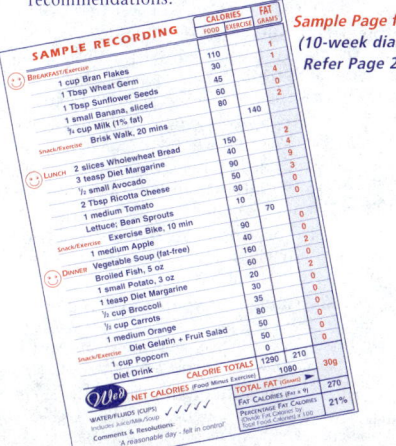

Sample Page from The Pocket Food & Exercise Diary
(10-week diary to record food and exercise)
Refer Page 256

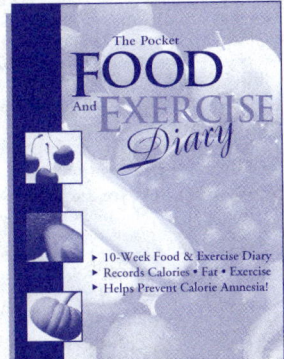

The Pocket
FOOD
And **EXERCISE** *Diary*

▶ 10-Week Food & Exercise Diary
▶ Records Calories • Fat • Exercise
▶ Helps Prevent Calorie Amnesia!

HEALTHY WEIGHT GAIN GUIDE

GENERAL NOTES

- **Slim people** usually find weight gain to be just as difficult as overweight persons find weight loss. Heredity and body build may have a lot to do with it - regardless of food and exercise habits.

- **If you are naturally slim**, yet healthy, eat well, sleep well, and have abundant energy, then you probably don't need to become obsessed with weight gain. Simply enjoy the envy of friends who wonder how you stay so slim!

- **A healthy weight gain means gaining muscle mass without excessive amounts of body fat.** To gain pounds of blubber around the waist may not only compromise health but does little for your looks.

Thus, healthy weight gain does not entail simply stuffing yourself with rich fatty foods. Dedication to a program of both **sensible eating and exercise** is required.

- Factors (apart from heredity) which may contribute to a person being **underweight** include: erratic eating habits, small meals with insufficient calorie intake, excessive exercise, tobacco smoking, and medical problems.

Medical conditions which may contribute to underweight include diabetes (Type-1), cancer, stroke, HIV infection, dysphagia (difficulty in swallowing), gastro-intestinal ailments, anorexia nervosa, nausea, vomiting, and stress.

Be sure to **check any unexplained weight** loss with your doctor.

- **Important keys for successful weight gain** include careful planning, motivation to change eating and exercise habits, professional and family support - and especially perseverance.

TEN HINTS TO GAIN WEIGHT

1. **Don't skip meals.** Establish a regular eating pattern. Eat three main meals - plus healthy snacks. Aim for 2000-3000 calories daily - more if very active. Eat foods you enjoy.

2. **The eating plan** (page 11) shows the types of foods that are ideal for healthy eating. Simply **increase** food quantities, particularly bread, breakfast cereals, potatoes, rice, pasta, baked beans, and fruits. **Avoid** filling up on low or no-calorie drinks and foods.

3. **Start the day right with a good breakfast.** It can be difficult to make up lost calories and nutrition during the course of a busy day. Cereals with extra fruit, wheatgerm, and milk are ideal.

4. **Snack on healthy foods** such as nuts, seeds, dried fruits, bananas, avocados, fat-reduced cookies, muffins, granola bars and sandwiches; as well as milk or soy drinks, shakes, yogurt and fruit juices. Nutritional sports shakes may also help.

5. **Avoid high-fat foods** that are also high in saturated fats - moreso, if your blood cholesterol is high. (See Fats/Cholesterol Guide)

6. **Quit smoking.** It wastes calories as the body has to work harder to rid itself of tobacco toxins. Your appetite, taste and smell will improve and heighten food appeal.

7. **For fitness and muscle gains,** a mixture of weight training and aerobics is recommended. Join a gym or work out at home. **Be patient** - allow 6-12 months for significant results to show.

8. **Chronic stress can reduce appetite.** Seek advice on managing stress. Learn relaxation techniques.

9. **Keep a diary of your eating and exercise.** Use *The Pocket Food and Exercise Diary* to help identify problem times, and meals where insufficient calories are consumed.

10. **Consult a dietitian** for extra ideas and meal planning if you have a medical problem or have a heavy sports.

HEALTHY WEIGHT GAIN GUIDE

EXTRA HINTS & NOTES

- While **vitamin/mineral supplements** may benefit many people, they contain no calories and cannot replace food.

Persons with anorexia and weight loss may benefit from a zinc supplement in addition to a general vitamin-mineral supplement. (A lack of B vitamins can also reduce appetite even when little food is being eaten). Check with your doctor.

- **Adolescent boys** aspiring to attain a Schwarzenegger look should realise that while weight training will help to strengthen and define existing muscles, extra muscle growth and bulking will not occur until the body's hormone system allows it - usually after 16 years of age, when near the end of their growth spurt.

Further, many muscle-men who pose in muscle magazines use steroids - a definite health hazard, both physically and mentally.

- **Athletes** need to eat sufficient food to prevent weight loss and energy fade-out - particularly teenagers who are still growing. A healthy breakfast is important.

Liquid nutritional supplements as well as milk, shakes and fruit juices will help to boost calorie and fluid intake. Weight loss from **dehydration** through sports should be corrected with adequate water and other fluids.

Although muscles are built of protein, excess protein will not build bigger muscles - it is converted and stored as fat. Muscles use carbohydrates and fats for fuel.

- **Elderly persons** may be underweight and malnourished due to lack of dentition and inability to prepare adequate meals. Some drug medications can reduce taste, saliva flow and appetite. Vitamin deficiencies can further reduce appetite. (Smoking and excess alcohol add to the problem.)

Choose nutritious soups and casseroles, omelets, shakes, fruit juices and nutritional supplements. Fluids between meals will prevent dehydration - a common problem.

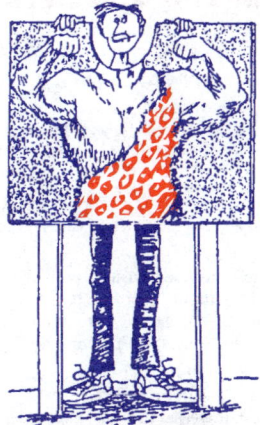

For healthy weight gain, eat regular meals, stop smoking, and include strength training in your exercise program.

EXTRA HINTS & NOTES (Cont)

Elderly persons (Cont):
If **nauseous**, avoid greasy, high-fat and spicy foods. Spread easily digested foods over six small meals.

- **Infants:** For healthy weight gains, do not overly restrict calories or fat in baby's food. When stopping breast-feeding or formula feed, use whole milk or soy for infants less than two years. Reduced-fat milks may have too few calories, as may high-fiber diets. Toddlers who are fussy eaters should not be allowed to fill up on fluids before or during meals.

- **Persons with HIV infection** have increased nutritional needs. Regular meals with supplementation of protein, vitamins and minerals are important. Seek professional advice.

DIABETES & WEIGHT CONTROL

WHAT IS DIABETES?

Diabetes is a disorder in which the body cannot make proper use of carbohydrates (sugar and starches).

- After digestion, sugar and starches are changed into **glucose** - the simplest form of sugar that is vital to body cells for energy and growth.
- **Insulin** is the hormone which acts like a key that opens the door to body cells and allows glucose to enter.
- **Without sufficient insulin**, unused glucose builds up in the blood and passes into the urine. This produces symptoms of frequent urination, continual thirst and tiredness.
- **Untreated diabetes** increases the risk of damage to nerves and blood vessels. This, in turn, increases the risk of heart disease, stroke, blindness, kidney damage, gangrene, impotence and other complications.

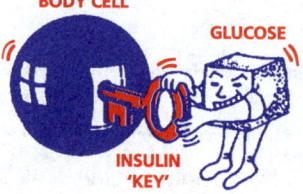

Insulin acts like a key. It opens the door to body cells and allows glucose to enter.

Some persons with diabetes (Type 1) have too few or no keys and require insulin injections.

Others (Type 2) have ample keys but 'mis-shapen' key holes (insulin resistant) - particularly if obese.

TYPE-1 DIABETES

Insulin-Dependent Diabetes

- Occurs in 10% of diabetes cases.
- Usually children and young adults.
- Pancreas gland produces little or no insulin. Daily insulin injections are necessary, plus:
- Regular meals with even carbohydrate distribution to match insulin dosage. Regular exercise and weight control are also important.

WARNING SIGNALS

- Frequent urination
- Continual thirst
- Rapid weight loss
- Unusual hunger
- Extreme weakness/fatigue
- Nausea, vomiting, irritability

TYPE-2 DIABETES

Non-Insulin Dependent

- Occurs in 90% of diabetes cases.
- Occurs mainly in adults - particularly in overweight and inactive persons.
- Insulin is produced but body cells resist its action and glucose cannot enter cells.
- Usually treated with diet and exercise. Sometimes requires medication (pills or insulin injections).

WARNING SIGNALS

- Any Type-1 symptom
- Blurred vision
- Excessive itching
- Skin infections with slow healing
- Tingling/numbness in feet

DIABETES & WEIGHT CONTROL

IMPORTANCE OF WEIGHT CONTROL

- **Type-2 diabetes** occurs 2-3 times more often in overweight and obese persons.
- Such persons do not usually lack insulin. Rather, their insulin is less effective. As fat cells in overweight persons enlarge, the cells may resist insulin in varying degrees. The resultant build-up of blood glucose may lead to diabetic symptoms.
- **Weight loss alone** often corrects this condition in Type-2 diabetes. If overweight, try a moderate diet of 1200-1500 calories **plus daily exercise**.

Within several weeks, the tissue cells can lose their resistance and become sensitive once again to the effects of insulin. Insulin and blood glucose levels may normalise, and diabetic symptoms may disappear.

Further, the need for oral antidiabetic drugs might be prevented or much lessened in dosage. **So, give diet and exercise a fair go** - and maintain them **to keep symptoms at bay.**

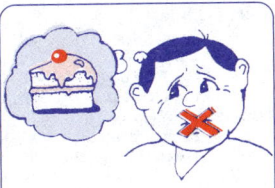

Simply losing weight and exercising daily can often control Type-2 diabetes in obese persons.

Give diet and exercise a fair go before resorting to oral antidiabetic drugs.

HINTS FOR MANAGING DIABETES

Don't battle diabetes alone. Establish a partnership with your doctor, dietitian, nurse educator and pharmacist. For extra information and support, contact the *American Diabetes Association*.
(Phone 1-800-232 3472 or your state affiliate)

Hints to keep blood glucose within safe limits:

▶ **Control your diet.** Know what and when you will eat. Seek referral to a dietitian for expert advice.

▶ **Exercise regularly.** It assists weight control and can improve sensitivity of body cells to insulin. Plan exercise into your daily routine.

▶ **Monitor your blood glucose** at home and work - ideally with a portable blood glucose meter. It will help you become familiar with your blood glucose patterns, and the effects of diet, exercise and medication.

▶ **Don't skip prescribed insulin or oral medication.** If on insulin, know what action to take if hypoglycaemia (low blood glucose) occurs. Also educate family and friends.

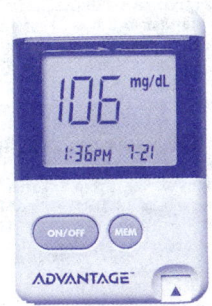

Blood glucose meters can aid the control of diabetes. (Available from Pharmacies)

MILK & SOY DRINKS

COW'S MILK

	C	F	%fc
Whole (3.5% fat):			
2 Tbsp, 1 fl.oz	20	1	48%
1 Glass, 6 fl.oz	110	6	48%
1 Cup, 8 fl.oz	150	8	48%
1 Pint, 16 fl.oz	300	16	48%
Reduced-fat (2% fat):			
2 Tbsp, 1 fl.oz	15	0.5	38%
1 Glass, 6 fl.oz	90	4	38%
1 Cup, 8 fl.oz	120	5	38%
1 Pint, 16 fl.oz	240	10	38%
Light/Lowfat (1% fat):			
2 Tbsp, 1 fl.oz	12	0.3	22%
1 Glass, 6 fl.oz	75	2	22%
1 Cup, 8 fl.oz	100	2.5	22%
1 Pint, 16 fl.oz	200	5	22%
Skim (Nonfat):			
2 Tbsp, 1 fl.oz	10	0	5%
1 Cup, 8 fl.oz	90	0.5	5%
1 Pint, 16 fl.oz	180	1	5%
Fat-Free (w/Replace Oatrim)			
Golden Jersey, 1 cup	85	0	0%
Protein-Fortified: 2% fat, 1 cup	140	5	32%
1% fat, 1 cup	120	3	22%
Skim, 1 cup	100	0.5	5%
Acidophilus (Borden), 1%, 1 c.	100	2	18%
Buttermilk: Regular, 1 cup	120	4	30%
Nonfat (Hood): Regular, 1 cup	90	0	0%
Lactose-Reduced:			
2% fat, Lactaid, 1 cup	130	5	35%
1% fat, Lactaid, 1 cup	110	2.5	20%
Nonfat, Lactaid/Lucerne, 1 cup	80	0	0%

CANNED & DRIED MILK

Average All Brands

	C	F	%fc
Condensed: Reg. 2 Tbsp, 1 fl.oz	130	3	23%
Lowfat (Eagle), 2 Tbsp	120	1.5	11%
Fat Free (Eagle), 2 Tbsp	110	0	0%
Evaporated: Whole, 2 Tbsp	40	3	68%
Whole, 1/2 cup	170	10	53%
Lowfat (Carnation), 2 Tbsp	25	1	25%
1/2 cup	110	3	25%
Light/Skim, 1/2 cup	100	0.5	5%
Dried: Whole, 1/4 cup, 1 oz	150	8	49%
Skim/Nonfat, 1 oz	80	0	0%
Made-up, 1 cup, 8 fl.oz	80	0	0%
Buttermilk, sweetcream, 1 oz	110	2	15%
Nonfat, 1 Tbsp	25	0	0%

GOAT'S & SHEEP'S MILK

	C	F	%fc
Goat's Milk (Meyenberg):			
Whole, 1 cup, 8 fl.oz	140	7	45%
Light/Lowfat (1%), 8 fl.oz	110	2.5	20%
Evaporated, 1/2 cup	143	8	52%
Sheep's Milk: Whole, 1 cup	265	17	58%

SOY & NON-DAIRY DRINKS

(Lactose & Cholesterol Free)
Per 1 Cup Serving (8 fl. oz)

	C	F	%fc
Better Than Milk: Natural	90	5	50%
Light	80	0	0%
Edensoy (Organic):			
Extra Original	130	5	35%
Extra Vanilla	140	3	19%
Vanilla	150	3	18%
Carob	150	4	24%
Soy Moo (Health Valley)	110	0	0%
Soy-Um: Original	100	3	27%
Vanilla	110	3	25%
Vitamite: Regular (2% fat)	110	5	45%
Fat Free	90	0	0%
Vitasoy: Creamy Original	160	7	26%
Light Original	90	2	20%
Vanilla Delite	190	6	28%
Light Vanilla	110	2	16%
Carob Supreme	210	6	26%
Rich Cocoa	210	6	26%
Light Cocoa	130	2	14%
Westsoy: Regular	120	2	15%
Plain Lite	100	2	18%
Cocoa	190	4	19%
Cocoa Lite	140	2	13%
Vanilla Lite	110	2	16%
Soy Powder Mix (1 oz makes 8 fl.oz)			
Soyagenl/Soyamel, 1 oz	130	6	42%
Soy Protein Isolate, 1 oz	95	1	1%

RICE DRINKS

	C	F	%fc
Amazake: Original, 1 cup	90	0	0%
Almond Shake, 1 cup	200	7	32%
Eden Rice	110	3	25%
Pacific Rice: 1 cup	100	2	18%
Rice Dream: Original, 1 cup	160	3	17%
Organic Original/Lite	120	2	14%
Vanilla Lite	130	2	14%
Carob Lite	150	3	18%

FLAVORED MILK DRINKS

C ~ CALORIES **F** ~ FAT (Grams) **%fc** ~ PERCENT FAT CALORIES

CHOCOLATE MILK

	C	F	%fc
QUICK QUIDE			
Average All Brands			
Chocolate Milk: Per Cup, 8 fl.oz			
Whole Milk (3.3%): 1 cup	225	9	36%
1 Pint	450	18	36%
2% Milk, 1 cup	190	5	24%
1% Milk, 1 cup	160	3	17%
BRANDS			
Ready-To-Drink (Per 8 fl.oz)			
Bodywise, nonfat	180	0	0%
Borden, lowfat	180	5	25%
Bosco	230	8	31%
Hershey's: Lowfat (2%) Choc Milk	200	4.5	20%
Chocolate Drink	130	1.5	10%
Hood, Lowfat (1%)	150	2	12%
Johanna Farms: Regular	200	5	23%
Lowfat	150	6	6%
Kroger (3.25% mild)	220	9	37%
Lactaid (1%)	160	3	17%
Land O'Lakes, lowfat (1/2%)	150	1.5	9%
Meadow Gold (3.5%)	210	8	34%
Nestle Choc. Milk	110	1.5	12%
Quik: (Nestle) Chocolate Milk	190	5	24%
Strawberry Milk	210	5	21%
Parmalat (2%)	180	5	25%
Yoo Hoo Choc Drink, 8 fl.oz	130	1	7%

SHAKES & SMOOTHIES

	C	F	%fc
SHAKES			
Regular: Chocolate, 10 fl.oz	360	11	28%
Vanilla/Strawberrry, 10 fl.oz	320	9	25%
McDonald's Reduced Fat,			
Small (14 fl.oz), all flavors	340	5	13%
Burger King: Vanilla, medium	430	9	18%
Chocolate w. Syrup	570	10	16%
SHAKE MIXES			
Weight Watchers Choc. Fudge	80	1	11%
Alba Dairy Shake (prep'd w. water):			
Double Fudge; Vanilla	70	0.5	6%
Diet Shake	30	0	0%
SMOOTHIES: (Milk/Soy + Fruit), Per 12 fl. oz			
Average all types			
with Whole Milk	300	8	24%
+ Icecream, 1 scoop	350	10	26%
with Nonfat Milk	240	0	0%

COCOA-CHOCOLATE MIXES

	C	F	%fc
Add extra cals/fat for milk			
Alba '66 Milk Choc, 1 pkt	60	0	0%
Carnation Cocoa Mixes:			
Chocolate Rich, 3 Tbsp/1 pkt	110	1	8%
Milk Chocolate, 3 Tbsp	110	1	8%
w/mini Marshmallows, 1 oz pkt	110	1	8%
Malted Milk Original, 3 Tbsp	90	2	20%
70 Calorie Cocoa Mix	70	0.5	6%
Fat-Free, 2 Tbsp/1 pkt	25	0	0%
No Added Sugar, 1 pkt	50	0.5	7%
Land O' Lakes (Per 1 1/4 oz pkt):			
Choc.Mint/Raspb./Supreme	160	5	28%
Nestle Hot Cocoa Mix, 1 oz	110	1	8%
w. Marshmallows, 1 oz	120	1	7%
Ghiradelli (Per 2 heaping tsp):			
Choc. Mocha/Hazelnut/Dble Choc	80	1.5	17%
Pralines & Creme, 2 Tbsp	90	0	0%
Ovaltine Cocoa Mixes, 4 tsp	80	0	0%
Swiss Miss Cocoa Mixes:			
Milk Chocolate, 1 oz pkt	110	1.5	12%
w. Marshmallows, 1.2 oz pkt	140	3	19%
Choc. Sensation, 1.25 oz pkt	150	4	24%
Lite, 1 pkt	70	0	0%
Diet Cocoa Mix, 1 pkt	20	0	0%
Sugar Free	60	0	0%
Fat Free, 0.53 oz	50	0	0%
Vending Machine, 1.34 oz pkt	145	2	12%

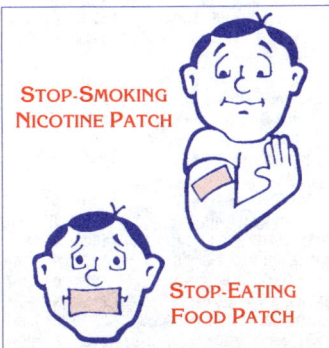

STOP-SMOKING NICOTINE PATCH

STOP-EATING FOOD PATCH

YOGURT

QUICK GUIDE

	C	F	%fc
Average All Brands: Per 8 oz			
Plain Yogurt: Whole, 8 oz	180	7	35%
Lowfat	140	4	26%
Nonfat	110	0	0%
Fruit Flavored: Whole, 8 oz	250	6	22%
Lowfat	230	3	12%
Nonfat, regular	150	0	0%
Nonfat, no sugar added	120	0	0%
Goat's Milk Yogurt-Same as Regular			

YOGURT BRANDS

	C	F	%fc
BORDEN: Light, 8 oz	120	<1	1%
Lite-Line: Plain, 8 oz	140	2	13%
Fruit Flavors, 8 oz	140	2	13%
Lowfat, fruit, 8 oz	225	4	16%
BREYERS: Average, 1% fat, 8 oz	250	3	11%
CABOT: Plain, 8 oz	140	4	26%
Flavors, 8 oz	220	3	12%
COLOMBO: Fruit Flavors, 8 oz	200	4	18%
Fat Free: Cappuccino, 8 oz	170	0	0%
Fruited Flavors, 8 oz	200	0	0%
Banana/Strawberry, 8 oz	220	0	0%
Light 100, all flavors, 8 oz	100	0	0%
CONTINENTAL: Plain, 1 cup	120	0	0%
100% Lactose Reduced, 1 cup	190	0	0%
Other varieties, 1 cup	190	0	0%
DANNON			
Chunky Fruit w. Frt Jce (NF), 6 oz	160	0	0%
Fruit on the Bottom (lowfat), 8 oz	240	3	11%
Minipack, 4.4 oz	130	1.5	11%
Blended Fruit (nonfat), 4.4 oz	120	0	0%
Danimals Lowfat, 4.4 oz	130	1	7%
Double Delights Lowfat:			
with fruit topping, 6 oz	170	1	5%
with chocolate topping, 6 oz	220	0	0%
Natural Flavoured Lowfat, 8 oz	210	3	13%
Light N/fat w. NutraSweet, 8 oz	100	0	0%
Light Duets w/fruit topping, 6 oz	90	0	0%
Light 'N Crunchy, all types 8 oz	140	0	0%
Sprinkl'ins: Rainbow, 116g	130	1.5	11%
Magic Crystals, 1 ctn, 116g	110	1	8%
FRIENDSHIP: Fruit Flavors, 6 oz	190	5	37%
HOOD: Fat Free, Plain, 8 oz	130	0	0%
Average all flavors, 8 oz	190	0	0%
JELL-O: Jigglers, 6 oz	215	1.5	6%
KNUDSEN: 70 Calories, 6 oz	70	0	0%
Free, average all flavours, 6 oz	170	0	0%

	C	F	%fc
LA YOGURT			
Latin Style, 6 oz	190	3	14%
French Style, regular, 6 oz	180	3	15%
Nonfat, 6 oz	70	0	0%
LIGHT N'LIVELY			
Free 50 Calories, 4.4 oz	50	0	0%
Free 70 Calories, 6 oz	70	0	0%
Free (Regular) 6 oz: Vanilla	160	0	0%
Strawb. Frt/Peach/Lem./Berry	170	0	0%
Strawberry/Raspberry	180	0	0%
Kidpack/Multipack, aver. 4.4 oz	140	1	6%
MEADOW GOLD: Plain, 8 oz	160	5	28%
Flavors, average, 8 oz	250	4	14%
MOUNTAIN HIGH			
Fruit Flavors, aver., 1 cup	220	6	25%
Plain: Light/Nonfat, 1 cup	120	0	0%
Flavors, average, 1 cup	170	0	0%
SNACKWELL'S			
Nonfat, all varieties, 6 oz	180	0	0%
WEIGHT WATCHERS			
Fat Free: Plain; Fruited, 8 oz	90	0	0%
YOPLAIT			
Original Cafe au Lait, 6 oz	170	2	11%
Coconut Creme Pie, 6 oz	200	3	14%
99% Fat Free, 6 oz	180	1.5	8%
4 oz mini cup	120	1	8%
Original Nonfat: Plain, 1 cup	130	0	0%
Vanilla, 1 cup	200	0	0%
Custard Style: All flavors, 6 oz	190	3	14%
4 oz mini cup	130	2	14%
Trix: All fruit flavors, 6 oz	160	2	11%
4 oz mini cup	110	1.5	13%
Light, all flavors, 6 oz	90	0	0%
Crunch 'n Yogurt Light:			
All flavors, average, 7 oz	140	2	13%
Fat Free: Per 6 oz,			
Fruit on the Bottom	160	0	0%

YOGURT DRINKS

	C	F	%fc
Alta Dena: Raspberry, 1 cup	180	0	0%
Other flavors, 1 cup	220	0	0%
Glen Oaks: All flav., aver., 1 cup	250	4	14%
Yonique: All flavors, aver., 6 oz	175	2	10%

FROZEN YOGURT

See Next Section
*(Colombo/Dannon/Dreyers/Frusen Gladje/
Haagen Dazs/I Can't Believe It's Yogurt))*

ICECREAMS & ICES

QUICK GUIDE | BRANDS

	C	F	%fc
Vanilla: *Average All Brands*			
Regular (10% fat):			
(Examples: *Borden/Breyers/Hood*)			
3 fl.oz scoop	100	5	48%
1/2 cup, 4 fl.oz	130	7	48%
1 Pint, 16 fl.oz	520	28	48%
1/2 Gallon (4 Pints)	2100	112	48%
Rich (16% fat): (*Baskin-Robbins*)			
3 fl.oz scoop	170	10	51%
1/2 cup, 4 fl.oz	230	13	51%
1 Pint	960	52	51%
Super-Rich (20% fat): (*Haagen-Dazs/Ben & Jerry's*)			
3 fl.oz scoop	200	14	60%
1/2 cup, 4 fl.oz	270	18	60%
1 Pint	1100	72	60%
Reduced Fat/Light (6% fat):			
(*Breyer's Light/Hood/Lucerne Light*)			
3 fl.oz scoop	100	3	26%
1/2 cup, 4 fl.oz	140	4	26%
1 Pint	560	16	26%
Low Fat (less than 4% fat):			
(*Healthy Choice/Weight Watchers*)			
3 fl.oz scoop	90	2	19%
1/2 cup, 4 fl.oz	120	2.5	19%
1 Pint	480	10	19%
Fat Free: (*Baskin-Robbins FF/Borden FF/ Breyers FF/Simple Pleasures*)			
3 fl.oz scoop	75	0	0%
1/2 cup, 4 fl.oz	100	0	0%
1 Pint	400	0	0%
Soft Serve, 1/2 cup	180	9	45%
Note: Above figures - Vanilla only.			
Other flavors ~ See Brand Listings.			

OTHER ICES - QUICK GUIDE

	C	F	%fc
Frozen Yogurt, average:			
Hard: Lowfat, 1/2 cup	140	3	19%
Nonfat, 1/2 cup	110	0	0%
Soft: Lowfat, 1/2 cup	120	2.5	19%
Nonfat, 1/2 cup	100	0	0%
(See Brands - Colombo/Dannon/Dreyers/Frusen Gladje/Haagen-Dazs/I Can't Believe It's Yogurt).			
Ice Milk: Average all flavors			
Hard (4% fat), 1/2 Cup	100	3	27%
Soft Serve (3% fat), 1/2 Cup	110	2	16%
Sherbet, average, 1/2 Cup	120	2	15%
Sorbet: Fruit (no fat), 1/2 Cup	110	0	0%

	C	F	%fc
ALTA DENA: *Per 1/2 Cup (4 fl. oz)*			
Touch Of Honey: Choc; Strawb.	80	1	11%
Classic Vanilla	170	11	58%
Pralines & Creme	110	2.5	20%
BASKIN-ROBBINS			
See Fast-Food & Restaurant Section ~ Page 144.			
BEN & JERRY'S: *Per 1/2 Cup*			
Butter Pecan	310	26	75%
Cherry Van./Cream Cherry Garcia	240	15	56%
Chocolate Chip Cookie Dough	270	17	57%
Chocolate Fudge Brownie	250	14	50%
Chonky Monkey	280	19	61%
Coffee Almond Fudge Chip	290	20	62%
Coffee/English Toffee Crunch, aver.	300	20	60%
Heath Bar Crunch	280	19	61%
Mint Chocolate Cookie	260	17	59%
New York Super Fudge Chunk	290	20	62%
Peanut Butter Cup	370	26	63%
Rain Forrest Crunch	300	23	69%
Smooth Deep Dark Chocolate	260	15	52%
Smooth Double Chocolate Fudge	280	16	51%
Vanilla	230	17	67%
Vanilla Caramel Fudge	280	17	55%
Wavy Gravy	330	24	65%
Fat Free: Strawberry	140	0	0%
Vanilla Fudge Swirl	150	0	0%
Pops: See Page 27			
BON BON'S			
Vanilla w. choc. coating, 4 pieces	160	12	65%
8 pieces	330	23	65%
BORDEN: *Per 1/2 Cup*			
Buttered Pecan (Lady Borden)	180	12	60%
Chocolate Swirl; Strawberry	130	6	42%
Olde Fashioned: Vanilla	130	7	48%
Dutch Chocolate	130	6	42%
Strawberries 'n Cream	130	5	35%
Fat-Free: All flavors, average.	90	0	0%
Ice Milk: Chocolate, 1/2 cup	100	2	18%
Strawberry/Vanilla, 1/2 cup	90	2	20%
Sundae Cone	210	12	51%

ICECREAMS & ICES CONT

BRESLER'S: *Per 1/2 Cup*	C	F	%fc
Icecream: All flavors, average.	230	12	63%
Royal Cremes, average	260	16	55%
Royal Lites, average	220	0	0%

BREYER'S: *Per 1/2 Cup*	C	F	%fc
Original: Butter Pecan	180	12	60%
Cherry Vanilla; Coffee	150	7	42%
Chocolate; French Vanilla	160	10	56%
Choc. Chip; Mint Choc. Chip	170	10	53%
Cookies 'n Cream	170	9	48%
Peach; Strawberry	130	6	42%
Vanilla; Van./Choc./Strawberry	150	8	48%
Van. & Choc.; Van. Fudge Twirl	160	8	45%
Breyers Light: Average, 1/2 c.	140	4	26%
Reduced Fat: Average	160	6	34%
Vienetta: All flavors, 1 slice	190	11	52%
Fat Free: Vanilla Fudge Twirl	110	0	0%
No Sugar Added: Vanilla	80	4	45%
Vanilla Fudge Twirl	90	3.5	35%
Vanilla Chocolate Strawberry	90	4	40%
Mint Chocolate Chip	100	5	45%
Sorbet: Average, 1/2 cup	160	7	39%
Frozen Yogurt: Average, 1/2 c.	140	4	26%

COLOMBO

Frozen Yogurt: *Per 1/2 Cup*	C	F	%fc
Banana Split; Caramel Fudge	140	1.5	10%
Chocolate Peanut Butter	140	3	19%
Pina Colada; Dble Choc Sundae	130	0	0%
Cherry Chunk; Vanilla	110	0	0%
Choc.; White & Dutch Choc.	110	0	0%
Choc. Capp./Strawb. Van. Twist	110	0	0%
Soft Serve: Nonfat varieties	100	0	0%
Slender Sensations varieties	70	0	0%
Cooler varieties	60	0	0%
Lowfat: Peanut Butter	120	2.5	19%
Other varieties	110	2.5	20%

DAIRY QUEEN/BRAZIER
See Fast-Foods Section ~ Page 158.

DANNON FROZEN YOGURT

	C	F	%fc
Light, all flavors, aver., 1/2 cup	90	1	10%
Light 'N Crunchy, all flavors, aver.	110	1	8%

DRYERS: *Per 1/2 Cup*	C	F	%fc
Grand Light: Vanilla	100	4	36%
No Sugar Added: Van. & Caramel	90	3	30%
Fat Free: All flavors	110	0	0%
Fat Free - No Sugar Added:			
Raspberry Vanilla/Swirl	90	0	0%
Frozen Yogurt:			
Health Bar Crunch	120	4	30%
Vanilla	100	2.5	23%
Fat Free: Choc./Silk Mousse	90	0	0%
Vanilla	100	0	0%

EDYS: *Per 1/2 Cup*	C	F	%fc
American Dream: Chocolate	90	1	10%
Choc. Chip, Cookies 'n Cream	100	1	9%
Mocha Alm. Fudge, Rocky Rd	110	1	8%
Strawberry	70	0	0%
Vanilla	80	0	0%
Edy's Light:			
Almond Praline, Butter Pecan	140	5	32%
Cafe Au Lait, Banana-Politan	110	4	33%
Candy Bar, Dreamy Crmel Crnch	140	5	32%
Choc. Chip, Marble Fudge	120	4	30%
Cookies 'n Cream	120	5	38%
Malt Ball 'n Fudge, Mocha Alm.	140	5	32%
P/nut Butter & Choc., Rocky Rd	130	5	35%
Strawberry, Van. Choc. Strawb.	110	4	33%
Vanilla	100	4	36%

FRUSEN GLADJE: *Per 1/2 Cup*	C	F	%fc
Butter Pecan	280	21	67%
Chocolate	240	17	64%
Chocolate Choc. Chip	270	18	60%
Mocha Chip, Praline & Cream	280	18	58%
Strawberry	230	15	59%
Swiss Almond Chocolate	270	19	63%
Vanilla	230	17	67%
Vanilla Swiss Almond	270	19	63%
Frozen Yoghurt: Strawberry	120	3	22%
Double Chunk Chocolate	160	5	28%
Vanilla	130	4	28%

GOOD HUMOUR

Light: *Per 1/2 Cup*	C	F	%fc
Choc. Chip, Toffee Bar Crunch	130	4	28%
Coffee	110	3	25%
Cookies n' Crm; Praline Alm. Crnch	130	3	21%
Vanilla, Vanilla Choc. Strawb.	110	3	25%
Bars/Ices/Sandwiches ~ Page 27.			

ICECREAMS & ICES CONT

HAAGEN-DAZS
Per 1/2 Cup

	C	F	%fc
Brownies a la Mode	280	18	58%
Butter Pecan	320	24	68%
Cappuccino, Caramel Cone	310	21	61%
Cherry Vanilla	240	15	56%
Chocolate, Coffee	270	18	60%
Choc. Choc. Chip, Cookie Dough	300	20	60%
Cookies & Cream, Rum Raisin	270	17	57%
Deep Choc Peanut Butter	370	25	61%
Macadamia/Spec. Mac Brittle	300	20	60%
Orange Vanilla; Raspberry Cream	190	9	43%
Pralines & Cream	290	18	56%
Strawberry	250	16	58%
Strawb. Cheesecake, Vanilla Fudge	280	18	56%
Vanilla	270	18	60%
Vanilla Chocolate Chip	310	20	58%
Vanilla Swiss Almond	310	21	61%
Lowfat: Coffee	150	2	12%
Strawberry; Vanilla	170	2.5	13%
Full Listings ~ See Fast Foods Section			
Sorbets ~ See Fast Foods Section			
Frozen Yogurt: Vanilla Fudge	160	0	0%
Vanilla Raspberry Swirl	130	0	0%
Other flavors	140	0	0%
See Full Listings - Fast Foods Section			

HEALTHY CHOICE
Per 1/2 Cup

	C	F	%fc
Black Forest, Butter Pecan Crunch	120	2	15%
Cappuccino Choc./ Mocha Fudge	120	2	15%
Cherry Triple Choc. Chunk	110	2	16%
Choc. Fudge Mousse	120	2	15%
Cookies 'n Cream	120	2	15%
Fudge Brownie/a la Mode	120	2	15%
Mint Choc. Chip, Strawb. Sh.cake	120	2	15%
Praline & Caramel/Cluster	130	2	14%
Rocky Road	140	2	13%
Vanilla	100	2	18%
Lowfat: All varieties, average	110	1.5	12%

ICECREAM CONES & CUPS

	C	F	%fc
Wafer Cone/Cup, average	20	<1	9%
Sugar Cone, average	40	<1	11%
Oreo Chocolate Cone	50	1	18%
Waffle Cone: Small	60	<1	8%
Large	100	1	9%

HOOD: *Per 1/2 Cup*

	C	F	%fc
Chocolate, Coffee	140	7	45%
Chocolate Chip, Maple Walnut	160	9	51%
Cookie Dough, Cookies 'n Cream	160	8	45%
Grasshopper Pie	160	7	39%
Heavenly Hash, Vanilla Fudge	140	6	39%
Strawberry	130	7	48%
Vanilla, Van. Choc. Strawberry	140	7	45%
Light: Alm. Praline, Carrib. Coffee	110	5	41%
Strawberry, Vanilla	110	4	33%
Other Flavors, average	140	5	32%
Lowfat: (No Added Sugar)			
Average all flavors, 1/2 cup	110	3	25%
Fat Free: Average all flavors	120	0	0%

I CAN'T BELIEVE IT'S YOGURT
See Fast-Foods Section ~ Page 177.

JERSEYMAID (VONS)
Per 1/2 Cup

	C	F	%fc
After Dinner Mint; Cookie Dough	170	9	37%
Chocolate	150	7	42%
Chocolate Chip; Chunky Brownie	160	9	50%
Cookies & Cream; Mint Choc. Chip	160	7	39%
Heavenly Hash; Nut Chunky Choc.	170	8	42%
Neopolitan; Real Strawberry	140	7	45%
Rocky Road	160	7	39%
Real Vanilla; French Vanilla	150	7	42%
Light: After Dinner Mint	110	5	41%
Heavenly Hash: Rocky Road	120	5	38%
Other varieties, average	110	4.5	37%
Fat Free: Pralines & Cream	110	0	0%
Vanilla	100	0	0%
Sherbets: All flavors	130	1.5	10%

LUCERNE (SAFEWAY): *Per 1/2 Cup*

	C	F	%fc
Regular: Average all flavors	140	8	51%
Light: Chocolate	115	4	31%
Cookie Cream	130	5	35%
Mocha Almond	125	4	29%
Rocky Road	130	4	28%
Strawberry Cream	105	3	26%

PASCAL'S: *Per 1/2 Cup*

	C	F	%fc
Sorbet: Chocolate	150	0	0%
Other flavors, average	120	0	0%
Real Fruit Sorbet: Lemon Peel	90	0	0%
Wild Berries	100	0	0%

ICECREAMS & ICES CONT

C ~ CALORIES **F** ~ FAT (Grams)
%fc ~ PERCENT FAT CALORIES

	C	**F**	**%fc**
McCONNELL'S: *Per 1/2 Cup*			
Choc Chip; Peppermint; Fr. Vanilla	270	18	60%
Bordeaux Strawb; Island Coconut	290	17	53%
Macadamia Nut	290	17	53%
ICE DREAM: *Per 1/2 Cup*			
Chocolate	150	7	42%
Strawberry	140	5	32%
Other flavors	150	6	36%
Supreme: Peanut Butter Cup	160	7	39%
Double Espresso Bean	180	8	40%
Pies: Mocha; Mint	320	18	40%
SEALTEST: *Per 1/2 Cup*			
American Glory, Strawberry	130	6	42%
Butter Pecan	160	9	51%
Chocolate, Coffee	140	7	45%
Choc. Butter Pecan, Choc. Chip	150	8	48%
French Vanilla	140	8	51%
Fudge Royale, Heavenly Hash	150	7	42%
Triple Chocolate Passion	160	7	39%
Vanilla, Vanilla Chocolate	140	7	45%
Free: All flavors, 1/2 cup	100	0	0%
SIMPLE PLEASURES *Per 1/2 Cup*			
Chocolate	140	0	0%
Chocolate Chip	150	3	18%
Coffee, Peach, Strawberry	120	0	0%
Cookies 'n Crm, Mint Choc. Chip	150	2	12%
Pecan Praline	140	2	13%
Rum Raisin, Toffee Crunch	130	0	0%
Vanilla	120	0	0%
Light: Average, all flavors	80	0	0%
STARBUCKS *Per 1/2 Cup*			
Dark Roast Espresso Swirl	220	10	41%
Italian Roast Coffee	230	12	47%
Java Chip	250	13	47%
Vanilla Mucha	270	14	47%
Lowfat: Latte	170	3	16%
Mattus: Caramel Crunch	180	3	15%
Chocolate; Coffee; Vanilla	160	3	17%
Other varieties	170	3	16%
TCBY ~ See Fast-Foods Section			

	C	**F**	**%fc**
THRIFTY DRUGSTORES *Per 1/2 Cup*			
Black Cherry	130	6	42%
Chocolate Brownie	170	9	48%
Chocolate Choc. Chip Light	130	6	42%
Chocolate Malted Crunch	160	8	45%
Pecan Praline, Rocky Road	160	8	45%
Strawberry; Rainbow	130	6	42%
Vanilla Light	110	5	41%
Other varieties, average	150	7	42%
Colosso: Cone w. 3 scoops, aver.	550	23	38%
Nonfat Sugar-Free: Cherry Van.	80	<1	6%
Frozen Yoghurt: aver., 3 fl. oz	90	2	20%
TURKEY HILL: *Per 1/2 Cup*			
Black Cherry	140	7	45%
Butter Pecan	170	11	58%
Choco. Mint Chip, Cookies 'n Crm	160	10	56%
Neapolitan, Vanilla & Choc.	150	8	48%
Rocky Road	170	8	42%
Vanilla, Vanilla Bean	140	8	51%
Lite: Choco Mint Chip	140	5	32%
Cookies 'n Cream	130	5	32%
Vanilla & Choc., Van. Bean	110	3	25%
WEIGHT WATCHERS: *Per 1/2 Cup*			
Cookie Dough Craze	140	3.5	23%
Oh! So Very Vanilla	120	2.5	19%
Postively Praline Crunch	140	3	19%
Reckless Rocky Road	140	3	19%
Triple Chocolate Tornado	150	3.5	21%
Bars: Page 28			

TOFU FROZEN DESSERTS

	C	**F**	**%fc**
Per 1/2 Cup			
Dreamy Tofu: Average	140	5	32%
It's Soy Delicious			
Choc. P'nut; Espresso Almond	140	4	26%
Espresso; Vanilla Fudge	120	2	15%
Chocolate Almond	150	5	30%
Raspberry	110	1	8%
Le Tofu: Average all flavors	180	9	45%
Tofulite: Average all flavors	150	7	42%
Tofutti: Butter Pecan	220	13	53%
Choc. Supreme; Vanilla, aver.	185	11	54%
Choc Cookie Crunch; Van. Alm.	210	11	47%
Wildberry Supreme	190	9	43%
Tofruzen: Strawberry	160	8	45%
Praline Pecan; Vanilla Almond	180	8	40%

ICECREAMS - BARS & CUPS

Per Bar/Serving	C	F	%fc
Baskin Robbins:			
Cappuccino Blast	100	1	9%
Sundae Bar: Pralines 'n Cream	280	17	55%
Tiny Toons Vanilla	140	12	77%
Ben & Jerry's: Vanilla Pop	360	28	70%
Choc Chip Cookie Dough Pop	450	28	56%
English Toffee Crunch Pop	340	23	61%
Borden: Light Dream Pops	30	0	0%
Ice Pop, regular	40	0	0%
Bounty: all varieties	70	5	64%
Carnation: Bon Bons, 5 piece	170	12	64%
Heaven, average	225	13	52%
Sundae Cup, Strawberry	200	8	36%
Chipwich Jr: Choc. Chip Cookie	240	17	64%
Creamsicle: Sugar-free pops	25	1	36%
Creme Pops	60	0	0%
Crystal Light: Cool 'n Creamy			
Average all bars	50	2	36%
Dole Bars: Fresh Lites	25	0	0%
Fruit 'n Juice: Pina Colada	90	3	30%
Lime; Raspberry, average	100	0	0%
Other Types	70	0	0%
No Added Salt, all varieties	45	0	0%
Fruit 'n Cream: Choc./Banana	175	9	46%
Chocolate/Strawberry	140	8	51%
Other Types	80	1	10%
Fruit & Yogurt: All types	75	<1	6%
Sun Tops: All types	40	0	0%
Dove Bar: Almond; Choc Milk	340	22	58%
Caramel Pecan:	350	35	90%
Vanilla Milk/Dark Choc	340	21	56%
Single Vanilla Dark	200	12	54%
Bite Size, 5 pces, 92g	330	21	57%
Coffee Cashew; Crunchy Cookie	340	22	58%
Drumstick varieties, average	350	19	49%
Peanut	380	25	59%
Dreyers: Peach Fruit Bar	140	0	0%
Grand Bars	260	17	59%
Raspberry Kiwi Fruit	100	0	0%
Sundae Cones: Average	250	12	43%
Drumstick: Original	340	19	50%
Cappuccino; Vanilla Chip	260	13	45%
Pralines 'n Creme	250	13	47%
Supreme Strawberry Swirl	230	10	39%
Eskimo Pie: Icecream S'wich, 66 g	160	4	23%
Bars, 52g: Pecan	190	15	71%
Original; Van; Milk Choc	160	11	62%
Butterscotch Crunch; Cherry,	170	11	58%

Per Bar/Serving	C	F	%fc
Eskimo Pie (Cont)			
Big Bar, 99g	300	20	60%
Reduced Fat: 49g Bar			
Praline; Butter Pecan	140	7	45%
Fudge Ripple; Choc M'mallow	130	4	28%
Neopolitan	110	4	33%
Sunday Cones	270	15	50%
Crispy Bar	130	8	55%
Reduced Fat	120	7	53%
Fi-Bar: All flavors	95	0	0%
Flintstones: Push Up	100	2	18%
Freezer Pleezer, choc-coated	150	10	60%
Froz-Fruit: Cherry	60	0	0%
Strawberry	80	4	30%
Fruit A Freeze: Coconut	130	5	35%
Lime	65	0	0%
Banana; Strawberry	90	1.5	7%
Dark Choc-Dipped Strawberry	90	3.5	35%
Fudgesicle: Fudge Pop	70	1	13%
Sugar-Free	40	0.5	11%
Fudgetastics: Sticks Sundae	220	15	61%
Giant: Sandwich, 5 fl. oz	180	9	45%
Good Humor: Candy Crunch	260	18	62%
Chocolate Eclair; Fat Frog	170	9	48%
Chocolate Fudge Cake	220	15	61%
Chocolate Taco	310	17	49%
Icecream Sandwich	165	5	27%
King Cone	290	12	37%
Strawberry Shortcake	160	7	39%
Supreme	380	25	59%
Vanilla Cup (3 fl. oz)	100	5	45%
Van.-Choc. Combo Cup (6 fl. oz)	200	9	40%
Vanilla w. Choc Coating	200	14	63%
Haagen-Daz Bars:			
Plain Choc; Coffee; Vanilla	200	13	59%
Choc/Vanilla & Dark Chocolate	400	27	60%
Multipack, each	320	22	62%
Coffee & Almond Crunch	360	26	65%
Multipack, each	290	21	65%
Strawberry & White Chocolate	270	19	63%
Vanilla & Almonds	370	27	66%
Multipack, each	300	22	66%
Vanilla & Milk Chocolate	330	24	65%
Multipack, each	280	20	64%
Icecream Sandwich, each	260	13	45%
Sorbet 'n Yogurt Bars, each	100	0	0%

ICECREAMS - BARS & CUPS CONT

Per Bar/Serving	C	F	%fc
Jell-O: Pop Bars	35	0	0%
Jigglers, all varieties, 6 oz	215	1.5	6%
Pudding Bars	80	2	22%
Snowburst	45	0	0%
Jerseymaid: Creamy Orange	60	0	0%
Fruit Juice flavors	70	0	0%
Fudge Bars	100	1	9%
Kreme Koolers	40	0.5	11%
Ice Cream Sandwich, aver.	180	6	30%
Klondike: Choco Tycos	310	17	49%
Original; Krispy Almond	310	21	61%
No Sugar, Reduced Fat	190	10	47%
Kool-Aid Pops	40	0	0%
Mama Tish's: Ice Cups	80	0	0%
Mars Almond Bar	210	14	60%
Matterhorn: 7 fl. oz	280	15	48%
Milky Way: Choc, Reduced Fat	140	7	45%
Snack Bar, Vanilla/Chocolate	70	4	51%
Minute Maid: Fruit Juice Pops	60	0	0%
Mrs Fields Icecream Bars:			
Brownies & Fudge	360	27	67%
Chocolate Chip Cookie	350	26	67%

Per Bar/Serving	C	F	%fc
Nestle: Alpine White Premium	350	25	64%
Bon Bons: Milk Choc, 38 pces	330	23	63%
Dark Chocolate, 38 pces	310	21	60%
Each, average	9	0.6	60%
Butterfinger Icecream Bar	190	13	62%
Crunch (Van./Choc.), average	200	14	63%
Reduced Fat	130	7	16%
Cool Creations, 1 cup	160	8	45%
Quik Fudge Pops, 2 pops	160	8	45%
Milk Chocolate Premium	300	20	60%
with Almonds Premium	350	23	59%
Vanilla w. chocolate coating	290	19	59%
Oreo: Choc; Vanilla	160	9	50%
Pascal: Lemon Sorbet	140	0	0%
Pathmark: Vanilla w/choc. coat.	150	10	60%
Polar Bar: Vanilla w/choc. coat.	240	18	67%
Pops: Vanilla	360	28	70%
Choc. Chip Cookie Dough	450	28	56%
English Toffee Crunch	340	23	61%
Popsicles: Fudgesicle Fudge Pop	90	1.5	15%
Sugar-free Ice Pop	15	0	0%
Reece's: Peanut Butter Icecream	160	11	62%
Rhondos: aver. all flavors, each	60	4	60%
Chocolate Chip, each	80	5	56%
Snackwell: Icecream Sandwich	90	1.5	15%
Yogurt Bars, 1 bar, 80g	120	2	15%
Snickers Ice Cream Bar, 52g	200	13	59%
Ice Cream Cones, 78g	135	15	99%
Starburst: Juice Bars	20	0	0%
Super Sundae Bar, 4 fl. oz	190	11	52%
3 Musketeers, 2 fl. oz bars	170	10	53%
Snack Bars, regular	60	4	60%
Trix: Pops, Original	40	0	0%
Vitari, soft serve, 4 fl. oz	80	0	0%
Welch's Fruit Juice Bars:			
All flavors, 54g bar	45	0	0%
No Sugar Added, 1 bar	25	0	0%
Real Fruit Chunky Sorbet, 1/2 cup	100	0	0%
Ultra Slim-Fast: Vanilla Sandwich			
with Oatmeal Cookies	150	3	18%
with Cookie Crush	90	4	40%
Weight Watchers Bars:			
Chocolate Dip	100	6	54%
Chocolate Mousse, 2 bars	70	1	12%
Chocolate Treat	100	1	9%
English Toffee Crunch	120	7	53%
Icecream Sandwich	150	3	18%
Orange Vanilla Treat, 2 bars	70	1	12%

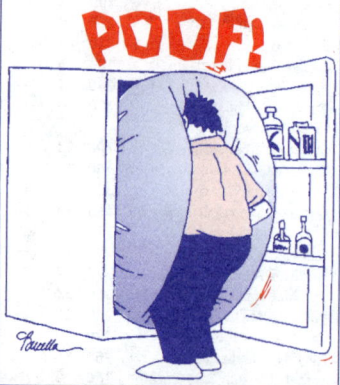

New Diet Aid - The Refrigerator Air Bag!

POOF!

FATS, SPREADS, OILS

BUTTER & MARGARINE

Butter, Margarine, Blends	C	F	%fc
Regular: 1 tsp (5g)	35	4	100%
1 Pat (5g)	35	4	100%
1 Tbsp, approx. 1/2 oz	100	11	100%
2 Tbsp, 1 oz	205	23	100%
1 Stick, 1/2 cup, 4 oz	810	92	100%
1 Pound, 2 cups, 16 oz	3240	368	100%
Whipped: 1 tsp (4 g)	27	3	100%
1 Tbsp (10g)	70	7.5	100%
1 Stick, 1/2 cup, 2 2/3 oz	570	60	100%
Unsalted: Same as Salted			
Clarified Butter, 1 Tbsp, 1/2 oz	130	15	100%

LIGHT & REDUCED FAT SPREADS

Per 1 Tbsp

	C	F	%fc
Blue Bonnet: Whipped Margarine	80	9	100%
Breakstone's Whipped Butter	60	7	100%
Chiffon: Whipped, 1 Tbsp	70	7	90%
Country Morning: Light	50	6	100%
Fleischmann's: Light Spread	80	8	90%
Extra Light/Diet	50	6	100%
'I Can't Believe It's Not Butter':			
Light	60	7	90%
Imperial: Diet, 1 Tbsp	50	6	90%
Kraft: 'Touch of Butter', bowl	50	6	100%
Land O'Lakes: Tub	80	8	90%
Honey Butter	90	8	80%
Light Whipped Butter	35	3.5	90%
Mazola: Diet	50	6	100%
Mother's Spread: 1 Tbsp	70	8	100%
Mrs Filbert's Spread: 1 Tbsp	70	8	100%
Miracle: Soft	60	7	100%
Stick	70	7	90%
Nucoa: HeartBeat Margarine	25	3	100%
Olivio: Vegetable Spread	80	8	90%
Parkay: Squeeze, 1 Tbsp	80	9	100%
Stick, 1/3 Less Fat	70	7	90%
Tub, 1 Tbsp	60	7	100%
Tub, Light/Soft Diet	50	6	100%
Whipped	70	7	90%
Promise: Regular	90	10	100%
Extra Light	50	6	100%
Ultra, w. canola oil	35	4	100%
Shedd's: Spread, Squeezable	80	9	100%
Country Crock	60	7	100%
Smart Beat: Tub	20	2	100%
Weight Watcher's: Light, all types	45	4	80%

COOKING FATS & OILS

ANIMAL FATS
Average All Types:
Beef Tallow/Drippings, Lard (Pork), Chicken, Duck, Goose, Turkey.

	C	F	%fc
1 Tbsp (13 g)	115	13	100%
2 1/4 Tbsp, 1 oz	255	28	99%
1 cup, 7 1/4 oz	1850	205	100%
1/2 pound, 8 oz	2040	227	100%
Ghee/Butter Oil: 1 Tbsp, 13 g	110	13	100%
2 1/4 Tbsp, 1 oz	250	28	100%

VEGETABLE SHORTENING
Average All Types (e.g. *Crisco*)

	C	F	%fc
1 Tbsp	113	13	100%
2 1/4 Tbsp, 1 oz	250	28	100%
1 cup, 7 1/4 oz	1810	205	100%

VEGETABLE OILS: All Types: (Includes almond, avocado, canola, corn, coconut, flaxseed, grapeseed, linseed, mustard, olive, palm, peanut, rice-bran, safflower, sesame, sunflower, soybean, wheatgerm)

	C	F	%fc
1 tsp, 5g	45	5	100%
1 Tbsp, 1/2 oz	120	14	100%
2 Tbsp, 1 oz	250	28	100%
1 cup, 7 3/4 oz	1930	218	100%

SPRAYS, BUTTER SUBSTITUTES

No-Stick Sprays (*Pam, Mazola, Weight Watchers, Wesson*):

	C	F	%fc
Per serving	2	0	100%
2-3 second spray	6	1	100%
Butter Buds: 1 serving, 1/2 tsp	4	0	0%
Butterlike Saute Butter, 1 Tbsp	35	2	50%
Butter Sprinkles (*Watkins*): 1 tsp	5	0	0%
Molly McButter: 1/2 tsp	4	0	0%
Mrs Bateman's Baking Buttter, 1 T.	35	1	20%

(Direct 800 574 6822)

FISH OILS: All Types: [a]Includes cod liver, herring, menhaden, salmon, sardine[o]

	C	F	%fc
1 Tbsp, 1/2 oz	125	14	100%

SPREADS COMPARISON

	C	F	%fc
Mayonnaise: Regular, 1 Tbsp	100	11	99%
Light, average, 1 Tbsp	50	5	90%
Fat Free (e.g. *Wt. Watcher's*), 1 T.	12	0	0%
(See Salad Dressings for extra listings)			
Peanut Butter, 1 Tbsp	100	8	72%
Avocado, mashed, 1 Tbsp	25	2.5	90%

CREAM & CREAMERS

QUICK GUIDE

CREAM
Average All Brands

	C	F	%fc
Half & Half Cream: 1 Tbsp	20	2	90%
2 Tbsp	40	4	90%
Light, coffee/table (20% fat): 1 T.	30	3	90%
2 Tbsp	60	6	90%
Medium (25% fat), 1 Tbsp	40	4	90%
Sour Cream: Regular, 1 Tbsp	30	3	90%
1 cup	490	48	88%
Light, 1 Tbsp	20	1	45%
Half & Half, 1 Tbsp	20	2	90%
Nonfat (*HeluvaGood*), 1 Tsbp	10	0	0%
Whipping Cream:			
Heavy (37% fat):			
1 Tbsp fluid/2 T. whipped	50	5.5	100%
1/4 cup whipped	100	11	100%
1/2 cup fluid/1 c. whipped	400	44	100%
Light (30% fat):			
1 Tbsp fluid/2 T. whipped	45	5	100%
1/2 cup fluid/1 c. whipped	350	37	100%

WHIPPED TOPPINGS

	C	F	%fc
Cream (Pressurized): Average,			
1 Tbsp	10	1	90%
1/4 cup	40	4	90%
Cream Toppings:			
Cool Whip: Regular, 2 Tbsp	25	1.5	55%
Regular, 1/4 cup/4 Tbsp	50	3	55%
Lite, 2 Tbsp	20	1	45%
Fat Free, 2 Tbsp	15	0	0%
Chocolate, 2 Tbsp	25	1.5	55%
Kraft: Fat Free, 2 Tbsp	15	0	0%
Real Cream, 2 Tbsp	25	1.5	55%
Reddi-Wip: Deluxe, 2 Tbsp	30	3	90%
1/4 cup/4 Tbsp	60	6	90%
Lite, 2 Tbsp	20	2	90%
Fat Free, 2 Tbsp	10	0	0%

COCONUT CREAM/MILK

CANNED

	C	F	%fc
Coconut Cream:			
Plain/unsweetened, 2 Tbsp, 1 oz	70	6	77%
1/2 cup	280	24	77%
Sweetened: *Coco Lopez*, 1 oz	120	5	38%
1/2 cup, 4 oz	480	20	38%
Coconut Milk, can, 1/2 cup	225	24	95%
Coconut Water (center), 1 cup	45	0.5	10%

COFFEE CREAMERS

POWDER

	C	F	%fc
Coffee-Mate: Regular, 1 tsp	10	0.5	50%
1 heaping tsp	15	1	50%
Fat Free, 1 tsp	10	0	0%
Flavors, 12g	60	3	45%
Fat Free, 12g	50	0	0%
Cremora: Same as *Coffee Mate*			
N-Rich: Same as *Coffee Mate*			

LIQUID/REFRIGERATED: *Per Tbsp*

	C	F	%fc
Coffee-Mate Coffee Creamer:			
Plain: Regular/Plain, 1 Tbsp	20	1	50%
Fat Free, 1 Tbsp	10	0	0%
Lite, 1 Tbsp	10	0.5	50%
Flavors: Amaretto/Fr.Vanilla	40	2	45%
Fat Free, all flavors	25	0	0%
Hood (Non Dairy), 1 Tbsp	25	0	0%
International Delight:			
Regular/Flavors	40	1.5	34%
Nonfat flavors	30	0	0%
Mocha Mix: Regular, 1 Tbsp	20	1.5	67%
Fat Free	10	0	0%
Lite	10	0.5	45%
Rich's Coffee Rich: Regular	25	1	36%
Light	15	0.5	30%
Rich's Farm Rich: Regular, 1 Tbsp	20	1	45%
Light/Fat Free	10	0	0%

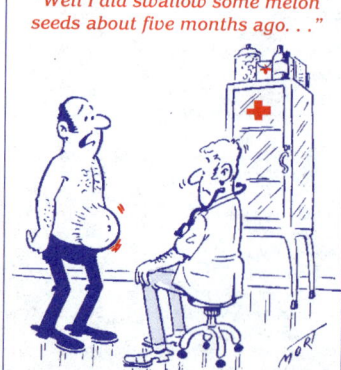

"Well I did swallow some melon seeds about five months ago..."

CHEESE

QUICK GUIDE

	C	F	%fc
FIRM/HARD CHEESES:			
(American, Cheddar, Colby, Coon, Swiss)			
Regular:			
1 oz slice/piece	110	9	74%
8 oz package	880	72	74%
16 oz (1lb) package	1760	144	74%
Cubes: 1" cube, $3/4$ oz	55	5	82%
$1^{1}/4$" cube, 2 oz slice	110	9	74%
Diced: 1 cup, $4^{1}/2$ oz	500	40	72%
Grated: 1 Tbsp, $1/4$ cup	27	2	67%
Shredded: $1/4$ cup, 1 oz	110	9	74%
1 cup, 4 oz	440	36	74%
Sliced: 1 thin ($3^{1}/2$" sq.), $3/4$ oz	85	7	74%
Rectangular (7"x 4"x $1/8$"), $1^{1}/2$ oz	165	14	76%
Round ($3^{1}/4$" diam. x $1/8$"), $3/4$ oz	85	7	74%
Semi-circular, $1^{1}/4$ oz			
($5^{1}/2$" long, $3^{1}/2$" radius, $1/8$"thick)	140	11	71%
Cholesterol Content: 30mg per 1 oz			
Sodium Content: 180mg per 1 oz			

CHEESES

Per 1 oz, Unless Indicated	C	F	%fc
American:			
Regular, 1 slice, 1 oz	110	9	74%
Kraft Deluxe, 0.7 oz slice	70	6	73%
Grated, 1 Tbsp, $1/4$ oz	23	2	73%
Light (*Borden*), 1 oz	70	4	40%
Land O'Lakes, 1 oz	70	5	64%
Smart Beat, 0.6 oz slice	35	2	50%
Fat Free: *Alpine Lace*, 1 oz	45	0	0%
HealthyChoice, Singles, 0.7 oz	30	0	0%
Weight Watchers, all types, $3/4$ oz	30	0	0%
Babybel (*Laughing Cow*), 1 oz	90	7	70%
Crumbled, $1/2$ cup, $2^{1}/2$ oz	250	20	72%
Dorman's Castello, 1 oz	135	12	80%
Bonbel (*Laughing Cow*), 1 oz	100	8	70%
Mini, $3/4$ oz	75	6	70%
Brick, 1 oz	110	8	65%
Brie, 1 oz	95	8	75%
Camembert, 1 oz	90	7	70%
Caraway, 1 oz	105	8	70%
Cheddar:			
Regular, 1 oz	110	9	74%
(Also see 'Quick Guide')			
Reduced Fat/Light, 1 oz	80	5	56%
Weight Watchers, 1 oz	80	5	56%
Fat Free: *Alpine Lace*, 1 oz	45	0	0%
Weight Watchers, 1 sl., $3/4$ oz	30	0	0%
Cheese Balls (*Kaukauma*),			
all types, 1 oz	100	7	60%
Cheese Nut, Average, 1 oz	100	7	60%
Cheese Logs, Average, 1 oz	100	7	60%
Cheshire, 1 oz	110	9	74%
Colby, Regular, 1 oz	110	9	74%
Reduced Fat (*Alpine Lace*), 1 oz	80	5	56%
Colby-Jack, 1 oz	110	9	74%
Cottage Cheese: *Average All Brands*			
Creamed: 2 Tbsp, 1 oz	30	1	30%
$1/2$ cup, 4 oz	120	5	30%
w. fruit, $1/2$ cup, 4 oz	130	4	27%
Reduced Fat (2%), 2 T., 1 oz	25	<1	18%
$1/2$ cup, 4 oz	100	2	18%
Low Fat (1%), 2 Tbsp, 1 oz	20	<1	11%
$1/2$ cup, 4 oz	80	1	11%
NonFat, 2 Tbsp, 1 oz	20	0	0%
$1/2$ cup, 4 oz	80	0	0%
Borden Dry Curd (0.5% Fat),			
$1/2$ cup, 4 oz	80	0	0%
Friendship : Low Fat P/apple, 4oz	120	1	7%
NonFat Plus Peach, $1/2$ c., 4 oz	110	0	0%
Pot Style, $1/2$ cup, 4 oz	90	3	30%
w. Pineapple, 4 oz	140	4	25%
Hood: 1% Fat Chive/Pppr Herb, 4oz	90	2	25%
1% Pineapple Cherry, 4 oz	110	1	7%
NonFat Pineapple, 4 oz	110	0	0%
Knudsen: 1.5% Fruit, 4 oz	110	2	15%
Free, $1/2$ cup, 4.3 oz	80	0	0%
Light N' Lively: Garden Salad, 4 oz	90	2	20%
Peach and Pineapple,			
$1/2$ cup, 4.3 oz	120	1	7%
Lite Line: Low Fat 1.5%, $1/2$ cup	90	2	20%
Weight Watchers: 1%, $1/2$ cup	90	1	10%
2%, $1/2$ cup	90	2	20%
Chevre: See Goat's Milk Cheese			
Cream Cheese: See Page 34.			
Danbo (*Dormans*): 20%, 1 oz	62	3	44%
45%, 1 oz	100	7.5	65%
Edam: Regular, 1 oz	100	8	70%
Farmer (*Friendship*), 2 Tbsp, 1 oz	50	3	55%
Feta: Regular, *Frigo*, 1 oz	100	8	70%
Crumbled, $1/2$ cup, $2^{1}/2$ oz	190	15	70%
Reduced Fat (*Alpine Lace*),	60	4	60%
Fontina (*Sargento/Classica*), 1 oz	110	9	74%
Gjetost (Goat's Milk, fresh), 1 oz	85	7	74%
Sargento, 1 oz	130	8	55%
Goat's Milk: Soft: *Chevre*, 1 oz	70	6	77%
Chavril, 3 Tbsp, 1 oz	60	4.5	65%

CHEESE CONT

Goat's Milk Cheese (Cont)	C	F	%fc
St, Loup Camembert, 1 oz	80	7	78%
SilverGoat, 1 oz	70	6	77%
Semi-Soft: 1 oz	100	8.5	75%
Hard: Sargento, 1 oz	130	10	70%
Gorgonzola: 1 oz	110	9	74%
Galbani Dolcelatte: 1 oz	95	8	75%
Gouda: 1 oz	100	8	70%
Gruyere, 1 oz	115	9	70%
Havarti, 1 oz	120	11	80%
Italian (*Classica Italiano*), 1 oz	110	9	74%
Jarlsberg, 1 oz	100	7	63%
Jarlsberg Lite shredded, 1 oz	70	4	50%
Kefir, 2 Tbsp, 1 oz	60	4	60%
Limburger, 1 oz	90	8	80%
Mascarpone, 1 oz	130	13	90%
Mexican (*Sargento* Recipe Blend), Shredded, 1/4 cup, 1 oz	110	9	74%
Monterey, 1 oz	105	8.5	71%
Monterey Jack: regular, 1 oz	110	9	74%
Light Naturals (Kraft), 1 oz	80	5	55%
Alpine Lace , Monti-Jack Lo, 1 oz	80	5	55%
Weight Watchers, 1 oz	80	5	55%
Mozzarella:			
Regular: *Kraft/Dorman's*, 1 oz	90	7	70%
Land O'Lakes/Polly-O, 1 oz	80	6	66%
Shredded, 1/4 cup, 1 oz	80	6	66%
Light: *Polly-O Lite*, 1 oz	70	4	50%
Kraft Light Naturals, 1 oz	80	4	45%
Sorrento Lite, 1 oz	60	3	45%
Part Skim (*Alpine Lace*), 1 oz	70	4	50%
Polly-O, 1 oz	70	5	64%
Fat Free: *Healthy Choice*, 1/4 c.,1 oz	45	0	0%
Polly-O, 1 oz	35	0	0%
Kraft, shredded, 1/4 cup, 1 oz	50	0	0%
Muenster: regular, 1 oz	110	9	74%
Reduced Fat: *Dorman's*, 1 oz	80	5	55%
Neufchatel: Regular, 1 oz	75	7	65%
Philadelphia, 1 oz	70	6	77%
Flavored: Fruit/Herbs	80	7	78%
Chocolate (*Hickory Farms*), 1 oz	110	8	65%
Parmesan: Fresh/Block, 1 oz	110	7	70%
Shredded/Grated, 1 Tbsp	22	1.5	57%
Grated (Packaged): 1 Tbsp	26	2	62%
1 oz quantity	130	9	62%
1/2 cup, 1 3/4 oz	230	16	62%
w.Romano (*Frigo*), grated, 1 oz	130	9	62%

Note: Packaged grated and shredded Parmesan have more calories than block Parmesan due to a lower moisture content.

Pizza, shredded:	C	F	%fc
Frigo, 1/4 cup, 1 oz	90	7	70%
1 cup, 4 oz	360	28	70%
Lowfat (*Frigo*), 1 oz	65	3	41%
Port Du Salut, 1 oz	100	8	72%
Port Wine (*Hickory Farms*), 1 oz	100	7	42%
Pot (*Sargento*), 1 oz	25	0	0%
Provolone: Regular, 1 oz	100	8	72%
Reduced Fat, *Alpine Lace*, 1 oz	70	5	64%
Pub (*Hickory Farms*), 1 oz	95	7	65%
Quark: 40% fat, 1 oz	47	3	57%
20% fat, 1 oz	32	1.5	45%
Skim, 1 oz	22	0	0%
Queso:			
Anego/Asadero/Blanco, 1oz	105	9	77%
Queso Chichuahua/De Papa, 1 oz	110	9	74%
Queso De Taco, 1 oz	105	9	77%
Ricotta Cheese:			
Whole Milk, 2 Tbsp, 1 oz	50	3.5	63%
1/2 cup, 4 1/2 oz	225	16	63%
Part Skim, 2 Tbsp, 1 oz	40	2.5	57%
1/2 cup, 4 1/2 oz	180	12	57%
Light/Low Fat, 2 Tbsp, 1 oz	30	1.5	40%
1/2 cup, 4 1/2 oz	140	6	40%
Fat Free (*Polly-O*), 1/2 cup, 4 1/2 oz	100	0	0%
Baked Ricotta, 2 oz portion	130	9	60%
Romano: Block/Loaf, 1 oz	110	8	65%
Grated (Pkg), 1 oz	120	9	67%
1 Tbsp	26	2	67%
Roquefort, 1 oz	105	9	77%
Slim Jack (*Dorman's*), 1 oz	90	7	54%
Sheep's Milk (*Hollow Rd Farm*)	45	3	60%
Smoked: *Sargents* Smokestick	100	7	50%
Hickory Farm, Smoky Lyte, 1 oz	80	6	67%
Stilton, 1 oz	118	10	76%
String (*Frigo/Kraft/Sargents*), 1 oz	80	5	56%
String Lite (*Frigo*), 1 oz	60	2	30%
Swiss: Regular, 1 oz	110	8	65%
Reduced Fat: *Alpine Lace*, 1 oz	90	6	60%
Dorman's, Kraft Light Naturals, 1oz	90	5	50%
Weight Watchers, 3/4 slice	30	0	0%
Taco, shredded (*Frigo/Kraft/Sargents*)	110	9	78%
Tilsit (*Sargents*), 1 oz	100	7	63%
Tybo (*Dorman's/Sargents*), 1 oz	100	7	63%
Vermont (*Churny*), 1 oz	110	9	78%
Wensleydale, 1 oz	108	9	79%
Whey Cheese, 1 oz	125	8	57%

CHEESE CONT

CHEESE PRODUCTS

	C	F	%fc
Alouette: French Onion/Garlic, 2 Tbsp, 0.8oz	70	7	90%
Light Garlic, 2 Tbsp, 0.8 oz	50	4	72%
Cheez Whiz: Regular, 2 T, 1.2 oz	90	7	70%
Light, 2 Tbsp, 1.2 oz	80	3	33%
Squeezable, 2 Tbsp, 1.2 oz	100	8	70%
Cracker Barrel, Cheddar, 1.1 oz	100	8	70%
Delico: Alouette Cajun, 2 T, 0.8 oz	70	7	90%
Garden Vegetable, 2 Tbsp, 0.8 oz	60	6	90%
Handi-Snacks			
Cheez 'n Breadsticks, 1 pkg	130	7	48%
Cheez'n Pretzels, 1 oz pkg	110	6	49%
Cheez'n Crackers, 1.1 oz pkg	130	8	55%
Mozzarella StIngchse Stick, 1oz	80	6	67%
Healthy Choice			
American Singles, 1 slice	30	0	0%
Heluva Good Cheese			
American, 1 slice	45	5	90%
Cheddar Sharp w. Horseradish, 2 Tbsp, 1oz	90	7	70%
Jalapeno: Aver., all brands, 1 oz	90	7	70%
Kraft: American grated,1T., 0.2 oz	25	2	70%
Singles, 1 slice, 3/4 oz	70	6	77%
Free Singles, 1 slice, 0.7 oz	30	3	90%
Pimento Spread, 2 Tbsp, 1.1 oz	80	6	67%
Roka Blue, 2 Tbsp, 1.1 oz	80	7	79%
Rondele: Soft Spreadable, 2 T, 1oz	100	9	80%
Light, 2 Tbsp, 0.9 oz	60	4	60%
SmartBeat: All flav., 1 sl., 0.6 oz	35	2	50%
Spreadery			
Vermont Cheddar, 2 Tbsp, 1oz	80	5	56%
Neufchatel, all flavors, 2 T, 1 oz	70	6	77%
Nacho Flavor, 2 T, 1 oz	70	4	50%
Velveeta: Cheese, 1 slice, 0.7 oz	80	5	64%
Light, 1 oz	60	3	45%
Shredded, 1/4 cup, 1.3 oz	130	9	62%
WisPride: Per 2 Tbsp, 1.1 oz			
Hickory Smoked Cup	100	7	63%
Port Wine Ball/Cup	100	7	63%
Port Wine Cup, Light	80	3	64%

CHEESE DIPS ~ See Next Page ~

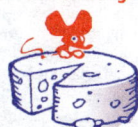

CHEESE SUBSTITUTES

	C	F	%fc
Per 1 oz Unless Indicated			
Almond Rella (Nu Soya)			
Cheddar; Garlic & Herb, 1 oz	60	3	45%
Borden: Taco-Mate, 1 oz	100	7	49%
Delicia: Amer. Ch. Subst.	80	6	65%
Colby Imitation Cheese	80	6	65%
Dorman's Lo Chol: Colby style	90	7	54%
Swiss/MuensterStyle	100	7	60%
Formagg: Cheddar, 1 slice, 0.7 oz	60	4	60%
American Wh./Yellow, 1 sl. 0.7 oz	60	4	60%
Cheddar, 1 slice, 0.7 oz	60	4	60%
Mozzarella (Old World), 1 oz	60	3	45%
Parmesan Grated, 1 Tbsp, 1/4 oz	22	1.5	60%
Provolone (Vintage), 1 oz	60	3	45%
Swiss White, 1 slice, 0.7 oz	60	4	60%
Fisher: Ched-O-Mate, shrd, 1 oz	90	7	54%
Pizza-Mate, shredded, 1 oz	90	7	54%
Frigo: Cheddar (Imitation), 1 oz	90	7	54%
Mozzarella (Imitation), 1 oz	90	7	54%
Georgio's: Imitation Cheddar; Mozzarella.,shredded, 1/4 c, 1oz	90	7	54%
Golden Image: Amer., 1 sl., 0.7oz	70	5	64%
Mild Cheddar, 1 slice, 0.7 oz	70	5	64%
Harvest Moon (Per 1/4 c., 1.3 oz):			
Shredded: American; Cheddar	120	9	67%
Mozzarella	110	8	65%
Nu Tofu: Cheddar Cheese Altern.	70	4	50%
Sargento: Classic Supreme:			
Cheddar, shredded, 1oz	90	6	60%
Mozzarella, shrd, 1/4 cup	80	6	65%
Smart Beat, all variet. 0.67 oz sl.	25	0	0%
Soya Kaas: American Style	70	5	64%
Garlic & Herb	70	5	64%
Jalapeno Mexi Kaas	70	5	64%
Mozzarella; Monterey Jack	70	5	64%
Fat Free, all varieties, 1 oz	40	2	45%
Tofutti Better Than Cream Cheese	80	8	90%
TofuRella: Cheddar, 1 oz	70	5	64%
Jalapeno; Mozzarella; Monterey	70	4.5	57%
Weight Watchers: Fat Free Slices, All varieties, 3/4 oz slice	30	0	0%
Grated Italian Topping, 1 Tbsp	20	0	0%
White Wave, *Soy A Melt:*			
Chedr/Mozz./Monterey Jack, 1 oz	80	5	55%
Fat Free, 1 oz	40	0	0%
Singles: Amer./Mozzrlla, 3/4 oz sl.	60	4	60%

CREAM CHEESE, DIPS, SPREADS

CREAM CHEESE

	C	F	%fc
CREAM CHEESE			
Regular/Soft, 2 Tbsp, 1 oz	100	10	90%
3 oz pkg	300	30	90%
w. Chives/Herbs/Pimento, 1 oz	90	9	90%
W. Fruit/Strawb./P'apple, 1 oz	90	8	80%
Lox, 1 oz	90	9	90%
Philadelphia Brand:			
Plain/Soft, 2 Tbsp, 1 oz	100	10	90%
1/3 Less Fat, 1 oz	70	6	77%
Light, 1 oz	70	5	64%
Fat Free, 1 oz	25	0	0%
Flavor./Herbs/Fruit/Salmon, 1 oz	90	9	90%
w. Smoked Salmon 1 oz	100	10	90%
Whipped, 3 Tbsp, 1 oz	110	11	90%
Alpine Lace: Fat Free, 2 T., 1 oz	30	0	0%
Weight Watchers, 2 Tbsp, 1 oz	40	2.5	55%

DIPS/SPREADS

Per 2 Tbsp (1 oz) Unless Indicated

	C	F	%fc
Avocado/Guacomole	50	4	65%
Baba Ghannouj (Eggplant/Sesame)	70	6	77%
Bagel Spread: Bacon Scallion	90	7	70%
Breakstone: Sour Cream, all flav.	50	4	65%
Chi-Chi's: Fiesta Bean,	35	2	50%
Fiesta Cheese	40	3	65%
Eagle: Bean	35	2	50%
Frito Lay: Chili Cheese	45	3	60%
French Onion	60	5	75%
Bean/Jalapeno Bean	35	1	26%
Jalapeno & Cheddar	50	3	54%
Guiltless Gourmet:			
Black Bean Dip	30	0	0%
BBQ Black/Pinto Bean Dips	35	0	0%
Nacho Dip	25	0	0%
Salsas, all varieties	10	0	0%
Heluva Good Cheese:			
Clam/French Onion	50	5	90%
Bacon/Homestyle/Ranch	60	5	75%
Light Fr. Onion/Jalapeno Cheddar	40	2	45%
French Onion Dip, aver., all brands	60	6	90%
Guacamole, 2 Tbsp, 1 oz	50	4	65%
Heluva Good Cheese: 'N Salsa	80	6	65%
'N Pretzel	80	6	65%
Hummus, 2 Tbsp, 1 oz	50	2.5	45%
1/2 cup, 4.5 oz	220	11	45%
Knudsen: Nacho Cheese	60	4	60%
Sour Cream Bacon & Onion	60	5	90%
Sour Cream Fench Onion	50	4	65%

DIPS/SPREADS (CONT)

	C	F	%fc
Kraft: Avocado/Clam	60	4	60%
French Onion/Jalapeno	60	4	60%
Jalapeno Chse, Bacon. H'radish	60	5	75%
Premium: Bac. & On./Nacho Ch.	60	5	75%
French Onion/Crmy Cucumber	50	4	65%
Blue Chse./Clam/Crmy Onion	45	4	80%
Philly flavors: Apple Cinnamon	100	8	72%
Chive & Onion	110	10	82%
Pineapple; Salmon	100	9	81%
Strawberry; Honey Nut	110	9	74%
Strawberry, Fat Free	45	0	0%
Garden Veges, Fat Free	35	0	0%
Lay's: Lowfat Sr. Cream, Onion	40	1	23%
Louise's: (Fat Free) Honey Mustard	40	0	0%
Sour Cream & Onion/Wh.Cheese	25	0	0%
Lucerne: French Onion	70	6	75%
Guacamole	80	6	90%
Marzetti: Blue Cheese	200	21	98%
Light Ranch Veggie	60	7	98%
Other flavors, average	140	14	90%
Nalley's: Bacon,Guacomole,			
Jalapeno	110	12	95%
Nacho Cheese Dip	120	13	95%
Nasoya: Vegi Dip	50	3	54%
Old Dutch: Cheddar, Nacho	35	0	0%
Old El Paso: Black Bean	20	0	0%
Cheese'n Salsa: Mild; Medium	40	3	68%
Lowfat, medium	30	1.5	45%
Chunky Salsa varieties	15	0	0%
Jalapeno Dip	30	1	30%
Olys Bagel Spread:			
Berry; Honey Cinnamon; Raisin	100	8	72%
Garden Veg; Garlic & Herb	90	9	90%
Parkers Farm: Garden Veggie	90	8	80%
Wildberry	80	5	56%
Rondele Bagel Temptations:			
Crispy Veg; New York Style	90	9	90%
Cinnamon & Honey; Very Berry	100	9	81%
Ruffles: Fr. Onion; Ranch	70	6	77%
Lowfat varieties	40	1	23%
Sealtest: French Onion	50	2	35%
Clam/Cucumber & Onion	50	4	70%
Snyder's Mustard Pretzel	90	4	40%
Taramosalata (Fish Roe Puree)	70	6	77%
Tztziki (Cucumber/Yoghurt Dip)	40	3	65%
Wise: Jalapeno Bean	25	0	0%
Taco	12	0	0%

EGGS & EGG DISHES

CHICKEN EGGS

C ~ CALORIES **F** ~ FAT (Grams) **%fc** ~ PERCENT FAT CALORIES

	C	F	%fc
FRESH			
Raw (weight with shell):			
Small, 40g	65	4	55%
Medium, 44g	70	4	55%
Large, 50g	75	4.5	55%
Extra Large, 56g	80	5	55%
Jumbo, 63g	90	5.5	55%
Egg Yolk, 1 extra large	63	5	71%
Egg White, 1 extra large	16	0	0%
DRIED EGG POWDER			
Whole Egg: 1/4 cup, 1 oz	170	12	64%
1 Tbsp	30	2	64%
Egg White, 1/4 cup, 1 oz	105	0	0%
Egg Yolk, 1/4 cup, 1 oz	195	18	83%
1 Tbsp	27	2.5	81%

EGG SUBSTITUTES

	C	F	%fc
1/4 Cup (Equivalent to 1 Egg)			
Better 'n Eggs (Papetti), 1/4 cup, 2 oz	30	0	0%
Egg Beaters (Fleischmann's):			
Regular, 1/4 cup	30	0	0%
Cheese Omelete, 1/2 cup	110	5	40%
Vegetable Omelete, 1/2 cup	50	0	0%
Egg Magic (Featherweight), 1/2 pkg	60	2	30%
Egg Watchers (Tofutti), 2 oz	50	2	36%
Eggstra, 1/2 envelope	50	2	36%
Healthy Choice, 1/4 cup, 2 oz	25	0	0%
Scramblers (Morn Star), 1/4 cup	35	0	0%
Second Nature: Regular, 1/4 cup	60	2	30%
Fat Free, 1/4 cup	40	0	0%
Simply Eggs, 1/4 cup	35	1	25%

OTHER EGGS

	C	F	%fc
Duck, 1 large, 2 1/2 oz	130	9.5	65%
Goose, 1 large, 5 oz	280	19	63%
Quail, 3 eggs, 1 oz	42	3	64%
Turkey, 1 large, 3 oz	135	9.5	63%
Turtle, 1 egg, 1 3/4 oz	75	5	60%

OMEGA-3 FAT ENRICHED

	C	F	%fc
Eggs Plus (Pilgrim's Pride): 1 large	80	5	55%

Note: Cholesterol content same as regular eggs, but Omega-3 fats inhibit blood cholesterol increase. (Also see Cholesterol ~ Page 221)

COOKED EGGS

	C	F	%fc
Boiled Egg: Same as raw egg			
Fried Egg: With fat, 1 large,	100	8	72%
2 small eggs	175	13	67%
no fat/nonstick pan, 1 lge	80	5.5	60%
Deviled Egg, 2 halves	145	13	80%
Eggs Benedict (2) on toast or English muffin	860	56	60%
Eggs Florentine (2) on toast or English muffin	890	59	60%
Omelets:			
1 Egg: Plain (w. 1 tsp fat)	125	10	72%
with 1/2 oz cheese	175	15	77%
w. 1/2 oz chse + 1/2 oz ham	200	16	72%
2 Eggs: Plain (w. 2 tsp fat)	250	20	72%
with 1 oz cheese	360	29	72%
w. 1 oz cheese + 1 oz ham	410	32	70%
3 Eggs: Plain (w. 1 Tbsp fat)	360	29	72%
w. 2 oz cheese	580	47	73%
w. 2 oz chse + 2 oz ham	680	53	70%
Extras: Tomato/Onion/Veges	20	0	0%
Egg Substitute (Eggbeaters):			
2 eggs (1/2 cup) + 1 tsp fat	100	4	36%
3 eggs (3/4 cup) + 2 tsp fat	160	8	45%
Extras: 1 oz cheese	110	9	74%
1 oz ham	50	3	54%
Tom./Onion/Veges	20	0	0%
Pickled Egg, 1 large	80	5.5	60%
Poached Egg: 1 large	80	5.5	60%
Scotch Egg, 1 egg	300	21	63%
Scrambled Eggs: 1 large egg:			
w. 1 Tbsp milk + 1 tsp fat	120	9	68%
w. 1 Tbsp skim milk/no fat	85	5.5	58%
2 large eggs:			
w. 2 Tbsp milk + 2 tsp fat	260	20	69%
w. 2 Tbsp skim milk/no fat	180	11	55%

EGG NOGS

	C	F	%fc
Per 1/2 Cup (4 fl. oz)			
Regular: Borden	160	9	50%
Crowley	190	9	43%
Hood (Goldeen)	180	8	40%
Light: Borden/Hood	120	2	16%
Fat Free: Hood	100	0	0%

EGGS & EGG DISHES

BREAKFAST SIDES

	C	F	%fc
Toast: Plain, 1 thick slice	85	1	10%
with 2 tsp butter/marg.	155	9	54%
with 3 tsp/1Tbsp	190	13	62%
English Muffin: Plain, 2 oz	130	1	6%
with 3 tsp fat	230	12	47%
Bacon, 2 strips	70	5	64%
Ham: Lean, 2 oz	100	3	27%
Hash Browns: 1/2 cup	125	6.5	47%
1 cup serving	250	13	47%
Sausages, 2 links (1 oz ea.)	180	16	80%

FROZEN EGG DISHES

	C	F	%fc
Downyflake: Scrambled Eggs			
w. Ham & Hash Browns, 1 pkg	360	26	65%
w. Ham & Pecan Twirl	470	28	54%
w/ Hash Browns & Saus.	420	34	73%
Swanson Great Starts			
Eggs, Canadian Bacon	290	15	47%
Scrambled Eggs:			
w. Cheese & Cinn. Pancakes	290	23	71%
w. Bacon & Home Fries	340	26	69%
w. Home Fries	200	12	54%
w. Sausages & Hash Browns	430	34	71%
Egg, Sausage & Cheese	460	28	55%
Omelets w. Cheese & Ham	390	29	67%
Reduced Cholesterol Eggs			
w. Mini Oatbran Muffins	250	12	43%
Sausage Egg Muffin	490	30	55%
Quaker Scrambled Eggs	490	30	55%
w. Cheese/Fried Potatoes	250	13	47%
w. Sausage & Hash Browns	290	20	62%
w. Sausage & Pancakes	270	14	47%
Weight Watchers			
Vegetable Omelet	210	6	26%
Ham & Cheese Omelet	220	5	20%

EGG ROLLS

	C	F	%fc
Average All Brands (Frozen)			
(Chun King/La Choy)			
Chicken Egg Rolls: Mini, 5 rolls	170	6	21%
Restaurant Style, 1 roll, 3 oz	170	5	26%
Pork & Shrimp Egg Rolls:			
Mini, 12 rolls	420	16	34%
Pork Restaurant Style, 1 roll	170	6	32%
Shrimp Egg Rolls: Mini, 5 rolls	160	3.5	20%
Restaurant Style, 1 roll	150	4	24%

FAST FOOD/RESTAURANTS

	C	F	%fc
Burger King:			
Bisc. w. Bacon/Egg/Cheese	510	31	55%
Croissan'wich Saus./Egg/Chse	600	46	69%
Carl's Jr: Scrambled Eggs	160	11	62%
Denny's: Country Scramble	800	50	57%
Eggs Benedict	860	56	60%
Omelette: Ham 'n Cheese	740	55	60%
Vegie Cheese	720	53	66%
Farmer's	890	71	72%
Steak & Eggs	885	66	67%
Hardees: Bacon & Egg	570	33	52%
Ham, Egg & Cheese	540	30	50%
Ultimate Omelet	570	33	52%
Jack in the Box:			
Scrambled Egg Pocket	430	21	44%
McDonald's: Egg McMuffin	290	12	37%
Bacon, Egg & Cheese Bisc.	440	26	53%
Scrambled Eggs (2)	160	11	63%
Perkins: Country Club Omelet	930	79	76%
Roy Rogers: Ham & Egg Bisc.	460	23	45%

"Were your eyes ever bigger than your stomach?"

MEAT - BEEF

BEEF

Note: Cooking reduces weight of meat by 20-45% due to water and fat losses. Average weight loss is 30%. Actual loss depends on cooking method and cooking time. Examples:

4 oz raw wt. = approx. 3 oz cooked wt.
4 oz cooked wt. = approx. 5 1/2 oz raw wt.

WHAT 3 OZ COOKED MEAT LOOKS LIKE
- Half the size of this book (4 1/4" x 3" x 3/8" thick)
- Rectangular piece (4" x 2 1/2" x 1/2" thick)
- Pack of cards (3 1/2" x 2 1/2" x 5/8" thick)

STEAK QUICK GUIDE

SIRLOIN (CHOICE GRADE) — C F %fc
External fat trimmed to 1/4"
BROILED, Edible Portion (no bone)
Small Serving, 3 oz
(3 oz cooked, from 4-4 1/2 oz raw)

	C	F	%fc
Lean + fat (1/4"), 3oz	230	14	55%
Lean + marbling, 3 oz	195	10	46%
(External fat trimmed **before** cooking)			
Lean only, 3 oz	170	7	37%
(No external fat or marbling)			

Medium/Regular Serving, 5 oz
(from approx. 7 oz raw)

Lean + fat (1/4"), 5 oz	470	29	55%
Lean + marbling, 5 oz	400	20	46%
Lean only, 5 oz	350	14	37%

Large Serving, 8 oz
(from 11-12 oz raw)

Lean + fat, 8 oz	610	38	55%
Lean + marbling, 8 oz	520	26	46%
Lean only, 8 oz	454	18	37%

Extra Large Serving, 12 oz
(from approx. 16-17 oz raw)

Lean + fat (1/4"), 12 oz	915	57	55%
Lean + marbling, 12 oz	780	39	46%
Lean only, 12 oz	680	27	37%

PAN-FRIED
Sirloin (choice), medium serving:

Lean + fat (1/4"), 5 oz	450	32	64%
Lean only, 5 oz	330	15	41%

> **HINT TO SAVE FAT & CALORIES**
> Save extra calories with broiled steak by trimming off the external fat **before** cooking. This prevents external fat liquefying and migrating into the lean meat.

OTHER STEAKS — C F %fc

Filet Mignon (Tenderloin):
1 medium steak, 6 oz raw wt.
Broiled, with 1/4" fat trim

	C	F	%fc
Lean + fat (1/4"), 4 oz	340	24	63%
Lean only, 3 1/2 oz	210	10	43%

Broiled, (1/4" fat removed before cooking)

Lean + marbling, 3 1/4 oz	220	12	49%
Lean only, 3 oz	180	8	40%

New York/Club Steak:
Top Loin/Short Loin
1 steak, regular (9 1/4 oz raw, 1/4" fat)

Broiled: Lean + fat (1/4"), 6 1/4 oz	510	35	62%
Lean + marbling, 5 1/2 oz	330	16	43%
Lean only, 5 1/4 oz	310	14	40%

Porterhouse Steak:
1 medium, 6 oz raw wt. (no bone)
Broiled:

Lean + fat (1/4"), 4 1/4 oz	370	27	66%
Lean only, 3 1/2 oz	220	11	45%

T-Bone Steak:
1 medium, 8 oz raw wt.

Broiled: Lean + fat	380	27	64%
Lean only	220	10	40%

AVERAGE ALL CUTS

Average all Retail Cuts: — C F %fc
Edible weight (no bone)

RAW
(1 lb raw yields approx. 11-12 oz cooked)

	C	F	%fc
Lean + fat (1/4" trim), 1 oz	70	5.5	70%
1/2 Pound, 8 oz	560	44	70%
Lean only, 1 oz	40	2	45%
1/2 Pound, 8 oz	320	16	45%
Fat only, 1 oz	190	20	95%

COOKED (No Added Fat)

Lean + fat (1/4"), 1 oz	86	6	63%
Small serving, 3 oz	260	18	63%
Lean + marbling, (no ext. fat), 1oz	78	5	58%
Small serving, 3 oz	235	15	58%
Lean only, 1 oz	60	3	45%
Small serving, 3 oz	180	9	45%
Fat only, 1 oz	193	20	93%

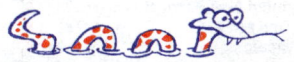

MEAT - BEEF

BEEF - INDIVIDUAL CUTS

	C	F	%fc
Average All Grades			
Edible Weight (no bone)			
Brisket, whole, braised:			
Lean + fat (1/4"), 3 oz	330	27	73%
Lean + marbling, 3 oz	250	17	61%
Lean only, 3 oz	205	11	48%
Chuck, blade, braised:			
Lean + fat (1/4"), 3 oz	290	22	68%
Lean + marbling, 3 oz	285	20	63%
Lean only, 3 oz	210	11	47%
Flank: Raw, 4 oz	200	12	54%
Braised, 3 oz	225	14	56%
Broiled, 3 oz	190	11	52%
Ribs, whole (ribs 6-12):			
Average all grades, roasted			
(1 lb raw yields 10 1/4 oz roasted)			
Lean + fat (1/4")			
(3.6 oz w. bone, 3 oz no bone)	300	25	75%
Lean only, 3 oz (no bone)	200	11	49%
Round, bottom, braised:			
Lean + fat (1/4"), 3 oz	235	14	54%
Lean only, 3 oz	180	7	35%
Round, eye/tip, roasted:			
Lean + fat (1/4"), 3 oz	200	11	49%
Lean, 3 oz	150	5	30%
Round, top, Per 3 oz:			
Braised, Lean + fat	210	10	43%
Lean only	175	5	26%
Broiled, Lean + fat	185	8	39%
Lean only	155	4	23%
Pan-fried, Lean + fat	235	13	50%
Lean only	190	7	33%

GROUND BEEF

	C	F	%fc
Raw: Reg. (73% lean), 4 oz	350	30	77%
Lean (80% lean), 4 oz	300	24	72%
Extra lean (85% lean), 4 oz	250	17	61%
Healthy Choice (97% lean), 4 oz	130	4	28%
Baked/Broiled: Reg., 3 oz	250	18	65%
Lean, 3 oz	230	16	63%
Extra lean, 3 oz	200	12	54%
Pan-fried: Regular, 3 oz	260	19	66%
Lean, 3 oz	230	16	63%
Extra lean, 3 oz	200	12	54%
Ground Beef Patties: Average			
Frozen, raw, 4 oz	320	26	73%
Broiled, 3 oz	240	17	64%

ROAST BEEF QUICK CHECK

	C	F	%fc
ROAST BEEF			
Round (Eye/Tip, average)			
Average All Cuts			
Small Serving, 3 oz			
(2 thin slices/1 thick slice)			
Lean + fat (1/4"), 3 oz	200	11	50%
Lean only, 3 oz	150	5	30%
Medium Serving, 5 oz, (3-4 thin slices)			
Lean + fat, 5 oz	330	18	50%
Lean only, 5 oz	250	8	30%
Large Serving, 8 oz, (3 thick slices)			
Lean + fat, 8 oz	530	29	50%
Lean only, 8 oz	400	13	30%

ROAST DINNER EXTRAS

	C	F	%fc
Gravy: Thin, 2 Tbsp	20	1	45%
Thick, 2 Tbsp	50	2	36%
1 Ladle/4 Tbsp	100	4	36%
Veges: Beans, green, 1/2 cup	20	0	0%
Cauliflower w. cheese sauce, 4 oz	135	9	60%
Corn, kernels, 1/4 cup	35	0	0%
Carrots, 1/4 cup	20	0	0%
Peas, 1/4 cup	35	0	0%
Pumpkin baked:w/fat, 4 oz	90	7	70%
No added fat, 2 pces, 4 oz	25	0	0%
Potato:			
Roasted w. fat, 1 small	155	8	46%
Baked in Jacket, 1 large	220	0	0%
with 1 Tbsp whipped butter	295	8	24%
with Sour Cream, 2 Tbsp	270	6	20%
Sweet Potato/Yam, 1 medium	80	0	0%

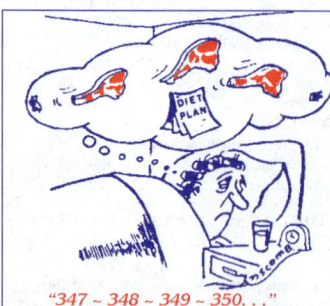

"347 ~ 348 ~ 349 ~ 350..."

MEAT - LAMB, VEAL, PORK

LAMB

	C	F	%fc
CHOICE GRADE			
Leg (Whole), roasted:			
Lean + fat, 3 oz	220	14	57%
Lean only, 3 oz	160	7	39%
Leg (Sirloin Half), roasted:			
Lean + fat, 3 oz	250	18	65%
Lean only, 3 oz	175	8	41%
Leg (Shank Half), roasted:			
Lean + fat, 3 oz	190	11	52%
Lean only, 3 oz	155	6	35%
Loin Chop, broiled:			
1 chop (raw wt., $4^{1}/4$ oz):			
Lean + fat ($2^{1}/4$ oz edible)	200	15	68%
Lean only (1.6 oz edible)	100	5	45%
Rib Chop, broiled:			
1 chop (raw wt., $3^{1}/2$ oz)			
Lean + fat ($2^{1}/2$ oz edible)	255	21	74%
Lean only ($1^{3}/4$ oz edible)	120	7	53%
Shoulder (Arm/Blade):			
Braised: Lean + fat, 3 oz	290	21	65%
Lean only, 3 oz	240	14	53%
Broiled: Lean + fat, 3 oz	240	16	60%
Lean only, 3 oz	180	9	45%
Roasted: Similar to Broiled			
Cubed Lamb (Leg/Shoulder):			
For stew or kabob			
Raw, lean only, 8 oz	310	12	34%
Braised, lean only, 3 oz	190	8	38%
Broiled, lean only, 3 oz	160	6	34%
New Zealand Lamb (Imported):			
Similar calories and fat to domestic.			

VEAL

	C	F	%fc
Edible Weights			
Leg (Top Round):			
Braised: Lean + fat, 3 oz	180	6	30%
Lean only, 3 oz	170	5	26%
Pan-fried, breaded:			
Lean + fat, 3 oz	195	8	37%
Lean only, 3 oz	175	6	31%
Pan-fried, not breaded:			
Lean + fat, 3 oz	180	7	35%
Lean only, 3 oz	155	4	23%
Roasted: Lean + fat, 3 oz	135	4	27%
Lean only, 3 oz	130	3	21%

VEAL (CONT)

	C	F	%fc
Loin Chop: 1 chop, 7 oz raw wt.			
Braised: Lean + fat	230	14	55%
Lean only	155	6	35%
Roasted: Lean + fat	175	10	51%
Lean only	125	5	36%
Rib, roasted: Lean + fat, 3 oz	195	12	55%
Lean only, 3 oz	150	7	42%
Shoulder, Arm/Blade, roasted:			
Lean + fat, 3 oz	155	7	40%
Lean only, 3 oz	145	6	37%
Sirloin, roasted:			
Lean + fat, 3 oz	170	9	47%
Lean only, 3 oz	145	6	37%
Cubed for Stew, braised:			
Leg/Shoulder, lean only, 3oz	160	4	23%
(1 lb raw yields approx. $9^{1}/4$ oz cooked)			

PORK

Figures based on NLMB data (1990)
FRESH PORK (Cooked Wt., no bone)
(4 oz raw wt. = approx. 3 oz cooked wt.)

	C	F	%fc
Blade Steak, broiled:			
Lean + fat, 3oz	220	15	61%
Lean only, 3oz	190	11	52%
Country Style Ribs, broiled:			
Lean + fat, 3 oz	270	22	73%
Lean only, 3 oz	205	13	57%
Leg (Ham), roasted:			
Lean + fat, 3 oz	250	18	65%
Lean only, 3 oz	180	9	35%
(Ham, cured — See Cold Meats)			
Loin Chops, broiled: Average			
(From 1 chop: 5 oz raw wt. w.bone			
or 4 oz raw wt., no bone)			
Lean + fat, 3 oz	200	11	50%
Lean only, 3 oz	165	7	38%
Rib Chops, broiled:			
Lean + fat, 3oz	215	13	54%
Lean only, 3 oz	180	7	35%
Rib Roast, roasted:			
Lean + fat, 3oz	210	13	56%
Lean only, 3 oz	175	9	36%
Loin Roast, roasted:			
Lean + fat, 3 oz	190	10	47%
Lean only, 3oz	160	7	39%
Back Ribs, broiled:			
Lean + fat	310	25	73%

MEATS CONT

PORK (Cont)

	C	F	%fc
Sirloin Chop, broiled:			
Lean + fat, 3 oz	175	8	41%
Lean only, 3 oz	155	6	35%
Sirloin Roast, roasted:			
Lean + fat, 3 oz	215	14	59%
Lean only, 3 oz	180	9	40%
Tenderloin, roasted:			
Lean + fat, 3 oz	140	4	26%
Lean only, 3 oz	135	4	27%
GROUND PORK			
Raw: Average, 1/4 lb, 4oz	300	24	72%
Broiled, 3 oz	245	18	66%
Pan-fried, drained, 3 oz	250	19	68%

BACON

	C	F	%fc
RAW: 1 med. slice (20 lb), 3/4 oz	125	13	93%
1 thick slice (12 lb), 1 1/3 oz	210	22	94%
(1 lb raw yields approx. 5 oz cooked)			
Broiled/Pan-Fried:			
1 medium slice, 6 g	36	3	75%
3 medium slices	110	9	74%
1 thick slice, 12 g	70	6	77%
Canadian-style Bacon:			
As purchased, 1 slice, 1 oz	45	4	80%
Cooked, 1 slice	43	4	84%
Bacon Bits, 1 Tbsp, 1/4 oz	20	1	45%
Breakfast Strips: Broil., 1 sl., 12 g	50	4	72%

HAM

	C	F	%fc
Boneless Ham, cooked:			
Regular, (approx. 11% fat):			
Unheated (as purch.), 1 oz	52	3	52%
Roasted, 3 oz	150	8	48%
Extra Lean (5% fat):			
Unheated, 1 oz	37	2	49%
Roasted, 3 oz	125	5	36%
Whole Ham, cooked:			
Lean + fat (as purchased)			
Unheated, 1 oz	70	5	64%
Roasted, 3 oz	345	26	68%
Lean only, unheated, 1 oz	40	2	45%
Roasted, 3 oz	135	5	33%
Canned Ham: Similar to boneless ham			
Chopped, canned, 3 oz	260	21	73%
Ham Patties, ckd, 1 pty, 2 1/4 oz	205	18	79%
Ham Steak, extra lean, 2 oz	70	2	26%
Luncheon Slices: See Cold Meats (Processed)			

GAME MEATS

	C	F	%fc
Antelope, roasted 3 oz	130	3	21%
Buffalo, roasted, 3 oz	160	6	34%
Boar (wild), roasted, 3 oz	140	4	26%
Caribou, roasted, 3 oz	140	4	26%
Deer/Venison, roasted 3 oz	135	3	20%
Rabbit: Roasted, 3 oz	130	6	42%
Stewed, 1 cup, diced, 5 oz	300	14	42%

VARIETY & ORGAN MEATS

Per 3 oz, Edible Weight

	C	F	%fc
Brains: Braised, 3 oz	130	9	62%
Pan-fried, 3 oz	200	14	63%
Chitterlings, pork, simmered	260	25	86%
Ears, pork, simmered, 1 ear	180	12	60%
Feet, pork: Simmered, 3 oz	165	11	60%
Cured, pickled	170	14	74%
Heart: Average, braised, 3 oz	140	5	32%
Jowl, pork, raw, 4 oz	750	80	96%
Kidneys, simmered, 3 oz	130	4	27%
Liver: Raw, 4 oz	160	5	28%
Braised, 3 oz	140	4	26%
Pan-fried, 3 oz	200	9	40%
Pancreas, braised, 3 oz	200	13	58%
Spleen, braised, 3 oz	130	4	27%
Stomach, pork, raw, 4 oz	180	11	55%
Sweetbreads: Beef, ckd., 3 oz	270	20	67%
Lamb, cooked, 3 oz	150	5	30%
Tail, pork, simmered, 3 oz	340	31	82%
Tongue, braised, 3 oz: Veal	170	9	48%
Beef/Lamb/Pork, aver.	240	17	64%
Tripe, beef, raw, 4 oz	110	5	41%

WILL POWER TONIC
~ RECIPE ~

1 Cup of Desire

1 Quart of Determination

1 Tbsp of Common Sense

1 Tbsp of Stick-to-itivness

1 Tbsp of Foresight

1 Cup of Energy

SAUSAGES

FRESH SAUSAGES

	C	F	%fc
PORK/BEEF: Average all types			
Small: Raw, 4" link, 1 oz	120	12	90%
Broiled/Pan-fried	50	4	72%
Medium: Raw, 2 oz	235	23	88%
Broiled/Pan-fried	100	8	72%
Large: Raw, 3 oz	360	36	90%
Broiled/Pan-fried	150	12	72%
Italian: Raw, 3.2 oz	315	28	80%
Cooked, 2.4 oz	215	17	71%

Note: Fat is lost in broiling/pan frying.
(Cooked wt. = approx. 60-70% raw wt.)

FRANKS & WEINERS

	C	F	%fc
Average All Brands			
Regular/Smoked: Per Frank			
2 oz link (8/16 oz pkg)	180	16	80%
1.6 oz link (10/16 oz pkg)	140	13	80%
1.5 oz link (8/12 oz pkg)	135	12	80%
1.2 oz link (10/12 oz pkg)	110	10	80%
1 oz link (16/16 oz pkg)	90	8	80%
Small/Cocktail (50/lb), each	30	3	80%
Light/Fat Reduced *(Osc. Mayer)*:			
2 oz link (8/16 oz pkg)	130	11	76%
1 oz link (16/16 oz pkg)	70	6	60%
Healthy Choice (Jumbo Frank)	60	2	30%
Pork: Eckrich, reg., 2 oz	260	26	90%
Brown 'n Serve *(Swift)*	95	8	85%
Jimmy Dean, cooked	140	13	84%
Little Friers *(Osc. Mayer)*	80	8	88%
Turkey Franks:			
Empire Kosher, 2 oz	90	6	60%
Louis Rich: Reg. (8/16 oz), 2 oz	130	11	76%
(8/12 oz pkg), 1 1/2 oz	100	9	81%
Shelton's: 1 frank, 1.2 oz	80	6	68%
Chicken Franks *(Shelton's)*, 1.2 oz	95	8	75%
Empire Kosher, 2 oz	100	7	49%

VEGETARIAN SAUSAGES

	C	F	%fc
LIGHTLIFE			
Lean Breakfast Links, 1 link, 35g	60	3	45%
Lean Italian Links, 1 link, 40g	60	2	30%
Smart Dogs, 1 link, 42g	45	0	0%
Tofu Pups, 1 link, 42g	60	2.5	38%
Wonderdogs, 1.5 oz	55	1	16%
YVES			
Vegetarian Chili Dogs, 1 dog	70	0	0%
Veggie Weiners, 1 pce	50	0	0%

HOT DOGS, CORN DOGS

	C	F	%fc
HOT DOGS, Ready-To-Go			
(Includes Ketchup/Relish)			
Small (1 oz frank/ 1 oz roll)	200	8	36%
Regular (1 1/2 oz frank/ 2 oz roll)	280	16	51%
Large (2 oz frank/ 2 oz roll)	330	24	65%
Super/Giant (3 oz frank/3 oz roll)	520	27	47%
CORN DOGS			
Beef/Pork frank, average	250	17	61%
Turkey: *Gobblers! (Shelton's)*	220	11	45%
WEINERSCHNITZEL (Franchise Outlets)			
Chili Dog, 1 serve	295	16	50%
w. Lowfat Frank	230	5	20%
Chili Cheese Dog	350	21	54%
w. Lowfat Frank	280	9	29%
Corn Dog	290	23	70%
Deluxe Dog	275	14	45%
w. Lowfat Frank	220	3.5	14%
Kraut Dog	265	14	46%
Mustard Dog	260	14	48%
Relish Dog	280	14	45%
Western Dog	380	23	55%
TOPPINGS/EXTRAS			
American Cheese, 1 slice, 1 oz	110	9	74%
Catsup, 1 Tbsp	16	0	0%
Chili (w. Beans), 1/4 cup	70	3.5	45%
Mustard, 1 Tbsp	20	0	0%
Pickle Relish, 1 Tbsp	20	0	0%
Sauerkraut, 1/2 cup	25	0	0%

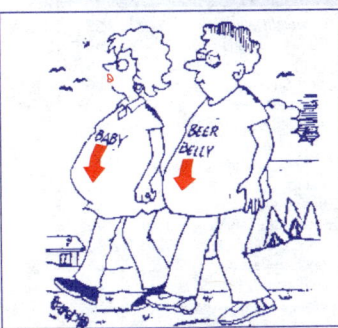

DELI & LUNCHEON MEATS

Item	C	F	%fc
Beef Jerky			
Denver Dan's, all flavors, 1 oz	80	1	11%
Frito Lay's: Regular, 0.21oz	25	1	30%
Tender, 0.7 oz	120	10	70%
Hickory Farms: Regular, 1oz	100	3	27%
Hormel: Lumberjack, 1oz	100	9	80%
Oberto, average, all flav., 1 oz	70	1	12%
Permican: Original, 1oz piece	80	2	22%
Tender Snacks, 1 oz	70	1	12%
SlimJim: Regular, 0.14 oz piece	20	1	30%
BigJerk, 0.25 oz	25	1	30%
GiantJerk, 0.63 oz	60	2	30%
Smokecraft Sticks, 1.1 oz	120	6	45%
Super Slim Jim Spicy, 1.28 pg	190	17	80%
Tombstone: 3 oz piece	110	3	25%
1 stick, 0.5oz	35	<1	5%
Vegetarian: Cajun Jerky, 0.5oz	50	2	36%
(Stonewalls) Jerquee, 0.5oz	50	2	36%
Beef Stick (Tombstone): 0.8oz	110	10	81%
Berliner (pork/beef), 1oz	65	4	55%
Beerwurst (Beef):			
Small (2.75"diam), 1/16" slice	20	2	80%
Large (4"diam), 1/8" slice	75	7	80%
Beerwurst (Pork):			
Small (2.75"diam), 1/16" slice	55	4	60%
Large (4"diam), 1/8" slice	15	1	60%
Bologna, Beef & Pork:			
1 thin slice, 1oz	90	8	80%
1 thick slice, 1.6oz	145	13	80%
Lite (Oscar Mayer), 1 slice, 1oz	60	4	60%
Red. Fat (Hebrew Nat.),1 oz	65	6	80%
Fat Free (Osc. M.), 2 sl., 1.6oz	35	0	0%
Healthy Choice, 1oz	30	1	30%
Weight Watchers, 2 sl., 3/4 oz	35	2	50%
Turkey, average, 1oz	60	5	75%
Chicken (Tyson), 1 slice	45	0.5	10%
Blood Sausage, 1 oz	100	9	80%
Bratwurst, 1oz	90	8	80%
Braunschweiger (Pork/Liver/Sausage),			
Oscar Mayer, 1 oz slice	100	9	85%
Chicken, Average All Brands			
1 thick or 2 thin slices, 1oz	30	1	30%
Chicken Roll, 1 slice, 1 oz	90	4	40%
Corned Beef, average, full fat, 1oz	70	5	64%
Healthy Choice, Hillshire Farm,1oz	30	1	30%
Hebrew National, 1oz	40	1.5	35%
Loaf, jellied, 1oz	45	2	40%
Hash, canned, average, 1oz	50	3	54%
Dutch Brand Loaf, average, 1oz	70	5	64%

Item	C	F	%fc
Ham, Luncheon:			
Baked/Boiled, sliced, 1oz	30	1	30%
Chopped: Eckrich, 1oz slice	45	2	30%
Eckrich (Lean Supreme), 1oz	35	2	40%
Hormel (Black Label), 1oz	70	6	75%
JM, 1 oz slice	80	7	78%
Kahn's, 1 slice	50	3	54%
Oscar Mayer, 1oz slice	40	2	45%
Armour, canned, 1oz	60	3	42%
Honey, average, 1oz	30	1	30%
Prosciutto, average, 1oz	70	5	64%
Ham & Cheese Loaf, aver., 1oz	70	5	64%
Head Cheese (Osc. Mayer), 1oz sl.	50	4	70%
Honey Loaf (Osc. Mayer), 1oz sl.	35	1	26%
Kielbasa (Polish Sausage), 1oz	85	7	74%
Knackwurst, 1oz	90	8	80%
Liverwurst, 1oz	95	8	75%
Liver Pate, fresh, average, 1oz	110	10	80%
Mortadella, 1oz	90	7	70%
Olive Loaf, average, 1oz	70	5	64%
Oscar Mayer, 1oz slice	70	2	25%
Pastrami (Beef), average, 1oz	40	2	45%
Healthy Deli, 1oz	34	1	27%
Hillshire (DeliSelect), 2 slices	20	0.5	20%
Turkey Pastrami, 1oz slice	30	1	30%
Peppered Beef, 1oz slice	40	2	45%
Pepperoni, 5 slices, 1oz	135	12	80%
Pickle Loaf, average, 1oz	80	6	65%
Pickle & Pimiento Loaf			
(Oscar Mayer), 1oz	70	2	25%
Proscuitti, average, 1oz	70	5	64%
Hormel, 1oz	90	7	70%
Roast Beef, lean, 1oz	40	1	20%
Salami: Beef, aver., 1oz	80	7	60%
Beer, average, 1oz	70	6	60%
Cotto: Echrich, 1oz slice	70	6	60%
Hormel, 'Club', 1oz	100	5	45%
'Perma-Fresh', 2 slices	105	7	60%
Kahn's 'Family Pack', 2 slices	90	6	60%
Oscar Mayer, 2 slices, 1.6oz	90	57	70%
Dry, Hard, aver. 3 slices, 1oz	110	10	80%
Oscar Mayer, 2 slices, 1.6oz	105	9	77%
Genoa, average, 1oz	110	10	80%
Turkey, average, 1oz	55	4	65%
Souse Loaf (Kahn's), 1 slice	90	7	70%
Spam: Original, 1oz	85	8	84%
Lite, 1oz	55	4	65%
Smoke flavoured, 1oz	85	8	85%
w. cheese chunks, 1oz	85	8	85%

42

DELI & LUNCHEON MEATS

	C	F	%fc
Spice Loaf: average, 1oz SLICE	70	6	60%
Hormel, canned, 1oz	90	9	85%
'Perma-Fresh', 2 slices	120	9	67%
Summer Sausage:			
Hillshire, 1oz	90	8	80%
Light, 1oz	75	6	56%
w. Cheddar Cheese, 1oz	100	9	90%
Oscar Mayer, 1 slice, 0.8oz	70	7	90%
Tongue, *Deli Express*, 1oz	60	5	75%
Treet *(Armour)*, canned, 1oz	100	9	90%
Turkey, average, 1oz slice	30	1	25%
¾ oz slice	22	0.5	25%
Turkey Ham, 1 slice, 1 oz	35	1.5	35%
Turkey Pastrami, 1oz	35	1.5	35%
Turkey Roll, 1oz	40	2	45%
Turkey Loaf, 1oz	30	1	30%

SPREADS

	C	F	%fc
Chicken, average, 1oz	70	4	40%
Ham Spread, devilled:			
Hormel, 2 Tbsp, 1oz	75	6	70%
Underwood, 1oz	80	7	78%
Ham & Cheese, 1oz	70	5	64%
Ham Salad, 1oz	60	4	60%
Roast Beef *(Underwood)*, 1oz	70	6	77%
Sandwich Spread *(Osc. Mayer)*, 1oz	70	5	64%
Turkey, 1oz	50	3	54%
Tuna, Lightly Seasoned *(Underwood)*	25	0.5	18%

PATE

CANNED:
Average All Brands

	C	F	%fc
Chicken Liver, 1 Tbsp, ½ oz	30	2	60%
2 Tbsp, 1oz	60	4	60%
Foie Gras, goose liver, 1oz	130	12	83%
Sells, liverpate, 2⅛ oz	190	16	76%

FRESH (Refrigerated):
Average all types, 1oz — 110 · 10 · 82%

	C	F	%fc
Marcel Henri, 2 oz serving	220	20	82%
Pate de Campagne, 1oz	105	9	77%
Chicken Liver w. Port Wine, 1oz	100	9	81%
Duck Truffle w. Port Wine, 1oz	120	12	90%
Coeur de France:			
Smoked Salmon Pate, 1oz	45	3.5	70%
Spinach Pate w. Roquefort	50	4	72%
Garden Fresh Vegetable Pate:			
Mushroom, Artichoke & Spinach in Puff Pastry, 2 oz	110	7	57%

LUNCH PACKS

	C	F	%fc
Per Package			
Lunch 'N Munch (Hillshire Farm)			
Bologna/American Chse/Crackers	480	37	70%
Bologna/American/Snickers with Hi-C (6 fl.oz)	490	34	62%
Cotto Salami/Monteray Jack Chse	440	32	65%
Pepperoni/American Cheese	570	46	73%
Smoked Turkey/Cheddar	350	21	54%
Turkey/Cheddar with Brownie	400	22	50%
Turkey/Cheddar/Brownie/Hi-C	500	22	40%
Lunchables (Oscar Mayer)			
Bologna/American Chse/Crackers	450	34	68%
Deluxe (Turkey/Ham)	360	19	48%
Dessert (Jello/Honey Tky/Cheddar)	320	16	45%
Fun Pack: Bologna/Wild Cherry	530	29	50%
Ham/Fruit Punch	450	20	40%
Turkey/Pacific Cooler	460	21	41%
Turkey/Sugar Cooler	440	16	33%
Ham/Swiss Cheese	320	17	48%
Pepperoni/American Cheese	480	36	68%
Turkey/Cheddar	360	22	52%
Turkey/Green Onion Cheese	380	20	47%
Turkey/Ranch & Herb Cheese	380	20	47%
Lunch Makers (Eckrich)			
Ham/Swiss Cheese/Crackers, 1 pce	40	2	45%
Turkey/Cheddar/Crackers, 1 piece	40	2	45%
Lunch Breaks (Louis Rich)			
Turkey/Cheddar/Crackers	410	26	57%
Turkey/Monterey Jack Cheese	400	25	56%
Turkey/Ham/Swiss Cheese	380	22	52%
Turkey Salami/Cheddar Cheese	430	29	60%

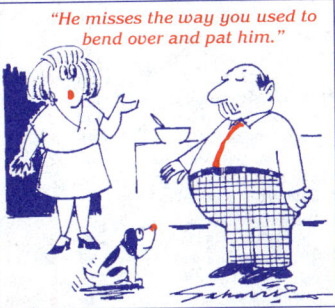

"He misses the way you used to bend over and pat him."

CHICKEN

QUICK GUIDE

From 3lb ready-to-cook chicken

	C	F	%fc
BREAST/WING QUARTER			
Roasted: With skin	300	15	45%
Without skin	190	5	24%
Fried, batter dipped	480	26	49%
LEG QUARTER			
Thigh & Drumstick			
Roasted: With skin	265	15	50%
Without skin	180	8	40%
Fried, batter dipped	430	26	54%
KFC ~ See Fast-Foods Section.			

AVERAGE - ALL MEATS

Average of Light & Dark Meats
Per 4 oz Serving (no bone)

	C	F	%fc
Roasted: With skin	270	15	50%
Without skin	215	8	33%
Stewed: With skin	250	14	50%
Without skin	200	8	36%
Fried: Batter-dipped	330	20	55%
Flour coated	305	17	50%

CHICKEN PARTS

BROILERS OR FRYERS
Edible Weights (no bone)
Breast: *Per 1/2 Breast*

	C	F	%fc
Raw: With skin, 5 oz	245	13	45%
Without skin, 4 1/4 oz	130	2	14%
Roasted: With skin, 3 1/2 oz	195	8	37%
Without skin, 3 oz	140	3	19%
Stewed: With skin, 4 oz	210	8	34%
Without skin, 3 1/4 oz	140	3	19%
Fried: Batter-dipped, 5 oz	370	19	46%
Flour coated, w. skin, 3 1/2 oz	220	9	37%

Drumstick: *Per Drumstick*

	C	F	%fc
Roasted: With skin, 2 oz	125	6	43%
Without skin, 1 1/2 oz	75	2	24%
Fried: Batter-dipped, 2 1/2 oz	195	11	51%
Flour coated, 1 3/4 oz	120	7	52%
Stewed: With skin, 2 oz	115	6	47%
Without skin, 1 1/2 oz	80	3	34%

Thigh Portion:
Edible Wt. (no bone)

	C	F	%fc
Raw: With skin, 3.3 oz (4 1/4 oz with bone)	200	14	63%
Without skin, 2.4 oz	80	3	34%
Roasted: With skin, 2 1/4 oz	155	10	58%
Without skin, 2 oz	110	6	49%
Thigh Portion (Cont)			
Stewed: With skin, 2 1/2 oz	160	10	56%
Without skin, 2 oz	105	5	43%
Fried: Batter-dipped, 3 oz	240	14	52%
Flour coated, 2 1/4 oz	165	9	49%

Wing: *Per Wing*
Raw Weight 3.2 oz (with bone)

	C	F	%fc
Raw: With skin	110	8	65%
Without skin	35	1	26%
Roasted: With skin	105	7	60%
Without skin	45	2	40%
Fried: Batter-dipped	160	11	62%
Flour coated	105	7	60%
Stewed: With skin, 4 oz	100	7	63%
Neck: Simmered, with skin	95	7	66%
Without skin	30	2	60%

Skin Only: *Skin from 1/2 Chicken*

	C	F	%fc
Raw skin, 2 3/4 oz	275	26	85%
Roasted skin, 2 oz	255	22	78%
Stewed skin, 2 1/2 oz	260	24	83%
Fried, Flour coated, 2 oz	280	24	77%
Fried, Batter-dipped, 6 3/4 oz	750	55	66%

ROASTERS
Average of Light & Dark Meat:

	C	F	%fc
Roasted: With skin, 4 oz	250	15	54%
Without skin, 4 oz	190	8	38%
Light Meat: Without skin, rst.	175	5	26%
Dark Meat: Without skin, rst.	206	10	44%

STEWING CHICKEN
Stewed: *Per 4 oz Serving*
Average of Light & Dark Meat:

	C	F	%fc
With skin	325	21	58%
Without skin	270	14	47%
Light Meat: Without skin	240	9	34%
Dark Meat: Without skin	295	17	52%

CAPON CHICKEN

	C	F	%fc
Roasted: With skin, 4 oz	260	13	45%
1/2 Chicken, with skin	1460	74	46%

MISCELLANEOUS & STUFFING

	C	F	%fc
Giblets, simmered, 1 cup	230	7	27%
Fried, flour-coated, 1 cup	400	20	45%
Gizzard, simmered, 1 cup	220	5	20%
Heart, simmered, 1 cup	270	12	40%
Liver: Raw, 4 oz	140	5	32%
Simmered, 1 cup	220	8	33%
Liver Pate, 1 Tbsp, 1/2 oz	60	8	100%
Stuffing: Average, 1/2 cup	200	2	10%

TURKEY

FRYER-ROASTERS

	C	F	%fc
Roasted: Per 3 oz Serving			
Light Meat: With skin	140	4	26%
Without skin	120	1	7%
Dark Meat: With skin	155	6	35%
Without skin	140	4	26%
1/2 of Whole Turkey: (Approx. 3 1/4 lbs raw wt. w/out neck and giblets; 2 lb 6 oz cooked wt.)			
Roasted: With skin	1400	46	30%
Without skin	1030	18	16%
Ground Turkey, Raw:			
Regular (85% lean), 4 oz	180	10	50%
Lean (90% lean), 4 oz	160	8	45%
Breast, no skin, 4 oz	115	1	8%
(4 oz raw wt. = 3 oz cooked wt.)			

TURKEY PARTS

Roasted, Edible Weights (no bone)

	C	F	%fc
Breast (1/2): (from 17 1/4 oz raw wt. w/bone)			
With skin, 12 oz (no bone)	525	11	19%
Without skin, 10 3/4 oz	415	2	4%
Back (1/2): With skin, 4 1/2 oz	265	13	44%
Without skin, 3 1/2 oz	165	5	27%
Leg (Thigh & Drumstick):			
(from 1 lb raw wt. w/bone)			
With skin, 8 1/2 oz (no bone)	420	13	28%
Without skin, 7 3/4 oz	355	8	20%
Wing: (from 7 1/4 oz raw wt. w/bone)			
With skin, 3 oz (no bone)	185	9	44%
Without skin, 2 oz	100	2	18%
Neck: Simmered, 1 neck			
(9 oz w. bone)	275	11	36%
Giblets, simm., 1 cup, 5 oz	240	7	26%

YOUNG HENS (ROASTED)

	C	F	%fc
Light Meat: With skin, 3 oz	175	8	41%
Without skin, 3 oz	135	3	20%
Dart Meat: With skin, 3 oz	200	11	49%
Without skin, 3 oz	165	7	38%
Young Toms — Similar to Young Hens			

DUCK, GOOSE, QUAIL

	C	F	%fc
Duck, roasted, with skin, 3 oz	285	24	76%
Without skin, 3 oz	170	10	53%
1/2 whole duck, with skin	1300	108	75%
Goose, roast, with skin, 3 oz	260	19	66%
Without skin, 3 oz	200	11	49%
Pheasant, 1/2 bird, raw	720	37	46%
Quail, 1 whole, raw	210	13	56%

POULTRY PRODUCTS

	C	F	%fc
***Armour*, Turkey:** Patty, 2 1/4 oz	170	11	58%
Breast Fillets w. cheese, 5 oz	300	16	48%
Turkey Sticks, 2 oz	150	10	60%
Banquet ~ Page 49.			
***Louis Rich* ~**			
Breast of Turkey, fully cooked:			
BBQ'd/Smoked/Rstd, 3 oz	105	3	26%
Fresh Turkey Cuts, cooked:			
Breast Cuts, 3 oz	120	3	23%
Drumsticks/Wings, 3 oz	165	8	44%
Luncheon Slices ~ See Cold Meats, Page 42			
Franks: Medium, 1 1/2 oz	100	9	81%
Large, 2 oz	130	11	76%
Smoked Sausage/Kielbasa, 1 oz	40	2	45%
Turkey Nuggets, cooked, each	60	4	60%
Turkey Patties, cooked, each	210	13	56%
Turkey Sticks, cooked, each	80	5	56%
***Shelton's*:** Gobblers! Corn Dog	220	11	45%
Turkey Sausage Patty, each	180	17	85%
Pot Pies (whole wheat): Turkey	350	12	31%
Chicken Pot Pie	430	20	42%
Turkey Jerky, 1/2 oz packet	45	<1	10%
Franks & Sausages ~ Page 41			
Swanson ~ Page 53			
Turkey Store:			
Breast Slices, 1 slice, 2 1/2 oz	70	1	13%
Breast Sirloins, each, 10 oz	285	3	9%
Drumstick Steaks, 3 1/2 oz	110	4	33%
Ground Turkey, lean, 1/4 lb	160	8	45%
Ground Turkey Breast, 1/4 lb	115	1	8%
Breakfast Sausage Links, 1 oz	70	6	77%
***Tyson*, Chicken Products:**			
Breast Chunks, 3 oz serving	240	17	64%
Breast Fillets: Regular, 3 oz	190	9	38%
Marinated, butter/garlic, 3 1/2 oz	160	7	39%
Other flavors, aver., 3 1/2 oz	125	2	14%
Breast Patties, each, 2 1/2 oz	220	15	61%
Brst. Tenders, Sthn. fried, 3 oz	220	15	61%
Chick'n Chunks/Chedd., 2 1/2 oz	220	15	61%
Chicken Pie, 6 oz	230	11	43%
Microwave Tenders, 3 1/2 oz	230	11	43%
Microwave Chunks, 3 1/2 oz	220	15	61%
M/wave S/wiches: Breast	275	12	39%
BBQ Chicken	210	4	17%
Wings: All flavors, 3 1/2 oz	220	14	57%
***Tyson* Frozen Dinners** ~ Page 54			

FISH - FRESH & CANNED

FRESH FISH QUICK GUIDE

LOW OIL (Less than 2.5% fat)
White/pale coloured flesh. Examples:
Cod, Flounder, Haddock, Halibut, Monkfish
Perch, Pike, Pollock, Snapper, Sole, Whiting.

Per 4 oz Edible Portion	C	F	%fc
Raw, 4 oz (no bones)	90	1	10%
Steamed, Broiled, Baked	130	1	7%
Fried: Lightly Floured	210	8	34%
Breaded	260	12	42%
In Batter	320	16	45%

MEDIUM OIL (2.5-5% fat)
Pale coloured flesh. Examples:
Bluefin Tuna, Catfish, Kingfish, Salmon (Pink),
Swordfish, Rainbow Trout, Yellowtail.

	C	F	%fc
Raw, 4 oz (no bones)	140	5	32%
Baked, Broiled, 4 oz	175	6	31%
Fried, 4 oz	230	11	43%

HIGH OIL (Over 5% fat)
Darker colored flesh. Examples:
Albacore Tuna, Bluefish, Herring, Mackerel,
Orange Roughy, Salmon (Atl./Chinook/Sockeye),
Sardines, Trout, Whitefish.

	C	F	%fc
Raw, 4 oz (no bones)	230	16	63%
Baked, Broiled, 4 oz	275	17	56%
Fried, 4 oz	340	23	61%

Cooking Yields (Fin Fish):
4 oz Raw wt. = 3 1/2 oz Cooked wt.
4 oz Cooked wt. = 5 oz Raw wt.

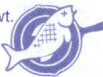

Calorie & Fat Variations
The amount of fat/oil in fish varies with the species, season and locality. Within the same fish, fat/oil content is generally higher towards the head.

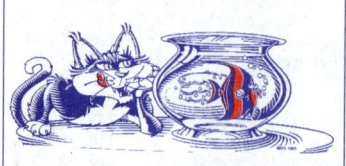

FISH & SHELLFISH

Edible Weights: (no bones/shell)	C	F	%fc
Abalone: Raw, 4 oz	120	1	7%
Anchovy: Paste, 1 Tbsp, 1/4 oz	15	1	60%
Cnd. in oil, drnd., 5 only, 3/4 oz	40	2	45%
Pickled, 1 oz	50	3	54%
Barracuda (Pacific), raw, 4oz	130	3	21%
Bass: Black, raw, 4 oz	105	1	8%
Striped, raw, 1 fillet, 5 1/2 oz	150	4	24%
Blue Fish, raw, 1 fillet, 5 1/4 oz	185	6	29%
Butterfish, raw, 4 oz	165	9	49%
Calamari, breaded/fried, 1 serving	360	21	53%
Carp, raw, 4 oz	145	6	37%
Catfish: Raw, 4 oz	130	5	35%
Fried, bread., 1 fillet, 3 oz	200	12	54%
Caviar: black/red, 1 Tbsp, 16g	40	3	68%
Clams: Raw, 3 oz (4 lge/9 sm)	65	1	14%
Fried, breaded, 3 oz	170	10	53%
Canned, 3 oz	125	2	14%
Minced, 1/4 cup, 2 oz	25	0	0%
Cod, Atl./Pacific: Raw, 4 oz	95	1	9%
Baked/Broil., 1 fill., 6 1/4 oz	135	2	13%
Canned, 3 oz	90	1	10%
Minced, 1/4 cup, 2oz	25	0	0%
Crab: Alaska King, raw, 4 oz	95	1	9%
1 leg, cooked, 4 3/4 oz	130	2	14%
Blue, raw, 1 crab (1/3 lb whole crab, 3/4 oz flesh)	18	<1	25%
Canned, 1/2 cup, 2 1/2 oz	65	<1	6%
Dungeness, 1 crab, 5 3/4 oz edible (from 1 1/2 lb whole crab)	140	2	13%
Imitation Crab Legs/Stix, 3 oz	80	1	11%
Crayfish, raw, 4 oz (edible)	100	1	9%
Croaker, raw, 4 oz	120	3	23%
Cuttlefish, raw, 4 oz	90	1	10%
Dolphinfish, raw, 4 oz	95	1	9%
Eel: Raw, 4 oz	210	13	56%
Smoked, 2 oz	190	16	76%
Flounder/Sole, raw, 4 oz	80	<1	5%
Gefilte Fish: See Jewish Foods ~ Page 136.			
Grouper, raw, 4 oz	105	1	8%
Haddock: Raw, 4 oz	100	<1	5%
Broiled, 1 fillet, 5 1/4 oz	170	1	5%
Smoked, 2 oz	22	<1	20%
Halibut, raw, 4 oz	125	3	22%
Herring: Atlantic, raw, 4 oz	180	10	50%
Pickled, 2 pieces, 1 oz	60	4	60%

FISH - FRESH & CANNED

	C	F	%fc
Herring Pickled **(Cont)**			
In Sour Cream, 1 oz	50	5	90%
Rollmops, 1 1/2 oz	110	8	65%
Canned: Plain w. liq., 4 oz	235	15	57%
in Tomato Sauce, 4 oz	200	12	54%
Smoked, kippered, 4 oz	245	14	51%
Jellyfish: Raw, 4 oz	30	<1	5%
Salted, 4 oz	40	<1	11%
Kingfish, raw, 4 oz	120	3.5	26%
Ling, raw, 4 oz	100	<1	5%
Lobster, Northern: Raw, 4 oz	105	1	8%
1 Lobster, 6 1/4 oz			
(from 1 1/2 lb whole lobster)	135	1.5	10%
Cooked, 1 cup, 5 oz	140	1	6%
Lobster Newberg, 3/4 cup	360	20	50%
Lobster Thermidor, 1 serv.	370	22	54%
Lobster Salads, 1/2 cup	220	13	53%
Lox, Regular/Nova, 2 oz	65	2	28%
Mackerel: Atlantic, raw, 4 oz	235	16	61%
Jack, can., 1/2 cup, 3 1/3 oz	150	6	36%
King, raw, 4 oz	120	2	15%
Pacific/Jack, raw, 4 oz	180	9	45%
Spanish, raw, 4 oz	160	7	39%
Mahi-Mahi, raw, 4oz	140	5	32%
Monkfish, raw, 4 oz	75	1	12%
Mullet, striped, raw	135	4	27%
Mussels: Raw, 4 oz (edible)	100	2	18%
1 cup, 5 1/4 oz (edible)	130	3	21%
Cooked, moist heat, 3 oz	150	4	24%
Ocean Perch, raw, 4 oz	90	1.5	15%
Octopus, common, raw, 4 oz	95	1	9%
Orange Roughy, raw, 4 oz	145	9	56%
(Cals may be much lower. Over 90% of total fat is waxester which may not be metabolized)			
Oysters: Common, raw, 3 oz	70	1	13%
Eastern raw:			
6 medium, 3 oz	60	2	30%
1 cup, 8 3/4 oz	170	6	32%
Fried/bread., 6 medium, 3 oz	170	11	58%
Pacific, raw, 1 med., 1 3/4 oz	40	1	23%
Oysters Rockfeller, 6 oyst.	220	13	53%
Perch, average, raw, 4 oz	105	2	18%
Pollock, raw, 4 oz	100	1	9%
Pompano, Florida, raw, 4 oz	190	10	47%
Porgy/Scup, raw, 4 oz	130	4	28%
Rockfish, Pacific, raw, 4 oz	110	2	16%
Roe, raw, 1 oz	40	2	45%
Sablefish, raw, 4 oz	220	18	74%

	C	F	%fc
Salmon, Raw:			
Chinook, 4 oz	205	7	31%
Atlantic; Coho/Silver, 4 oz	160	7	39%
Chum; Pink, 4 oz	135	4	27%
Red/Sockeye, 4 oz	190	10	47%
Smoked Salmon: Average, 2 oz	65	1	14%
Pacific Supreme, 2 oz	100	4	36%
Salmon, Canned: Average All Brands.			
Pink: 1 oz	40	2	45%
1/4 cup, 63g (2.2 oz)	90	5	45%
3 3/4 oz can, whole	155	8.5	45%
7 1/2 oz can, whole	300	17	45%
Skinless/boneless, 1/4 c., 2 oz	70	2	45%
Red Sockeye: 1 oz	50	3	55%
1/4 cup, 63g (2.2 oz)	110	7	55%
3 3/4 oz can, whole	190	12	55%
Atlantic, 1/2 cup, 3 1/2 oz	230	14	55%
Chinook/King, 1/2 cup	210	14	60%
Chum, 1/2 cup, 3 1/2 oz	140	5	32%
Coho/Silver, 1/2 cup	155	5	29%
Salmon Cake, take-out, 3 oz	240	15	56%
Sardines, Canned: Average All Brands			
In Oil, undrained, 1 oz	85	7	74%
Drained of oil, 1 oz	60	3	45%
3 3/4 oz can, drained, (3 1/4 oz)	190	11	52%
1 lrg/2 med. 3"/5 small, 0.8 oz	50	3	54%
In Tom./ Mustard Sce, 1 oz	45	3	60%
3 3/4 oz can (8 sardines)	170	11	58%
Scallop: Raw, 6 lg./14 sm., 3 oz	75	<1	6%
Breaded/fried, 6 lge, 3 oz	200	10	45%
Shark: Raw, 4 oz	150	6	36%
Batter-dipped, fried, 4 oz	260	16	55%
Shrimps: Raw, in shell, 1/2 lb	140	2	13%
Raw, shelled, 3 oz (12 lge)	90	1.5	15%
Bread./fried, 3 oz (11 lge)	210	11	47%
Canned, 2 oz	60	1	15%
Smelt, Rainbow, raw, 4 oz	115	3	23%
Snapper, raw, 4 oz	115	1	8%
Sole, Lemon, raw, 4 oz	90	1	10%
Squid, raw, 4 oz	105	1	8%
Surimi, Imt. Crablegs/Shrimp, 4 oz	110	1	8%
Swordfish, raw, 4 oz	140	5	32%
Trout, Rainbow, raw, 4 oz	135	4	27%
Smoked, 2 oz	110	6	50%
Tuna: Raw, Bluefin, 4 oz	165	6	33%
Skipjack, Yellowfin	120	1	8%

FISH - FRESH/CANNED/FROZEN PRODUCTS

FISH - FRESH/CANNED

	C	F	%fc
Tuna (Cont)			
Canned: (Average all brands)			
In Water, drained:			
Chunk/Solid, 2 oz can	60	0.5	10%
3 oz can	90	1	10%
6 oz can	150	1.5	10%
In Oil, drained:			
Chunk Light, 2 oz	110	5.5	45%
6 oz can, drained	275	14	45%
Solid White, 2 oz	90	2.5	27%
6 oz can, drained	225	6.5	27%
Tuna Salad:			
Deli Style, 1/2 cup, 4 oz	300	24	72%
Canned: *Starkist* w. Crackers	180	6	30%
Bumble Bee w. Crackers	250	15	54%
Fat Free, 2 3/4 oz	70	0	0%
Whitefish, raw, 4 oz	155	7	41%
Whiting, raw, 4 oz	100	1.5	14%

FROZEN FISH PRODUCTS

FISHER BOY
	C	F	%fc
Fish Sticks: Regular, 6 sticks, 3 oz	200	11	50%

GORTON'S
Fish Sticks: Crunchy, 6, 3 1/2 oz	260	14	48%
Fish Fillets: Breaded (Per Fillet)			
Lemon Pepper	135	9	60%
Garlic & Herb	125	6.5	47%
Grilled: It. Herb; Lemon Pepper	130	6	42%
Fish Portions: 1 portion, 2 1/2 oz	170	11	58%

MRS FRIDAY'S
Butterfly Shrimp, 3 shrimp, 4 oz	180	1	5%
Gourmet Shrimp, 6 shrimp, 4 oz	180	1	5%

FROZEN PRODUCTS (Cont)

	C	F	%fc
MRS PAUL'S			
Battered: Fish Sticks, 4	210	12	51%
Fish Portions, 2	300	19	57%
Batter Dipped: Fish Sticks, 2	330	17	67%
Crispy Crunchy: Fish Sticks, 4	190	8	38%
Fish Fillets, 2	230	10	39%
Breaded Fish Portions, 2	230	15	59%
Crunchy Batter: Fish Fillets, 2	280	14	45%
Flounder Fillets, 2	220	9	37%
Haddock Fillets, 2	190	5	24%
Healthy Treasures:			
Fish Sticks, breaded, 3	110	3	25%
Light Fillets 'N Sauce, 1 fillet	140	6	39%
Deviled Crabs, 1 cake, 3 oz	180	9	45%
Fish Cakes, 2 cakes, 4 oz	190	7	33%
Fish Scallops, 1/2 pkg, 3 oz	160	7	39%
Fried Clams, 1/2 pkg, 2 1/2 oz	200	9	41%
Light Seafood Entrees:			
Fish Dijon	200	5	23%
Fish Florentine	220	8	33%
Fish Mornay	230	10	39%
Seafood Lasagne	290	8	25%
Seafood Rotini	240	6	23%
Shrimp & Clams w. Linguini	240	5	19%

SEA-PAK
Clams, 1 pack, 5 oz	410	23	50%
Scallops, 13 pce, 3 oz	190	6	28%
Crunchy Popcorn Shrimp, 5 shrimp, 1 oz	70	4	40%
Crunchy Shrimp Poppers, 7 shrimp, 1 oz	70	4	40%

VAN DE KAMP'S
Fish Sticks: Breaded, each, 0.7 oz	50	3	54%
Battered Fillets: *Per Fillet*			
Halibut, 1.3 oz	110	7	57%
Fish Fillets, 2.6 oz	180	11	55%
Crunchy Baked: Garlic & Herb, 1 fillet, 2 3/4 oz	150	5	30%
Lemon Pepper, 1 fillet, 2 3/4 oz	140	5	32%
Crisp & Healthy: Breaded, 1 fillet, 1 3/4 oz	75	1	12%
Grilled: Italian Herb, (1), 4 oz	130	6	42%
Garlic Butter, (1), 4 oz	130	6	42%
Light Bread: Cod, 1 fillet, 6 oz	220	10	41%
Country Cornmeal: 1 fillet, 3 oz	180	11	55%

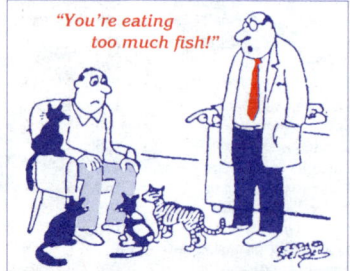

"You're eating too much fish!"

FROZEN ENTREES & MEALS

ARMOUR

	C	F	%fc
Classics: Per Serving			
Chicken: & Noodles	280	9	29%
Mesquite Chicken	280	13	42%
Parmigiana	360	18	45%
w. Wine & Mushroom Sce	260	11	38%
Glazed Chicken	280	14	45%
Meat Loaf	300	10	30%
Salisbury Steak	330	18	49%
Swedish Meatballs	300	17	51%
Turkey w. Dressing & Gravy	270	7	23%
Veal Parmigiana	400	22	50%
Lite: Per Serving			
Beef Pepper Steak	210	4	17%
Chicken Burgundy	210	5	21%
Salisbury Steak	260	7	24%
Shrimp Creole	220	1	4%
Sweet & Sour Chicken	220	1	4%

BANQUET

	C	F	%fc
Meals: Per Meal			
BBQ Style Chicken	320	12	34%
Beef Enchilada	380	12	28%
Beef Enchilada & Tomato Combo	400	13	29%
Beef Patty w. Country Style Veg.	300	20	60%
Boneless Pork Fillet	400	19	43%
Cheese Enchilada	340	6	16%
Chicken & Dumplings w. Gravy	260	8	28%
Chicken Chow Mein w. Egg Rolls	210	7	30%
Chicken Enchilada	360	10	25%
Chicken Fried Beef Steak	400	20	45%
Chicken Nugget	410	21	46%
Chicken Parmigiana	290	15	47%
Chicken Pasta Primavera	300	12	36%
Chimichanga	470	23	44%
Enchilada Combo Meal	350	9	23%
Fettuccine Alfredo	330	16	44%
Lasagne with Meat Sauce	260	6	28%
Macaroni & Cheese	320	11	31%
Meat Loaf Gravy	280	16	51%
Oriental Style Chick. w. Egg Rolls	260	9	31%
Our Original Fried Chicken	470	27	52%
Pasta w. Italian Saus.& Peppers	300	12	36%
Pork Cutlet Meal	410	24	53%
Salisbury Steak Dinner, 9.5 oz	340	19	50%
Sliced Beef	240	7	26%
Southern Fried Chicken	520	31	54%

BANQUET (CONT)

	C	F	%fc
Meals: Per Meal (Cont)			
Turkey Mostly White Meat	290	10	31%
Veal Parmigiana	320	14	39%
Western Style Beef Patty	350	20	51%
White Cheddar & Broccoli	320	11	31%
White Meat Fried Chicken	470	28	54%
Pot Pies			
Beef, 1 pie	330	15	41%
Chicken, 1 pie	350	18	46%
Macaroni & Cheese, 1 pie	200	3	14%
Turkey, 1 pie	370	20	49%
Vegetable Cheese, 1 pie	390	18	42%

BUDGET GOURMET

	C	F	%fc
Dinner			
Beef Sirloin	240	3.5	13%
Beef Sirloin Salisbury Steak	260	5	17%
Chicken in Mesquite BBQ Sauce	270	6	20%
Chicken Parmigiana	280	7	23%
Herbed Chicken Breast w. Fettucini	280	4	13%
Honey Mustard Chicken Breast	310	6	17%
Roast Chick. Breast w. Herb Gvy	250	5	18%
Shrimp Mariner	270	8	20%
Sirloin of Beef in Wine Sauce	220	3.5	14%
Special Recipe Sirloin Beef	270	5	17%
Stuffed Turkey Breast	240	3	11%
Teriyaki Beef	320	5	14%
Teriyaki Chicken Breast	300	4.5	14%
Yankee Pot Roast	250	5	18%
Italian Style Originals			
Four Cheese, Rice & Chicken	330	13	35%
Italian Style Meatballs & Vege.	280	12	39%
Pasta & Italian Sausage	440	21	43%
Pasta in Wine Sauce & Chicken	290	7	22%
Potatoes Mozzarella w. Chicken	390	19	44%
Light Entrees			
Beef Sirloin Salisbury Steak	240	5	19%
Beef Stroganoff	290	7	22%
Chicken Oriental & Vege.	300	5	15%
French Recipe Chicken	180	7	35%
Glazed Turkey	250	4	14%
Lasagna w. Meat Sauce	250	6	22%
Mandarin Chicken	270	5	17%
Orange Glazed Chicken Breast	300	2	6%
Oriental Beef	250	7	25%

FROZEN ENTREES & MEALS CONT

BUDGET GOURMET (CONT)

Regular Entrees

	C	F	%fc
Cheese Manicotti w. Meat Sauce	420	22	47%
Chicken & Egg Noodles	360	21	53%
Chicken Marsala	270	7	23%
Chicken w. Fettucini	380	19	45%
Italian Sausage Lasagna	450	21	42%
Linguini w. Bay Shrimp & Clam Marinara	270	9	30%
Pepper Steak w. Rice	290	8	25%
Roast Sirloin Supreme	300	13	39%
Sirloin Cheddar Melt	370	21	51%
Sirloin Tips w. Country Style Vege.	250	13	47%
Swedish Meatballs	550	34	56%
Sweet & Sour Chicken	330	5	14%
Three Cheese Lasagna	390	16	37%

Special Selections

	C	F	%fc
Chinese Style Vege. & Chicken	260	6	21%
Escalloped Noodles & Turkey	430	21	44%
Fettuccini Alfredo w. Four Cheeses	480	22	43%
Italian Style Vege. & Chicken	240	6	23%
Lasagna Alfredo w. Broccoli	360	13	32%
Lasagna Bolognese w. Meat Sce	340	12	32%
Lasagna Mozzarella	360	11	28%
Linguini w. Tom. Sce. & Ital. Saus.	380	14	33%
Macaroni & Chse w. Ched.& Parm.	310	7	20%
Penne Pasta w. Italian Sausage	290	8	25%
Rigatoni in Cream Sce & Chicken	230	5	20%
Spagh. w.Chnky Tom. & Meat Sce.	320	7	20%
Spicy Szechuan Style Vege. Chick.	330	10	27%
Wido Ribbon Pasta w. Ricotta & Tom. Sce.	430	23	48%

Value Classics

	C	F	%fc
Homestyle Macaroni & Cheese	360	13	33%
Spaghetti Marinara	290	6	19%
Stir Fry Rice & Vegetables	410	18	40%
Wild Rice Pilaf w. Vegetables	400	16	36%
Ziti Parmesano	350	10	26%

CHUN KING

	C	F	%fc
Chicken Egg Rolls: Mini, 5 rolls	170	6	21%
Restaurant Style, 1 roll, 3 oz	170	5	26%
Pork & Shrimp Egg Rolls:			
Mini, 12 rolls	420	16	34%
Pork Restaurant Style, 1 roll	170	6	32%
Shrimp Egg Rolls: Mini, 5 rolls	160	3.5	20%
Restaurant Style, 1 roll	150	4	24%

HEALTHY CHOICE

Entrees

	C	F	%fc
Beef Macaroni	210	2	10%
Beef Pepper Steak Oriental	250	4	14%
Beef Tips Francais	280	5	16%
Cheddar Broccoli Potatoes	310	5	15%
Cheese Ravioli Parmigiana	260	5	17%
Chicken & Vegetable Marsala	230	1.5	6%
Chicken Con Queso Burrito	360	3	8%
Chicken Enchiladas Suiza	270	4	13%
Chicken Fettuccine Alfredo	260	4.5	16%
Chicken Imperial	230	4	16%
Country Glazed Chicken	210	2	9%
Country Rst Turkey w. Mush.	220	4	16%
Fettuccine Alfredo	250	5	18%
Fiesta Chicken Fajitas	260	4	14%
Garden Potato Casserole	210	5	21%
Garlic Chicken Milano	240	4	15%
Honey Mustard Chicken	260	2	7%
Lasagna Roma	390	5	20%
Macaroni & Cheese	290	5	16%
Mandarin Chicken	280	2.5	8%
Manicotti with 3 Cheeses	260	4.5	16%
Penne Paste w. Tomato Sauce	230	5	20%
Sesame Chicken	240	3	11%
Spaghetti & Sce w. Seasoned Beef	260	3	10%
Swedish Meatballs	280	9	29%
Vegetable Pasta Italiano	240	1.5	6%
Zucchini Lasagna	330	1.5	4%

Meals

	C	F	%fc
Beef & Peppers Cantonese	270	6	29%
Beef Broccoli Beijing	300	4.5	14%
Beef Stroganoff	310	6	17%
Charbroiled Steak Patty	280	6	19%
Cacciatore Chicken	250	2.5	9%
Chicken Broccoli Alfredo	300	6	18%
Chicken Cantonese	260	2	7%
Chicken Dijon	270	5	17%
Chicken Enchilada Supreme	270	4	13%
Chicken Francesca	330	6	16%
Chicken Parmigiana	300	4	12%
Chicken Picante	260	6	21%
Chicken Teriyaki	230	3	12%
Country Breaded Chicken	360	9	23%
Country Herb Chicken	310	4	12%
Country Inn Roast Turkey	250	4	14%
Ginger Chicken Hunan	350	2.5	6%
Grilled Glazed Pork Patty	280	4	13%

FROZEN ENTREES & MEALS CONT

HEALTHY CHOICE (CONT)

Meals (Cont)

	C	F	%fc
Herb Baked Fish	340	7	19%
Lemon Pepper Fish	290	5	16%
Mesquite Beef w. BBQ Sauce	310	8	23%
Mesquite Chicken BBQ	270	2.5	85%
Pasta Shells Marinara	380	6	14%
Roasted Chicken	220	3	12%
Sesame Chicken Shanghai	310	2.5	7%
Shrimp & Vegetables Maria	270	3	10%
Shrimp Marinara	220	0.5	2%
Southwestern Grilled Chicken	200	3	14%
Sweet & Sour Chicken	330	5	14%
Traditional Beef Tips	260	6	21%
Traditional Breast of Turkey	280	3	10%
Traditional Meat Loaf	320	5	14%
Traditional Salisbury Steak	320	6	17%
Yankee Pot Roast	280	5	16%

Hearty Handfuls

	C	F	%fc
Chicken & Broccoli	320	5	14%
Chicken & Mushrooms	300	4	12%
Garlic Chicken	330	5	14%
Philly Beef Steak	290	5	16%
Roast Beef; Turkey & Vegetables	310	4.5	13%

KID CUISINE

Per Meal

	C	F	%fc
Big League Hamburger, Pizza	400	11	25%
Buckaroo Beef Patty S'wich w. Chse	410	15	33%
Circus Show Corn Dog	450	15	30%
Cosmic Chicken Nuggets	440	16	33%
Funtastic Fish Sticks	370	12	29%
High Flying Fried Chicken	440	19	39%
Magical Macaroni & Cheese	410	13	29%
Pirate Pizza w. Cheese	430	11	23%
Raptor Ravioli w. Cheese	310	5	15%
Rip-Roaring Macaroni & Beef	370	9	22%

LA CHOY

Egg Rolls - See Chun King Page 50.

LEAN CUISINE

Entrees:

	C	F	%fc
Angel Hair Pasta	260	3	10%
Baked Chicken w. Whipped Potatoes & Stuffing	250	6	22%
Baked Fish w. Cheddar Shells	260	8	28%
Beef Pot Roast & Whip. Potatoes	210	7	30%
Cheese Cannelloni	230	4	16%

LEAN CUISINE (CONT)

Entrees (Cont)

	C	F	%fc
Cheese Ravioli	240	7	26%
Chicken a l'Orange	250	2	7%
Chicken & Vegetables	250	6	22%
Chicken Chow Mein w/Rice	240	4	15%
Chicken Enchilada Suiza	280	5	16%
Chicken Fettucini	300	7	21%
Chick. Oriental w. Veg.. & Vermicelli	250	5	18%
Chicken Pie	310	9	26%
Classic Cheese Lasagna	290	6	19%
Country Veges. & Beef	220	4	16%
Fettucini Alfredo	300	7	21%
Fettucini Primavera	280	9	29%
Fiesta Chick. w. Rice & Veges	250	5	18%
Five Cheese Lasagna	230	5	20%
Glazed Chick. w. Vege. Rice	240	6	23%
Homestyle Turkey	240	5	19%
Lasagna w. Meat Sauce	290	8	25%
Macaroni & Beef	280	8	26%
Macaroni & Cheese	290	7	22%
Meatloaf & Whipped Potatoes	240	7	26%
Roast Turkey Breast, & Stuffing, Cinnamon Apples	290	3	9%
Salisbury Stk w. Macaroni & Chse	290	9	28%
Spaghetti w. Meat Sauce	300	4	12%
Spaghetti w. Meatballs	280	6	19%
Stuffed Cabbage w. Whipped Potatoes	180	5	25%
Swedish Meatballs w. Pasta	280	6	19%
Three Bean Chilli w. Rice	260	6	21%
Turkey & Country Vege. Pie	320	10	28%
Vegetable Lasagna	270	7	23%

Cafe Classics:

	C	F	%fc
Cheese Lasagna w. Chicken Scaloppini	290	9	28%
Chicken Breast in Wine Sce.	220	6	25%
Chicken Carbonara	280	8	26%
Chicken Mediterranean	230	4	16%
Chicken Parmesan	240	7	26%
Chicken Piccata	270	6	20%
Chicken w. Basil Cream Sce.	260	7	24%
Glazed Turkey	250	6	22%
Grilled Chicken Salsa	270	8	27%
Grilled Fish w. Vegetables	170	5	26%
Herb Roasted Chicken	210	5	21%
Honey Mustard Chicken	270	5	17%
Mesquite Beef w. Rice	280	7	23%
Sirloin Beef Peppercorn	220	7	29%

51

FROZEN ENTREES & MEALS CONT

LEAN CUISINE (CONT)

Lunch Classics

	C	F	%fc
Alfredo Pasta Primavera	300	7	21%
Bow Tie Pasta & Creamy Tom. Sce.	290	7	22%
Cheese Lasagna Casserole	280	7	23%
Macaroni & Cheese w. Broccoli	240	6	23%
Mandarin Chicken	260	5	17%
Penne Pasta w. Tomato Basil Sce.	290	4	12%
Roasted Potatoes w. Broccoli & Ched. Chse Sce.	210	5	21%
Teriyaki Stir-Fry	270	4	13%

MARIE CALLENDER'S

Meals & Dinners

	C	F	%fc
Angel Hair Pasta w. Sausage & Breadstick, 1 cup	460	16	31%
Baked Ham Steak w. Macaroni & Chse, 1 dinner	450	9	18%
Beef Stroganoff & Noodles, 1 cup	440	27	55%
Breaded Chicken Parmigiana	620	27	39%
Cheese Ravioli in Marinara Sauce w. Spirals & garlic bread, 1 c. + 1oz bread	370	14	34%
Chicken & Dumplings, 1 cup	260	12	42%
Chicken Cordon Bleu, 1 dinner	590	25	38%
Chicken Fried Beef Steak & Gravy	650	31	43%
Chicken Marsala, 1 dinner	450	17	34%
Country Fried Chick. & Gvy,1 din.	610	27	40%
Country Fried Pork Chop, 1 dinner	550	27	44%
Escalloped Noodles/Chicken, 1 c.	270	16	53%
Extra Cheese Lasagna, 1 cup	330	16	44%
Family Size: Chick. & Dumplings.	310	15	44%
Chicken Fried Steak & Gvy w. mashed potato, 1 cup	480	23	43%
Country Fried Chicken, w. mashed potato, 1 cup	520	22	38%
Meatloaf & Gvy w. Potato,1 c.	420	21	45%
Lasagna w. meat sauce, 1 cup	350	16	41%
Rigatoni Parmigiana, 1 cup	320	14	39%
Turkey & Gvy w. mashed Pot., 2 pces + 1/2 cup potatoes	280	9	29%
Fettucine Alfredo & Garlic Bread, 1 cup + 1 oz bread	460	27	53%
Fettucine Primavera w. Tortellini,1c.	310	19	55%
Fettucine w. Broccoli & Chick.,1 c.	410	24	53%
Grilled Chick. on Mushroom Sce	480	15	28%
Lasagna Primavera, 1 cup	260	12	42%
Lasagna w. Meat Sauce, 1 cup	370	18	44%
Macaroni & Beef	590	18	27%

MARIE CALLENDER'S (CONT)

Meals & Dinners (Cont)

	C	F	%fc
Meatloaf & Gvy w. Mashed Pot.	540	30	50%
Old Fashioned Beef Pot Roast & Gravy, 1 cup	250	6	22%
Pasta Primavera w. Chicken, 1 c.	340	20	53%
Salisbury Steak & Gravy, 1 dinner	550	25	41%
Spaghetti & Meat Sauce w. Garlic Bread, 1 cup + 1 oz bread	260	10	35%
Spaghetti Marinara w. Cheese Garlic Bread, 1 cup + 1 3/8 oz bread	270	10	33%
Sweet & Sour Chicken, 1 dinner	530	9	15%
Turkey with Gvy/dress., 1 dinner	530	17	29%

Pot Pies: Per 10 oz Pie

	C	F	%fc
Chicken; Yankee	680	44	58%
Turkey	710	46	58%
Chicken & Broccoli	780	48	55%
Chicken Au Gratin	720	48	60%

MICHELINA'S

Per Serving

	C	F	%fc
Spicy Spiral Pomodoro	280	2.5	8%
Wheels & Cheese	290	8	25%
Lasagna Primavera	300	10	30%
Rigatoni Pomodora	210	2.5	11%
Penne Pasta Mushroom Sce	320	9	25%
Spagh. w. Tomato & Basil Sce	240	3.5	13%
Fettucine Alfredo	430	18	37%
Spaghetti Bolognese	310	4	12%
Macaroni Cheese	360	14	35%
Meatloaf, Gravy, Mash. Potato	290	16	50%
Chicken Tetrazini w. Fettucine	310	12	35%
Lasagne w. Meat Sauce	320	10	28%
Linguini w. Clams & Sauce	310	4.5	13%
Chicken Cacciatore	260	6	21%
Italian Meat w. Sauce	200	8	36%
Salisbury Steak Mashed Potato	300	13	39%
Pepper Steak & Rice	260	4.5	16%
Lean & Tasty: Macaroni & Chse	290	6	19%
Southwestern Chicken & Pasta	200	2.5	11%
Fettucini Creamy Pesto	260	6	21%
Black Bean Chili w. Rice	410	5	11%

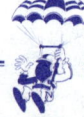

FROZEN ENTREES & MEALS CONT

STOUFFER'S

Entrees	C	F	%fc
Beef Pie	450	26	52%
Beef Stroganoff	390	20	46%
Cheddar Pasta w. Beef & Tom.	450	19	38%
Chse Enchilada & Mex. Style Rice	370	14	34%
Cheese Manicotti	380	17	40%
Cheese Ravioli	380	13	31%
Chicken a la King	350	13	33%
Chicken Chow Mein w. Rice	260	5	17%
Chick. Enchilada & Mex. Style Rice	370	14	34%
Chicken Enchiladas	230	11	43%
Chicken Pie, 10 oz	560	36	58%
Chili w. Beans	270	10	33%
Creamed Chicken	260	19	66%
Creamed Chipped Beef	160	11	62%
Creamy Chicken & Broccoli	320	15	42%
Escalloped Chick. & Noodles, 10 oz	450	28	56%
Larger package sizes, 1 c., 8 oz	360	22	55%
Fettucini Alfredo	520	28	48%
Fettucini Primavera	430	20	42%
Five Cheese Lasagna	360	13	33%
Glazed Chicken	100	3.5	32%
Green Pepper Steak	330	9	25%
Grilled Chick. & Angel Hair Pasta	380	13	31%
Ham & Asparagus Bake	520	36	62%
Homestyle:			
Baked Chicken, Gravy . Potato	270	12	40%
Beef Pot Roast	250	8	29%
Chicken Fettucini	390	15	35%
Chick. Monterey w. Mex. Rice	410	20	44%
Chick. Parmigiana w. Spaghetti	460	16	31%
Fish Fillet w. Macaroni & Chse	430	21	44%
Fried Chicken & Potato	310	12	35%
Meatloaf & Potato	330	16	44%
Rst. Turkey, Gravy, Stuff, Potato	320	13	37%
Salisbury Steak & Gravy			
& Macaroni & Cheese	350	16	41%
Veal Parmigiana w. Spaghetti	430	17	36%
Lasagna Bake	370	12	29%
Lasagna w. Meat Sauce, $10^{1}/2$ oz	370	14	34%
Larger pack sizes, 1 c., 8 oz	270	10	33%
Macaroni & Beef	420	20	43%
Macaroni & Chse, $^{1}/2$ of 12 oz pkt	320	16	45%
Larger pack sizes, 1 c., 8 oz	380	17	40%
Macaroni & Chse w. Broccoli	360	17	43%
Noodles Romanoff	490	25	46%
Pasta Shells & American Chse.	260	10	35%

STOUFFER'S (CONT)

Entrees (Cont)	C	F	%fc
Spaghetti w. Meatballs	440	15	31%
Spaghetti w. Meat Sauce	350	12	31%
Stuffed Pepper, 10 oz	200	8	36%
Swedish Meatballs	480	24	45%
Tuna Noodle Casserole	320	10	28%
Turkey Pie	530	33	56%
Turkey Tetrazzini	360	17	43%
Vegetable Lasagna, $10^{1}/2$ oz	440	20	41%
Larger package sizes, 1 c., 8 oz	340	17	45%
Side Dishes			
Corn Souffle	170	7	37%
Creamed Spinach	160	12	68%
Escalloped Apples	180	3	15%
Green Bean Mushroom Casserole	140	8	51%
Potatoes au Gratin	130	6	42%
Scalloped Potatoes	140	6	39%
Spinach Souffle	150	10	60%
Welsh Rarebit	120	9	68%

SWANSON

Homestyle Recipe: Entrees - Per Serving	C	F	%fc
Chicken Cacciatore	260	8	28%
Chicken Nibbles	340	20	53%
Chicken Pie	410	21	46%
Chili Con Carne	270	10	33%
Fish & Fries	340	16	42%
Fried Chicken	390	21	48%
Lasagna w. Meat Sauce	400	15	34%
Macaroni & Cheese	390	19	44%
Salisbury Steak	320	16	45%
Scalloped Potatoes & Ham	300	13	39%
Seafood Creole w. Rice	240	6	23%
Sirloin Tips in Burgundy Sce.	160	5	28%
Spag. w. Ital. Style Meatballs	490	18	33%
Swedish Meatballs	360	20	50%
Turkey w. Dressing/Potatoes	290	11	34%
Veal Parmigiana	330	13	35%
Hungry Man Dinners			
Boneless Chicken	700	28	36%
Chopped Beef Steak	640	37	52%
Fried Chicken, white/dark meat	870	46	48%
Mexican	820	41	45%
Salisbury Steak	680	41	54%
Sliced Beef	450	12	24%
Turkey	550	18	29%
Veal Parmigiana	590	26	40%

FROZEN ENTREES & MEALS CONT

SWANSON (CONT)

	C	F	%fc
Hungry Man Pot Pies			
7 oz Pie: Beef	370	19	46%
Chicken; Turkey	380	22	52%
Macaroni & Cheese	200	8	36%
16 oz Pie: Beef	610	31	46%
Chicken; Turkey	650	36	50%
Kids Fun Feast			
Fairly Bustin' Beef Patties	440	19	39%
Frazzlin' Fried Chicken	690	34	44%
Roarin' Ravioli	530	13	22%

TYSON

	C	F	%fc
Entrees: Beef Champignon	370	15	36%
Chicken Picante	250	4	14%
Chicken Supreme	230	6	23%
Francais	280	14	45%
Glazed Chicken	240	4	15%
Grilled Chicken	220	3	12%
Grilled Italian Chicken	210	3	13%
Honey Roasted Chicken	220	4	16%
Chicken: Kiev	450	18	36%
Marsala; Picatta	200	4	18%
Mesquite	320	8	23%
Roast Chicken	200	2	9%
Sweet & Sour Chicken	420	15	32%
Turkey w. Gravy	320	12	34%

TYSON (CONT)

	C	F	%fc
Healthy Portions:			
BBQ Chicken	400	8	18%
Chicken Marinara	340	7	19%
Chicken Mesquite; Herb Chicken	330	5	14%
Honey Mustard; Sesame Chicken	390	6	14%
Italian Style Chicken	310	4	12%
Salsa Chicken	370	6	15%
(Other Chicken Products ~ Page 45)			
Breakfast: Classic Omelet S'wich	220	6	33%
English Muffin Sandwich	210	5	21%
Glazed Cinnamon Rolls	200	5	23%
Ham & Cheese Omelet	220	5	20%
Sausage Biscuit	230	11	43%

WEIGHT WATCHERS

	C	F	%fc
Entrees: Per Meal			
Bow Tie Pasta & Mushr. Marsala	280	9	29%
Broccoli & Cheese Baked Potato	250	7	25%
Cheese Manicotti	260	7	24%
Chicken Cordon Bleu	230	4.5	18%
Chicken Enchiladas Suiza	270	9	30%
Chicken Fettucini	290	7	22%
Fettucini Alfredo w. Broccoli	230	6	23%
Garden Lasagna	270	7	23%
Grilled Salisbury Steak	250	9	32%
Hunan Style Rice & Veges.	250	7	25%
Italian Cheese Lasagna	300	8	24%
Kung Pao Noodles & Veges.	260	10	35%
Lasagna w. Meat Sauce	270	7	23%
Lasagna: Alfredo/Bolognese	300	7	21%
Macaroni & Cheese	280	7	23%
Paella Rice & Vegetables	280	7	23%
Parisian Style White Beans/Veges	220	9	37%
Pasta & Spinach Romano	240	8	30%
Pasta w. Tomato Basil Sce.	260	9	31%
Peking Style Rice & Vegetables	270	6	20%
Penne Pasta w. Sun-Dried Tom.	290	9	28%
Penne Pollo	290	5	16%
Pepper Steak	240	4.5	17%
Pilaf Florentine/ Risotto	290	7	22%
Santa Fe Style Rice & Beans	290	9	28%
Spaghetti Marinara, 9 oz	280	7	23%
Spaghetti w. Meat Sauce	290	6	19%
Spicy Penne Pasta & Ricotta	280	6	19%
Stuffed Turkey Breast	230	5	20%
Swedish Meatballs	280	8	26%
Tuna Noodle Casserole	270	7	23%
Ziti Mozzarella, 9 oz	280	6	26%

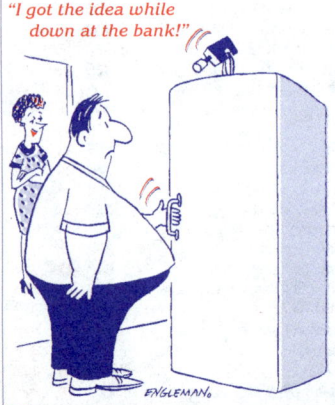

"I got the idea while down at the bank!"

FROZEN PIZZA

	C	F	%fc
AMY'S			
Cheese; Spinach, 13 oz	320	11	31%
Roasted Vegetable, 12 oz	270	8	27%
Pizza Pockets: Regular, 4½ oz	290	9	28%
Pepperoni Style, 4½ oz	220	7	29%
CELESTE			
Large Pizza: Per ¼ Pizza			
Cheese; Zesty Four Cheese	320	16	45%
Deluxe; Pepperoni	350	20	51%
Suprema w. Meat, ⅕ pizza	290	16	50%
Whole Pizza: Per Serve			
Cheese	540	25	42%
Deluxe; Original Four Cheese	540	30	50%
Hot & Zesty 4 Cheese	530	27	46%
Pepperoni; Saus.; Zesty 4 Cheese	530	27	46%
Suprema w. Meat	580	31	48%
Suprema Vegetable	480	23	43%
Italian Bread: Deluxe	290	11	34%
Garlic & Herb Zesty Chicken	260	8	28%
Pepperoni; Zesty 4 Cheese	320	13	37%
DI GIORNO			
Rising Crust Pizza:			
Large: Per ⅙ Pizza			
Pepperoni	320	11	31%
Four Cheese	380	16	38%
Three Meat	370	16	39%
Individual Size:			
Pepperoni; Suprema, ⅓ pizza	300	13	39%
1 whole pizza	900	39	39%
HEALTHY CHOICE			
French Bread Pizza:			
Cheese (1)	320	3	8%
Pepperoni (1)	340	5	13%
Sausage; Supreme	310	3	9%
Vegetable	270	2.5	8%
JENO'S			
Crisp 'n Tasty: Per Pizza			
Canadian Style Bacon	430	18	38%
Cheese	450	19	38%
Combination; Supreme	520	28	48%
Hamburger; Pepper.; Three Meat	500	26	47%
Sausage	510	27	48%
Microwave For One			
Cheese	240	11	41%
Combination	310	18	52%
Pepperoni; Sausage	280	16	51%
LEAN CUISINE			
French Bread Pizza: Cheese	320	6	17%
Deluxe, Pepperoni	320	8	23%
PAPPALO'S			
Pizzeria Style Crust, 12": Per ¼ Pizza			
Four Meat; Sausage	380	17	40%
Pepperoni; Saus.& Pepper.; Supr.	390	18	42%
Three Cheese	340	12	32%
Pizzeria Style Crust 9": Per 1/42 Pizza			
Pepperoni; Saus.; Saus. & Pepper.	440	20	41%
Three Cheese	400	15	34%
Supreme, ⅓ pizza	300	13	39%
Deep Dish: Per 1/45 Pizza			
Four Meat; Sausage	330	14	38%
Pepperoni; Saus. & Pepperoni	340	14	37%
Supreme	350	15	39%
Three Cheese	370	12	29%
For One: Three Cheese	500	20	36%
Pepperoni; Supreme	520	26	45%
Sausage & Pepperoni	530	27	49%
For One Deep Dish			
Pepperoni; Supreme	540	25	42%
Sausage & Pepperoni	550	26	43%
Three Cheese	540	20	33%
PEPPERIDGE FARM			
Croissant & Pastry Pizza:			
Cheese	430	23	48%
Deluxe	440	23	47%
Pepperoni	420	22	47%
PILLSBURY			
Microwave: Cheese, ½ pizza	240	10	38%
Pepperoni, Combination, ½ pizza	310	15	44%
Sausage, ½ pizza	280	13	42%
French Bread Pizza: Cheese (1)	370	15	36%
Pepperoni, 1 pizza	430	19	40%
Sausage, 1 pizza	410	16	35%
Sausage & Pepperoni	450	21	42%
RED BARON			
Large: 4 Cheese, ¼ pizza	430	21	44%
Pepperoni, ¼ pizza	450	24	48%
Supreme, ⅕ pizza	350	18	46%
Deep Dish Singles: 1 pizza	490	26	48%

FROZEN PIZZA CONT

STOUFFER'S

French Bread Pizzas: 1/2 Pkg

	C	F	%fc
Bacon Cheddar/Deluxe Pizza	430	21	44%
Cheese; Vegetable Deluxe	360	16	40%
Dble Cheese/Cheeseburger	420	20	43%
Pepperoni & Mushr./Sausage	440	21	43%
Pepperoni; Three Meat	450	24	48%
Sausage & Pepperoni/White Pizza	460	23	45%

TOMBSTONE

12" Pizza: Per Slice, 1/5 Pizza

	C	F	%fc
Canadian; Extra Cheese	370	17	41%
Cheese/Sausage & Pepperoni	340	18	48%
Other varieties, average	320	16	45%

12" Special Order: Per 1/5 Pizza

	C	F	%fc
Four Cheese	400	19	43%
Other varieties, average	350	18	46%

9" Pizza: Per 1/3 Pizza

	C	F	%fc
Extra Cheese	420	19	41%
Pepperoni & Sausage	360	21	53%
Other varieties, average	320	17	48%

9" Special Order: Per 1/3 Pizza

	C	F	%fc
All varieties, average	400	21	47%

Double Top:

	C	F	%fc
All Types, 1/6 Pizza	350	20	51%
Light: Supreme, 1/5 pizza	270	9	30%
Vegetable, 1/5 pizza	240	7	26%
Thin Crust Italian: 3 Cheese (1/4)	380	22	52%
Pepperoni	420	27	58%
Other varieties	410	25	55%

Thin Crust Mexican: 1/4 Pizza 380 23 54%

For One: Chse/Saus. Pepp; Sprme 590 37 56%
Extra Cheese; Italian Sausage 550 32 52%

For One (1/2 Less Fat)

	C	F	%fc
Cheese; Vegetable	360	10	25%
Pepperoni; Supreme	400	13	29%

TOTINO'S

Party Pizza: Per 1/2 Pizza

	C	F	%fc
Cheese	320	14	39%
Canadian Bacon; Vegetable	320	15	42%
Sausage; Bacon; Pepperoni	380	21	50%
Hamburger, Mexican	370	20	49%
Combination; Zesty Italiano	390	21	48%
Sausage; Supreme	380	20	47%
Three Meat	360	19	48%

Party Pizza Family Size

	C	F	%fc
Cheese, 1/3 pizza	360	16	40%
Combination, 1/4 pizza	300	16	48%
Pepperoni, 1/3 pizza	410	22	48%
Sausage, 1/4 pizza	300	16	48%

Select Pizza: Per 1/3 Pizza

	C	F	%fc
Sausage & Pepperoni; Supreme	360	19	48%
Three Cheese	300	14	42%
2 Cheese & Canadian Style Bacon	310	14	41%
2 Cheese & Pepperoni/Sausage	360	20	50%

Big & Hearty Stuffed Sandwich: Each

	C	F	%fc
Chicken Fajita Grande	270	10	33%
Mega Meat Pizza	330	15	41%
Packed w. Pepperoni Pizza	350	17	44%
Piled High Ham & Cheese	310	14	41%

Pizza Rolls: Per 6 Rolls

	C	F	%fc
Combination; Spicy Italian Style	220	11	45%
Hamburger & Chse; Saus. & Mush.	200	9	41%
Pepperoni & Cheese	230	12	47%
Sausage & Cheese; Three Meat	210	10	43%
Supreme; Three Cheese	210	9	39%

Microwave: Pizza For One

	C	F	%fc
Cheese	240	11	41%
Combination	380	18	43%
Pepperoni; Sausage	280	16	51%
Supreme	290	17	53%
Zesty Mexican Style	280	16	51%

WEIGHT WATCHERS

	C	F	%fc
Deluxe Combo, 1 pizza	380	11	26%
Pepperoni, 1 pizza	390	12	28%
Extra Cheese Pizza	390	12	28%

WOLFGANG PUCK

11 oz Pizza: Per 1/2 Pizza

	C	F	%fc
Pepperoni & Mushroom	320	15	42%
Grilled Vegetable	200	0	0%
Spicy Chicken	360	16	40%
Turkey Sausage	320	13	37%

CANNED & PACKAGED MEALS

B & M
Baked Beans: *Per 1/2 Cup, 4 1/2 oz*

	C	F	%fc
Barbeque; Vegetarian	170	1	5%
Other varieties, average	180	2	10%

BETTY CROCKER
Made As Directed: *Per Serving*

	C	F	%fc
Potato Buds: Plain, 2/3 cup	160	8	45%
Other varieties, 2/3 cup	190	11	52%
Specialty Potatoes: Hash Browns, 1/2 cup	200	8	36%
Other varieties, 1/2 cup	120	2.5	19%
Mashed, 1/2 cup	160	8	45%
Potato Shakers: 2/3 cup	140	4	26%
Seasoned Fries, 7 fries	120	4	30%
Twice Baked Potatoes, 2/3 cup	210	11	47%

CAMPBELL'S

	C	F	%fc
Barbecue Beans (Per 8 oz)	210	4	17%
Home Style Beans	230	4	16%
Old Fashioned Beans in Molasses	230	3	12%
Pork & Beans in Tomato Sauce	190	3	14%
Ranchero Beans	180	4	20%

CHEF BOYARDEE: *Per 7 1/2 oz*

	C	F	%fc
Beef Ravioli	190	3.5	17%
Lasagna	210	2	9%
Spaghetti & Meatballs	200	6	27%
Spaghetti Rings & Meatballs	230	7	27%

DENNISON'S: *Per 7 1/2 oz*

	C	F	%fc
Chili Con Carne w. Beans	300	12	36%

DR. McDOUGALL'S: *Per Cup*

	C	F	%fc
Ramen Noodles; Chicken; Beef	140	1	6%
Tamale Pie w. Baked Chips	190	2	9%
Pinto Beans & Rice, Sthwestern	190	1	5%
Pasta w. Beans, Mediterranean	180	1	5%
Rice & Pasta Pilaf	210	0.5	2%

EDEN: *Per 1/2 Cup, 4 1/2 oz*

	C	F	%fc
Baked Beans w. Sorghum, Mustard	150	0	0%
Ginger Blacks w. Ginger, Lemon	120	0	0%
Chili Beans w. Jalapeno & Peppers	130	0	0%
Lentils w. Onion, Bay Leaf	90	0	0%

FARMHOUSE
Rice Mix: *Per 2 oz*

	C	F	%fc
Broc. au Gratin; Herb/Butter Rice	210	2	9%
Chicken Pilaf	190	2	9%
Herb & Butter Wild Rice	200	2	9%
Mexican; Red Beans/Spanish Rice	180	2	5%

FEATHERWEIGHT

	C	F	%fc
Chicken Dumplings (Per Pkg)	160	5	28%
Beef Ravioli	220	4	16%
Chili with Beans	280	10	32%
Spagh./Meatballs; Beef Stew	160	3	17%
Chicken Stew; Spanish Rice	140	1	6%

HAMBURGER HELPER
Made As Directed: *Per 1 Cup Serving*

	C	F	%fc
Beef Pasta/Stew	270	10	33%
Beef Taco; Cheddar Melt	310	11	32%
Cheddar 'n Bacon; Cheeseburger Macaroni	350	16	41%
Cheesy Italian/Shells	340	14	37%
Fettuccini Alfredo; Mushroom Wild Rice	310	13	38%
Hamburger Stew; Lasagne; Italian Herb	270	10	33%
Italian Rigatoni	180	10	50%
Meatloaf	280	15	48%
Nacho Cheese	320	13	37%
Pizzabake, 1/6 pan	270	10	33%
Pizza Pasta w. Cheese	290	10	31%
Potatoes Au Gratin/Stroganoff	290	14	43%
Rice Oriental; Spaghetti; Southwestern Beef	310	10	29%
Stroganoff; Swedish Meatballs	320	13	37%
Three Cheese	340	15	40%
Zesty Italian; Zesty Mexican	310	11	32%

HORMEL: *Per Cup*
Dinty Moore:

	C	F	%fc
Beef Stew, 10 oz	260	13	45%
Chicken & Dumplings	200	6	27%
Corned Beef Hash	350	22	57%
Turkey Stew	130	2.5	17%

Kid's Kitchen: *Per Cup*

	C	F	%fc
Beans 'N Wieners	310	13	38%
Beef/Cheesy Macaroni	190	6	28%
Cheezy Mac 'N Cheese	260	11	38%
Mini Ravioli	260	7	24%
Noodle Rings w. Chicken	150	4	24%
Spaghetti Rings w. Franks	240	9	34%
Spaghetti Rings w. Meatballs	230	7	27%

Microwave Cup:

	C	F	%fc
Beef Stew	180	9	45%
Beef Vegetable, Low Calorie	90	1	10%
Chicken & Noodles	200	9	41%
Low Calorie	110	2.5	20%
Chile w. Beans	250	11	40%
Chili con Carne, no Beans	290	17	53%
Scalloped Potatoes & Ham	260	16	55%

CANNED & PACKAGED MEALS CONT

KAN TONG
Per 1 Cup

	C	F	%fc
Fried Rice: Chicken; Traditional	190	3.5	17%
Pork; Spicy Chicken	190	1	5%

KNORR
Per 1 Cup Prepared

Broccoli au Gratin Risotto	260	2.5	9%
Chicken Flavor Pilaf	210	1	4%
Lemon Herb Jasmine Pilaf	260	2	7%
Original Recipe Pilaf	220	0.5	1%
Rice Mix Risotto Mushroom	280	1	3%
Risotto Primavera	290	1	3%
Spanish Pilaf	230	1	4%

KRAFT
Side Dishes: *Made As Directed (1 Cup)*

Cheddar Cheese Egg Noodles	430	21	44%
Chicken Egg Noodle	330	12	33%
Macaroni & Cheese:			
Deluxe Original; Thick 'N Creamy	320	10	28%
Other varieties	390	17	39%
Pasta Salad, 3/4 cup: Light Italian	190	2	9%
Garden Primavera	280	12	38%
Other varieties	360	24	60%
Velveeta: Shells & Cheese	360	13	33%
Rotini Cheese Broccoli	400	16	36%
Amer./Tangy Italian Spaghetti	270	4.5	15%
Spaghetti w. Meat Sauce	330	11	30%

MELTING POT FOODS
Per 1/2 Cup

Calypso Cranberry Couscous	200	0	0%
Wild Mushroom Couscous	190	0	0%
Lentil Curry Couscous	170	0	0%
Sundried Tomato Couscous	190	1	5%
Lucky 7 Vegetable Couscous	190	0.5	2%

NISSAN FOODS: *Per Serving*

Top Ramen, all varieties	190	7	33%
Cup Noodles: Shrimp Picante	310	15	44%
Other varieties	300	14	42%

OLD EL PASO: *Per 1/2 Cup*

Refried Beans: Reg, Black	110	2	16%
Veget.; w. Green Chilies	100	1	9%
w. Cheese	130	3.5	24%
w. Sausage	200	13	59%
Fat Free varieties	100	0	0%
Mexe/Pinto Beans	110	0.5	4%
Black/Garbanzo Beans	110	1.5	12%

OLD EL PASO (Cont)
One Skillet Mexican:

	C	F	%fc
Nacho Cheese, prep. (2)	490	19	35%
Salsa; Taco, aver. prep. (2)	450	16	32%

Side Dishes: *Per Serving*

Canned: Chili with Beans, 1 cup	200	7	32%
Spanish Rice, 1 cup	130	1	7%
Tamales in Chili Gravy (3)	320	19	53%
Boxed: Cheesy Mexican Rice	420	3.5	8%
Spanish Rice	410	2	4%

PROGRESSO

Beef Ravioli, 1 cup, 9 oz	260	5	17%
Cheese Ravioli, 1 cup, 9 oz	220	2	8%
Italian Style Zucchini, 1/2 c., 4.2 oz	50	2	36%

RICE-A-RONI
Rice Mix - *Per Serving*

Chicken	510	1	2%
1/3 Less Salt Chicken	280	1	3%
Beef; Family Chicken	310	1	3%
Broccoli au Gratin	370	6	15%
Chicken Mushroom	360	2	5%
Chicken Vegetable	280	1	3%
Fast Cook: Broccoli, 1/2 cup	300	2	6%
Chicken, 1/4 cup	250	1	4%
Spanish, 1/2 cup	240	0.5	2%
Fried Rice	320	2	6%
Herb & Butter; Pilaf, 2 oz	310	1	3%
Long Grain & Wild Rice	240	0.5	2%
Spanish	270	1	3%
White Cheddar & Herbs	340	5	13%

SKILLET CHICKEN HELPER
Per 1 Cup

Stir Fried Chicken, prep.	270	9	30%

TUNA HELPER
Per 1 Cup (Prepared)

Tuna au Gratin; Tuna Tetrazzini	310	12	35%
Creamy: Broccoli/Pasta	310	12	35%
Fettuccino Alfredo	310	14	40%
Cheesy Pasta	280	11	35%
Garden Cheddar	310	12	35%
Pasta Salad, 2/3 cup	380	27	64%
Tuna Pot Pie	440	24	49%
Tuna Romanoff	280	8	34%

VEGETARIAN MEALS & PRODUCTS

AMY'S

	C	F	%fc
Frozen - Per Serving			
Pot Pie: Country, 1 pie, $7^{1}/2$ oz	370	16	39%
Broccoli, $7^{1}/2$ oz	430	22	46%
Vegetable, $7^{1}/2$ oz	360	18	45%
Non-Dairy Vegetable, $7^{1}/2$ oz	320	9	11%
Shepherd's Pie, 8oz	160	4	23%
Pasta: Macaroni & Cheese, 9 oz	450	9	18%
Macaroni & Soy Cheese, 9 oz	360	14	35%
Cheese Ravioli w. Sauce, $9^{1}/2$ oz	340	12	32%
Vegetable Lasagne			
w. Cheese, $9^{1}/2$ oz	300	10	30%
Tofu-Vegetable Lasagne, $9^{1}/2$ oz	300	10	30%
Burgers: California Veggie, $2^{1}/2$ oz	100	3	27%
Chicago Veggie, $2^{1}/2$ oz	160	5	28%
Mexican Favorites:			
Cheese Enchilada, $4^{3}/4$ oz	210	9	39%
Bl. Bean & Vege. Enchilada, $4^{3}/4$ oz	130	4	28%
Bean & Rice Burrito, 6oz	250	5	18%
Bean Rice & Cheese Burrito, 6oz	280	8	26%
Breakfast Burrito, 6oz	230	5	20%
Black Bean Burrito, 6oz	320	8	23%
Mexican Tamale Pie, 8oz	220	3	12%
Whole Meals:			
Country Dinner, 11 oz	380	12	28%
Cannelloni Dinner, 10 oz	260	11	38%
Enchilada Dinner, 10 oz	250	8	29%
Veggie Loaf Dinner, 10 oz	260	5	17%
Family Size Meals:			
Vegetable Lasagna, 7 oz	200	8	36%
Cheese Enchilada, 4.4 oz	200	8	36%
Black Bean Enchilada, 4.4 oz	120	4	30%
Pockets: Pizza, $4^{1}/2$ oz	290	9	12%
Pepperoni Style Pizza, $4^{1}/2$ oz	220	7	29%
Spinach Feta, $4^{1}/2$ oz	200	7	32%
Vegetable Pot Pie, 5 oz	230	6	23%

B & M

	C	F	%fc
Baked Beans: Per $^{1}/2$ cup ($4^{1}/2$ oz)			
Bacon & Onion w. Brown Sugar	190	2	9%
Baked Beans w. Pork	180	2	10%
Barbeque; Vegetarian	170	1	5%
w. Natural Honey; Red Kidney	170	2	11%
Yellow Eye Baked Beans	180	3	15%

TOFU & TEMPEH PRODUCTS
~ See Page 62 ~

BEAN CUISINE

	C	F	%fc
Made As Directed: Per 1 Cup			
Ital. Market Beans w. Mafalda	190	3	14%
Basque Beans w. Basil Fettuccine	200	3.5	16%
13 Bean Bouillabaisse	240	4.5	17%
Other varieties	210	4	17%

CELENTANO

	C	F	%fc
Catavelli, $^{2}/3$ cup, 3.2 oz	400	1.5	4%
Eggplant Parmigiana,			
10 oz size, 1 tray	420	27	76%
14 oz size: $^{1}/2$ tray (7 oz)	320	21	59%
25 oz size: 1 cup, 8 oz	360	25	64%
Lasagne, 1 tray, 10 oz	400	14	32%
14 oz size: $^{1}/2$ tray (7 oz)	280	10	32%
Manicotti: 2 pces, 10 oz size	450	21	42%
14 oz size: 2 pces (7 oz)	310	15	42%
no Sauce, 2 pces, 7 oz	410	19	41%
Ravioli: 6 pces, $6^{1}/2$ oz	400	9	20%
Mini, 12 pces, 4 oz	270	6	19%
Stuffed Shells: 3 pces, 10 oz	400	20	45%
12.5 oz size (no Sauce):			
4 pces, $6^{1}/4$ oz	330	15	42%
14 oz size: 2 pces (7 oz)	300	14	43%
9 Slice Pizza, 1 slice, $2^{1}/2$ oz	340	11	29%
Vegetarian Selects: Per Tray, 10 oz			
Broccoli Stuffed Shells	300	6	17%
Lasagne Primavera	280	5	21%
Manicotti Florentine	280	6	18%
Non-Dairy: Per Tray, 10 oz			
Eggplant Rollettes	220	13	55%
Lasagne Primavera	230	4	15%
Spinach & Broccoli Manicotti	230	4	15%
Spinach & Broc. Stuff. Shells	210	4	17%

GARDENBURGER
(Wholesome & Healthy Foods Inc.)

	C	F	%fc
Gardenburger: Original, $2^{1}/2$ oz	140	2.5	16%
3.4 oz patty	190	3	14%
Gardenburger Veggie: 3.4 oz	260	0	0%
Gardenburger Veggie Medley:			
$2^{1}/2$ oz patty	100	0	0%
Gardenburger Zesty Bean: $2^{1}/2$ oz	120	3	23%
Gardenburger Mexi: $2^{1}/2$ oz pat.	215	2.5	10%
3.4 oz patty	290	3	9%
Garden Sausage: $1^{1}/4$ oz patty	120	1	7.5%
$2^{1}/2$ oz patty	240	2.5	9%

VEGETARIAN MEALS & PRODUCTS cont

HARVEST BURGER
(Green Giant) Per Patty:

	C	F	%fc
Harvest Burger: Regular	140	4	26%
Italian	140	4.5	29%
Southwestern	140	4	26%

HEALTH VALLEY
Fat-Free Beans & Chili:

	C	F	%fc
Honey Baked Beans, 1/2 cup	110	0	0%
Chili in a Cup, all types, 3/4 cup	120	1	8%
Mild/Spicy Vegetarian Chili: all flavors, 1/2 cup	80	0	0%
Chili Burrito/Enchilada, 1/2 cup	80	0	0%
Chili, Fajito flavored, 1/2 cup	80	0	0%

LA LOMA

	C	F	%fc
Big Franks, each	110	6	49%
Corn Dogs, each	190	8	38%
Nuteena, 1/2" slice, 2 1/4 oz	160	12	67%
RediBurger, 1/2" slice, 2 1/3 oz	130	6	42%
Savory Meatballs, 7 balls, 2 1/2 oz	190	8	38%
Sizzle Burgers, each	220	12	49%
Sizzle Franks, 2 franks	170	13	69%
Swiss Steak, 1 pce, 3 1/4 oz	170	10	53%
Tender Bits, 4 pieces, 2 oz	80	3	34%
Tender Rounds, 6 pieces, 2 1/2 oz	120	4	30%
VegeBurger, 1/2 cup, 4 oz	110	2	16%
Vita-Burger Chunk, 1/4 cup, 3/4 oz	70	0	0%

LIGHTLIFE

	C	F	%fc
Gimme Lean Saus./Beef, 2 oz	70	0	0%
Grills: Lemon, 1 patty, 78g	140	5.5	35%
Barbecue, 1 patty, 78g	120	3.5	26%
Tamari, 1 patty, 78g	120	5	38%
Lean Breakfast Links, 1 link, 35g	60	3	45%
Lean Italian Links, 1 link, 40g	60	2	30%
Meatless Lightburger, 2 1/2 oz	110	3	25%
Savory Seitan, 4 oz	160	2	11%
Smart Deli Slices, 3 slices	50	0	0%
Smart Dogs, 1 link, 42g	45	0	0%
Tofu Pups, 1 link, 42g	60	2.5	38%
Wonderdogs, 1.5 oz	55	1	16%
Dinners: Country French Stew	340	3	8%
Meanloaf	300	5	15%
Moroccan Lentil Stew	400	2	5%
Penne Pasta Bolognese	410	3	7%
Thai Tofu	400	10	23%

LONGA LIFE

	C	F	%fc
Notchicken, 2 slices, 3/4 oz	50	2	36%
Notham, 2 slices, 3/4 oz	50	2	36%
Notbacon, 1 strip, 1/2 oz	43	3	63%
Notpepperoni, 4 slices, 1 oz	65	4	55%
Notchicken Nuggets, (4), 2 oz	130	5	35%

Distributor: United Specialty Foods Inc
PH: (800) 772 2218

LOMA LINDA

	C	F	%fc
Chik Nuggets, 5 pieces, 3 oz	240	16	60%
Corn Dogs, 1 corn dog	220	9	37%
Fried Chik'n, 1 piece, 2 oz	180	15	75%

Canned & Dry Products

	C	F	%fc
Big Franks, 1 link	110	7	57%
Chick.Supreme Mix, 1/3 cup mix	90	1	10%
Dinner Cuts, 2 slices, 3 1/4 oz	90	1.5	15%
Fried Chik'n/Gravy, 2 pcs, 3 oz	210	17	73%
Gravy Quik: Aver.,1 Tbsp mix	20	0	10%
Linketts, 1 link	70	4.5	58%
Little Links, 2 links	90	6	60%
Nuteena, 3/8" slice, 2 oz	160	13	73%
Ocean Platter, 1/3 cup dry mix	90	1	10%
Patty Mix, 1/3 cup dry mix, 1 oz	90	1	10%
RediBurger, 5/8" slice, 3 oz	170	10	53%
Sandwich Spread, 1/4 cup, 2 oz	80	4.5	51%
Savory Dinner Loaf, 1/3 cup, drain.	90	1.5	2.5%
Soyagen, all varieties. 1/4 c. drain.	130	6	42%
Swiss Stake, 1 piece, 3 1/4 oz	120	6	45%
Tender Bits, 6 pieces, 3 oz	110	4.5	37%
Tender Rounds, 6 pieces, 2 3/4 oz	120	5	37%
Vege Burger, 1/4 cup, 2 oz	70	1.5	19%
Vita Burger Chunks, 1/4 cup	70	1	13%
Vita Burger Granules, 3 Tbsp	70	1	13%

MORNINGSTAR FARMS

	C	F	%fc
Better'n Burger, 1 pattie	70	0	0%
Better'n Eggs, 1/4 cup, 2 oz	20	0	0%
Breakfast Links, 2 links	60	2.5	37%
Breakfast Patties, 1 pattie	70	3	39%
Breakfast Strips, 2 strips	60	4.5	67%
Chik Patties, 1 pattie	170	10	53%
Deli Franks, 1 link	110	7	57%
Garden Grain Patties, 1 pattie	130	2.5	17%
Garden Vege patties, 1 pattie	100	2.5	22%
Grillers, 1 pattie, 2 1/4 oz	140	7	45%
Ground Meatless, 1/2 cup, 2 oz	60	0	0%
Homestyle Noodles, 1/2 cup, 2 oz	160	0	0%
Prime Patties, 1 pattie, 2 3/4 oz	110	2	16%

VEGETARIAN MEALS & PRODUCTS cont

MORNINGSTAR FARMS (Cont)

	C	F	%fc
Roasted SoyButter., 2 Tbsp, 1 oz	170	11	58%
Scramblers, 1/4 cup, 2 oz	35	0	0%
Spicy Bl.Bean Burger, 1 pattie	100	1	9%
Breakfast Scramblers - Per Sandwich			
Bagel/Scramblers/Pattie/Cheese	320	4.5	13%
Engl.Muf./Scramblers/Pat./Chse	280	3	10%
English Muffin/Scramblers/Pattie	240	2.5	9%
Dry Products			
Garden Vegie Burger Kit, 1/4 pkg	80	0	0%
Sth.West.Veggie Burger, 1/4 pkg	90	0	0%

NATURAL TOUCH

Frozen Products

	C	F	%fc
Dinner Entree, 1 pattie, 3 oz	220	15	61%
Garden Vege pattie, 1 pattie	100	2.5	22%
Lentil Rice Loaf, 1" slice, 3 oz	170	9	48%
Nine Bean Loaf, 1" slice, 3 oz	160	8	45%
Okara Pattie, 1 pattie, 2 1/4 oz	110	5	41%
Spicy Bl.Bean Burger, 1 pattie	100	1	9%
Vegan Burger, 1 pattie, 2 3/4 oz	70	0	0%
Vegan Burger Crumbles, 1/2 cup	60	0	0%
Vegan Saus.Crumbles, 1/2 cup	60	0	0%
Vege Burger, 1 pattie, 2 1/4 oz	140	6	39%
Vege Frank, 1 link	100	6	54%

Canned & Dry Products

	C	F	%fc
Kaffree Roma, 1 rounded tsp, 2g	10	0	0%
Roma Cappuccino, 3 Tbsp, 10g	50	3	54%
Loaf Mix, 4 Tbsp dry mix, 1 oz	100	0.5	4.5%
Original Veggie Burger, 1/4 pkg	80	0	0%
Sthwestern Veggie Burger, 1/4 pkg	90	0	0%
Roasted Soy Butter, 2 Tbsp	170	11	58%
Stroganoff Mix, 4 Tbsp dry mix	90	3.5	35%
Taco Mix, 3 Tbsp dry mix, 0.6 oz	60	1	15%
Vegetarian Chili, 1 cup, 8 oz	270	12	40%

NEW MENU (*Vitasoy*)

	C	F	%fc
VegiBurgers, 3 oz	110	1	8%
VegiDogs, 1 frank, 1.5oz	45	0	0%
Tofumate (Seasoning Mixes):			
Average all varieties, 1/4 pkg	25	0	0%

SOY DELI

	C	F	%fc
Veggie Burgers, 3 oz	230	14	55%
Tempeh Burger: Marinated, 3 oz	130	4	28%
BBQ; Original, 3 oz	230	13	51%

WHITE WAVE

Meat Substitutes:

	C	F	%fc
Sandwich Slices, 2 slices	90	0	0%
Pastami/Turkey Style, 45g	90	0	0%
Burgers: Veggie Life, 3 oz	130	4	28%
Tempeh, 3 oz	110	3	25%
Teriyaki Tempeh, 3 oz	110	2	16%
Prime, 3 oz	110	0	0%
Chick'n Burger, 3 oz	220	0	0%
Tempeh: Five Grain, 1/3 pkg	140	4	26%
Sea Veggie, 1/3 pkg	120	3	23%
Soy Rice, 1/3 pkg	140	5	32%
Tofu: Baked: Italian, 2 oz pce	120	6	45%
Oriental (Teriyaki), 2 oz pce	120	6	45%
Hard (Organic), 1/5 pkg, 3.2 oz	90	6	60%
Soft, 1/5 pkg, 3.2 oz	90	6	60%
Fat-Reduced, 1/5 pkg, 3.2 oz	90	4	40%
Vegetarian Sloppy Joe, 1 cup	320	10	28%

WHOLESOME & HEARTY FOODS

	C	F	%fc
Garden Dog, 1 frank, 2 oz	120	2.5	19%

WORTHINGTON

Frozen Products

	C	F	%fc
Beef Style Meatless, 3/8" slice	110	7	57%
Bolono, 3 slices, 2 oz	80	3.5	39%
Chic-Ketts, 2 slices (3/8"), 2 oz	120	7	52%
Chick., Sliced or Roll, 2 sl., 2 oz	80	4.5	51%
ChikStiks, 1 piece, 1 1/2 oz	110	7	57%
Corn Beef Meatless, 4 sl., 2 oz	140	9	58%
Crispy Chic Patties, 1 pattie	170	9	48%
Dinner Roast, 3/4" slice, 3 oz	180	12	60%
Fillets, 2 pieces, 3 oz	180	10	50%
FriPats, 1 pattie	130	6	42%
Golden Croquettes, 4 pieces	210	10	43%
Grnd. Meatless Burger, 1/2 cup	80	2.5	28%
Ground Meatless Saus., 1/2 cup	110	6	49%
Leanies, 1 link	110	8	65%
Prosage Links, 2 links	60	2.5	37%
Prosage Patties, 1 pattie	100	3	27%
Prosage Roll, 5/8" slice, 2 oz	140	10	64%
Salami, Meatless, 3 slices, 2 oz	130	8	55%
Smkd Beef, Meatless, 6 sl., 2 oz	120	6	45%
Smkd Turkey., Meatless, 3 sl, 2 oz	140	10	64%
Stakelets, 1 piece, 2 1/2 oz	140	8	51%
Stripples, 2 strips, 1/2 oz	60	4.5	67%
Tuno, 1/2 cup (drained), 2 oz	80	6	67%
Veelets, 1 pattie, 2 1/2 oz	180	9	45%
Vegetarian Egg Rolls, 1 roll	180	8	40%
Wham, 2 slices, 1 1/2 oz	80	5	56%

VEGETARIAN MEALS & PRODUCTS cont

WORTHINGTON (Cont)
Canned & Dry Products

	C	F	%fc
Chili, 1 cup, 8 oz	290	15	47%
Low Fat Chili, 1 cup, 8 oz	170	1	5%
Choplets, 2 slices, 3 1/4 oz	90	1.5	15%
Country Stew, 1 cup, 8 1/2 oz	210	9	39%
Cutlets, 1 slice, 2 1/4 oz	70	1	13%
Diced Chik, 1/4 cup, 2 oz	60	3.5	52%
FriChik, 2 pieces, 3 oz	120	8	60%
Low Fat FriChik, 2 pcs, 3 oz	80	3	34%
GranBurger, 3 Tbsp, 0.6 oz	60	0.5	7.5%
Multigrain Cutlets, 2 sl., 3 1/4 oz	100	2	18%
Numete, 3/8" slices, 2 oz	130	10	69%
Prime Stakes, 1 piece, 3 1/4 oz	140	9	58%
Protose, 3/8" Slice, 2 oz	130	7	48%
Saucettes, 1 link	90	6	60%
Savory Slices, 3 slices, 3 oz	150	9	54%
Sliced Chik, 3 slices, 3 oz	90	6	60%
Super Links, 1 link	110	8	65%
Turkee Slices, 3 slices, 3 1/4 oz	190	14	66%
Vegetable Skallops, 1/2 c., 3 oz	90	1.5	15%
Vegetable Steaks, 2 pieces	80	1.5	17%
Vegetarian Burger, 1/4 c., 2 oz	60	2	30%
Veja Links, 1 link, 1 oz	50	3	54%
Low Fat Veja Links, 1 link	40	1.5	34%

YVES

	C	F	%fc
Burger Burgers, 3 oz	83	0	0%
Canadian Bacon, 3 slices	76	0	0%
Vegetable Patties, 3 oz	102	0	0%
Vegetarian Chili Dogs, 1 dog	70	0	0%
Vegetarian Deli Slices, 52g	70	0	0%
Veggie Pepperoni, 52g	78	0	0%
Veggie Weiners, 1 pce	50	0	0%

ZOGLO'S

	C	F	%fc
Crispy Vegn. Cutlets,(1), 3.5oz	200	10	45%
Savory Vegn. Kebabs,(1),2.8oz	135	5	33%
Tender Vegn. Burgers,(1),2.6oz	150	7	42%
Vegetarian Patties,(1), 2.6oz	130	5	35%
Vegetarian Franks,(1), 2.6oz	125	5	36%

"Being cheerful keeps you healthy. It is a slow death to be gloomy all the time."
~ Proverbs 17:22

SOYBEAN PRODUCTS, TOFU

	C	F	%fc
Cheeses (Soy): See Page 33.			
Miso, 1/2 cup, 5 oz	280	8	26%
Natto, 1/2 cup, 3oz	190	10	47%
Tempeh, 1 piece, 3 oz	170	6	32%
Fried, 3 oz	250	14	50%
Tofu: Mori-Nu Tofu (Silken):			
Soft, 4 oz	60	3	45%
Firm, 4 oz	70	3	39%
Extra Firm, 4 oz	70	2	26%
Hinoichu Tofu: Soft, 4 oz	60	3	45%
Reg. (Japanese), 4 oz	80	4	45%
Firm (Chinese), 4 oz	90	5	50%
Nasoya Tofu: Soft, 4 oz	70	6	77%
Premium Soft, 4 oz	80	4	45%
Silken, 4 oz	50	5	90%
Firm, 4 oz	100	8	72%
Extra Firm, 4 oz	140	8	51%
Chinese 5 Spice Tofu, 5 oz	150	8	48%
Azumaya Tofu:			
Soft (Silken), 3 oz	45	2	40%
Firm, 3 oz	60	2.5	38%
Extra Firm, 3 oz	80	3.5	39%
Age (Tofu Puff), 1/2 oz	40	1.5	34%
Nama-Age (Fried Tofu), 3 oz	130	5	35%
Tofu Stir Fried, 4 oz	120	8	60%
Dried Tofu, (Eden), 1 block	140	0	0%
Soybean Protein (TVP), 1 oz	90	0	0%
Soy Drinks ~ See Page 20.			

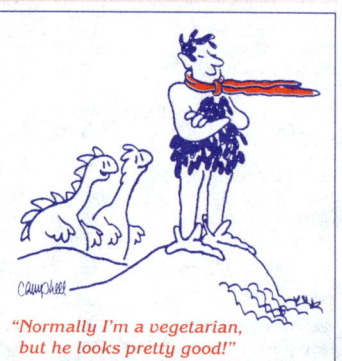

"Normally I'm a vegetarian, but he looks pretty good!"

SOUPS

HOMEMADE & RESTAURANT

	C	F	%fc
Homemade Soups:			
Calculate calories and fat from ingredients.			
Restaurant & Take-Out: Per 8 fl.oz			
Beef Consomme	30	0	0%
Borscht (w/ Cream)	130	8	55%
Bouillabaisse	350	11	28%
Chicken & Corn	290	14	43%
Chicken Consomme	50	0	0%
Chicken Jambalaya	160	7	39%
Chicken Noodle	80	2	23%
Chicken Soup	80	2	23%
Chili with Beans	250	12	43%
Clam Chowder	240	15	56%
Corn & Crab	120	3	23%
Cream of Broccoli	200	12	54%
Cream of Potato	220	12	49%
Cream of Mushroom	290	21	65%
Creamy Pumpkin	210	10	43%
Fish Chowder	220	15	61%
French Onion	420	10	21%
Gazpacho	60	0	0%
Lentil Soup	250	9	32%
Lobster Bisque	320	15	42%
Matzo Ball (w./1 large ball)	180	7	35%
Minestrone	250	6	22%
Mulligatawny	300	15	45%
Pea & Ham	240	10	38%
Potato & Bacon	170	7	37%
Shark Fin Soup	220	6	25%
Split Pea Soup	150	6	36%
Vegetable (Fat Free)	75	0	0%
Vegetable Beef	80	2	23%
Vichyssoise	210	15	64%

- Ethnic & Restaurant Section: Pages 134-138
- Fast Foods/Restaurant Section: Pages 139-218

(Arby's, Au Bon Pain, Boston Market, Dunkin' Donuts, Denny's, Sizzler, Souplantation, Sweet Tomatoes)

CAMPBELL'S

Red & White Label
Made as Directed: Per 8 oz Serving

	C	F	%fc
Bean & Bacon	180	5	25%
Beef Broth	15	0	0%
Beef Noodle	70	2.5	32%
Beef w. Vegetable & Barley	80	2	23%
Broccoli Cheese	110	7	57%
Californian Style Vegetable	60	1	15%

BOUILLON CUBES & POWDERS

Bouillon Cubes: Aver. all types

	C	F	%fc
Regular, 1 cube	8	0	0%
Low Sodium (LiteLine)	12	0	0%
Powders: Average, 1 tsp	8	0	0%

Herb-Ox:
Instant Broth & Seasoning:

Beef, 1 envelope	10	0	0%
Chicken, vegetarian	10	0	0%
Herbs, Spices: 1 tsp	5	0	0%

SOUP OYSTER CRACKERS

40 small/20 large, 1/2 oz	60	2	30%

CAMPBELL'S

Red & White Label (Cont)

	C	F	%fc
Cheddar Cheese	130	8	55%
Chicken & Dumplings	80	3	34%
Chicken & Wild Rice	70	2	26%
Chicken Alphabet	80	2	23%
Chicken Broth	30	2	60%
Chicken Gumbo	60	1.5	23%
Chicken Noodle	70	2.5	32%
Chicken Vegetable	80	2	23%
Chicken w. Stars	70	2	26%
Chicken Won Ton	45	1	20%
Clam Chowder, Manhattan	60	0.5	8%
Clam Chowder, New England	100	2.5	23%
Cream of Asparagus; Celery	110	7	57%
Cream of Broccoli; Shrimp	100	6	54%
Cream of Chicken/Broccoli	130	8	55%
Cream of Mushroom	110	7	57%
Cream of Potato	90	3	30%
Creamy Chicken Mushroom	130	9	62%
Double Noodle	100	2.5	23%
French Onion	70	2.5	32%
Golden Mushroom	80	3	34%
Italian Tomato	100	0.5	5%
Italian Vegetable	70	1	13%
Minestrone	100	2	18%
Old Fashioned Vegetable	70	2.5	32%
Split Pea w. Ham; Green Pea	180	3.5	18%
Tomato & Rice	120	2	15%
Tomato	100	2	18%
Turkey Noodle	80	2.5	28%
Vegetable & Beef	80	2	23%
Vegetable	80	1.5	17%

SOUPS CONT

CAMPBELL'S (CONT)

Healthy Request	**C**	**F**	**%fc**
Per 10 3/4 oz Can		
Average all varieties	80	2	23%
16 oz can - Per 1/2 Can Serving		
Chicken & Rice	100	2	18%
Chicken Broth	20	0	0%
Hearty Chicken Noodle	160	3	17%
Hearty Chicken Vegetable	120	2	15%
Hearty Vegetable & Beef	140	2.5	16%
Minestrone	120	2	15%
New England Clam Chowder	120	3	23%
Southwest Vegetable	140	1	6%
Split Pea & Ham	170	2	11%
Zesty Penne and Vegetables	90	0.5	5%

98% Fat Free: *Per 10 3/4 oz Can* | | |
---|---|---|---
Broccoli Cheese | 80 | 3 | 34%
Cream of Broccoli | 70 | 2 | 26%
Cream of Celery/Mushroom | 70 | 3 | 34%
Cream of Chicken | 80 | 4 | 45%

Home Cookin': *19 oz Can* | | |
---|---|---|---
Per 1/2 Can Serving | | |
Chicken Rice | 110 | 1.5 | 12%
Chicken Vegetable | 130 | 3.5 | 24%
Chicken w. Egg Noodle | 100 | 3.5 | 32%
Country Mushroom & Rice | 80 | 0.5 | 6%
Country Vege., 10 3/4 oz can, (1/2) | 130 | 2 | 14%
Creamy Potato | 180 | 9 | 45%
Fiesta | 130 | 2.5 | 17%
Italian Vegetable | 100 | 4 | 36%
Minestrone | 120 | 2 | 15%
New England Clam Chowder | 200 | 13 | 59%
Tomato Garden | 130 | 3 | 21%
Vegetable Beef | 120 | 2 | 15%

Chunky | | |
---|---|---|---
Per 10 3/4 oz Can - Ready to Serve | | |
Classic Chicken Noodle | 160 | 3.5 | 20%
New England Clam Chowder | 300 | 18 | 54%
Sirloin Burger | 230 | 11 | 43%
Vegetable | 160 | 4 | 23%
19 oz Can - Per 1/2 Can (9 1/2 oz) | | |
Cheese Tortellini | 110 | 1.5 | 12%
Chicken Broccoli Cheese | 200 | 12 | 54%
Chicken Chowder Mushroom | 210 | 12 | 51%
Chicken Corn Chowder | 250 | 15 | 54%
Classic Chicken Noodle | 130 | 3 | 21%
Hearty Chicken & Vegetable | 90 | 2 | 20%
Hearty Vegetable & Pasta | 130 | 3 | 21%
Potato Ham Chowder | 220 | 14 | 57%

Campbell's Chunky (Cont)	**C**	**F**	**%fc**
Savory Chicken & Rice	140	3	19%
Spicy Chicken & Vegetable	90	1	10%
Vegetable Beef	150	5	30%

Campbell's Cup | | |
---|---|---|---
Beef Noodle | 130 | 2 | 14%
Chicken Noodle | 140 | 3 | 19%
  w. White Meat | 90 | 2 | 20%
Creamy Chicken | 90 | 4 | 40%
Hearty Noodles w. Vegetables | 180 | 2 | 10%
Noodle w. Chicken Broth | 90 | 2 | 20%

Campbell's Microwave | | |
---|---|---|---
Bean with Bacon 'n Ham, 7 1/2 oz | 230 | 5 | 20%
Chicken Noodle | 100 | 4 | 40%
Chicken w. Rice | 100 | 4 | 40%
Chili Beef | 190 | 4 | 19%
Vegetable Beef | 100 | 2 | 18%

Cup-A-Soup | | |
---|---|---|---
Chicken Broth, 6 oz | 20 | 1 | 45%
Chicken Vegetable, 6 oz | 50 | 1 | 18%
Cream of Mushroom | 70 | 3 | 38%
Creamy Broccoli & Cheese | 70 | 3 | 39%
Green Pea | 115 | 4 | 31%
Hearty: Chicken & Noodles | 110 | 2 | 16%
  Creamy Chicken Lots-A-Noodles | 180 | 8 | 40%
Onion | 30 | 1 | 30%
Tomato | 105 | 1 | 8%

DR. McDOUGALL'S

	C	F	%fc
Minestrone & Pasta, 1 cup	180	1	5%
Split Pea w. Barley, 1 cup	200	2	9%
Tortilla Soup w. Baked Chips	180	1.5	8%

HAIN

Canned: *Per Serving* | | |
---|---|---|---
Chicken Broth | 70 | 6 | 77%
Chicken Noodle | 120 | 4 | 30%
Creamy Mushroom | 110 | 4 | 33%
Italian Vegetable Pasta | 160 | 5 | 28%
Minestrone | 170 | 2 | 11%
Mushroom Barley | 100 | 2 | 18%
New England Clam Chowder | 180 | 4 | 20%
Split Pea | 170 | 1 | 5%
Turkey Rice | 100 | 3 | 27%
Vegetable Broth | 45 | 0 | 0%
Vegetable Chicken | 120 | 4 | 30%
Vegetable Split Pea | 170 | 1 | 5%
Vegetarian Lentil | 160 | 3 | 17%
Vegetarian Vegetable | 140 | 4 | 26%

SOUPS CONT

HAIN (CONT)

No Salt Added varieties:
Same as Regular

	C	F	%fc
Soup Mixes: Per 3/4 cup (6 oz)			
Cheese & Broccoli	310	22	64%
Cheese Savory	250	16	58%
Savory Lentil	130	2	14%
Savory Minestrone	110	1	8%
Savory Mushroom	210	15	64%
Savory Mushroom, No Salt Added	250	20	72%
Savory Onion, all types	50	2	36%
Savory Potato Leek	260	18	62%
Savory Split Pea	310	10	29%
Savory Tomato	220	14	57%
Savory Vegetable, all types	80	1	11%

HEALTHY CHOICE

Per Cup	C	F	%fc
Bean and Ham, 1 cup	180	3	15%
Beef and Potato	120	2	15%
Chicken Corn Chowder	150	3	18%
Chicken with Pasta	120	3	23%
Chicken with Rice	100	3	30%
Chili Beef	190	1	5%
Country Vegetable	100	1	9%
Garden Vegetable	110	1	8%
Hearty Chicken	140	3	19%
Lentil	140	1	6%
Minestrone; Tomato Garden	110	2	16%
New England Clam Chowder	130	3	21%
Old Fashioned Chicken Noodle	130	2	14%
Split Pea with Ham	160	2	11%
Turkey w. White & Wild Rice	110	3	25%
Vegetable Beef	170	2	11%

HEALTH VALLEY

	C	F	%fc
Bean Vegetable (Per Cup)	140	0	0%
Beef Broth	20	0	0%
Black Bean/Vegetable	110	0	0%
Chicken Broth	45	1.5	30%
Country Corn & Veg.; Potato Leek	70	0	0%
Italian Plus Carotene	80	0	0%
Lentil/& Carrots; Minestrone	90	0	0%
Mushroom Barley	60	0	0%
Pasta Rotini & Vegetable	100	0	0%
Pasta Fagioli	120	0	0%
Pasta Primavera/Cacciatore	110	0	0%
Pasta Bolognese/Romano	100	0	0%
Split Pea/& Carrots	110	0	0%

Health Valley (Cont)

	C	F	%fc
Super Broccoli Carotene	70	0	0%
Tomato; Vegetable Barley	90	0	0%
Tomato/Vegetable, all types	80	0	0%
Vegetable Power Carotene	70	0	0%
Dry: Per 1/3 Cup Serving			
Average all varieties	120	0	0%

HORMEL

Micro Cup Hearty Soup, 1 cup, 7 1/2 oz	C	F	%fc
Bean and Ham	190	4	19%
Beef Vegetable	90	1	10%
Broccoli Cheese w. Ham	170	13	69%
Chicken & Rice Noodle	110	3	25%
New England Clam Chowder	130	5	35%
Potato Cheese with Ham	190	13	62%

KNOOR'S CUP-A-SOUP

Soup Mixes: Per 8 fl oz	C	F	%fc
Broccoli	160	8	45%
Bouillon, all types	15	1	60%
Cauliflower; Wild; Mushroom	100	3	27%
Chicken Noodle	25	0	0%
Chick 'n Pasta	90	2	20%
Fine Herb	130	6	42%
French Onion	50	1	18%
Mushroom; Spinach	100	4	36%
Oriental Hot and Sour	50	1	18%
Oxtail Hearty Beef	70	2	26%
Spring Vegetable w. Herbs	30	0	0%
Tomato Basil	90	3	30%
Tortellini in Brodo	60	1	15%
Vegetable	35	1	26%
Vegetarian Vegetable	15	1	60%

LIPTON

8 oz Serving	C	F	%fc
Beef Mushroom	40	1	23%
Beefy Onion	25	1	36%
Chicken Noodle	80	2	23%
Country Vegetable	80	1	11%
Giggle Noodle	70	2	26%
Hearty Noodle w. Vegetables	75	2	24%
Instant Oriental Noodle: Beef	175	1	5%
Chicken	180	2	10%
Onion	20	0	0%
Onion Golden	60	2	30%
Onion Mushroom; Vegetable	40	1	23%
Ring-O-Noodle	70	2	26%

SOUPS CONT

MANISCHEWITZ

	C	F	%fc
8 fl oz Serving			
Borscht Low calorie	20	0	0%
Borscht with Beets	80	0	0%
Soup Mixes, average, 6 fl oz	50	0	0%

MARUCHAN

	C	F	%fc
Per Pkt			
Instant Lunch Oriental Noodles:			
all flavors, average	280	13	42%
Instant Wonton, all flavors	200	12	54%
Oriental Noodle, all flavors	290	15	47%
Ramen flavors, 1/2 pkt, 1 1/2 oz	190	9	43%
Wonton flavors, 1/3 pkt	90	5	50%

NILE SPICE

	C	F	%fc
Per Pkt			
Couscous: Average all varieties	200	3	14%
Homestyle: Black Bean	190	2	9%
Chicken; Sweet Corn; Flav. Veg.	120	3	23%
Lentil	180	2	10%
Minestrone	160	2	11%
Red Beans & Rice; Split Pea	190	2	9%
Other Cup Soups: Potato Leek	150	6	36%
Potato Romano; Italian Tomato	140	5	32%

PROGRESSO

	C	F	%fc
19 oz Can - Per 1/2 Can Serving (9 1/2 oz)			
Bean & Ham	160	2	11%
Beef Barley	130	4	28%
Beef Minestrone	140	4	26%
Beef Noodle	140	3.5	23%
Beef Vegetable & Rotin	130	2.5	17%
Black Bean	170	1.5	8%
Chickarina	120	5	38%
Chicken & Wild Rice	90	2	20%
Chicken Barley	100	2	18%
Chicken Broth	20	0.5	23%
Chicken Minestrone	100	1.5	14%
Chicken Noodle	80	1.5	17%
Chicken Rice & Vegetable	100	3	27%
Chicken Vegetable	100	2	18%
New England Clam Chowder	200	10	45%
Cream of Mushroom	130	8	55%
Escarole in Chicken Broth	25	1	36%
Hearty Black Bean	170	1.5	8%
Hearty Chicken & Rotini	80	2	23%

PROGRESSO (Cont)	C	F	%fc
Hearty Penne In Chicken Broth	80	1	11%
Hearty Tomato	100	2	18%
Hearty Vegetable & Rotini	110	1	8%
Home Style Chicken	90	2	20%
Lentil/& Shells	140	2	13%
Macaroni & Bean	160	4	23%
Manhattan Clam Chowder	110	2	16%
Meatballs & Pasta Pearls	140	7	45%
Minestrone	120	2	15%
Minestrone & Shells	110	1.5	12%
Split Pea	170	3	16%
Split Pea with Ham	150	4	24%
Tomato Basil	100	2	18%
Tomato Vegetable; Vegetable	90	2	20%
Tortellini in Chicken Broth	70	2	26%
Pasta: Broccoli & Shells	80	1	11%
Hearty Chicken & Rotini	90	2	20%
Hearty Minestrone & Shells	110	1.5	12%
Hearty Penne in Chicken Broth	90	1	10%
Hearty Tom.Rotini; Lentil/Shells	130	1.5	10%
Hearty Vegetable & Rotini	110	1	8%
Spicy Chicken & Penne	110	3	25%
Tomato Tortellini	120	5	38%
99% Fat Free: Beef Barley	140	2	13%
Beef Vegetable	160	2	11%
Chicken Noodle/Rice w. Veges	90	1.5	15%
Creamy Mushroom Chicken	90	2	20%
Lentil; Minestrone	130	1.5	10%

OLD EL PASO

	C	F	%fc
Black Bean w. Bacon, 1 cup	160	2	11%
Chicken Vegetable; Garden Veg.	110	3	25%
Chicken w. Rice	90	3	30%
Hearty Beef	120	3	23%

RAMEN NOODLE

	C	F	%fc
Regular varieties, 8 oz	190	7	33%
Lowfat Pork, Oriental, 8 oz	150	1	6%
Other Lowfat varieties, 8 oz	160	1	6%
CUP-A-RAMEN: Reg., 8 oz	270	10	33%
Lowfat varieties, 8 oz	220	2	8%

SNOW'S

	C	F	%fc
Made as Directed, 7 1/2 fl oz			
Manhattan Clam Chowder	70	2	26%
New England: Clam/Corn Chowder	140	6	39%
Fish/Seafood Chowder	130	6	42%

SOUPS CONT • HERBS & SPICES

TABATCHNICK

	C	F	%fc
Barley Mushroom, 1 cup	70	0	0%
Cabbage	60	0	0%
Chicken w. Dumplings	70	2	26%
Corn Chowder; N. England Potato	150	6	36%
Cream of: Broccoli; Spinach	90	4	40%
Minestrone	150	1	6%
New York Chicken	35	0	0%
Old Fashion Potato	70	0	0%
Pea	180	2	10%
Vegetable	110	1	8%
Wisconsin Cheddar Vegetable	140	9	58%
Yankee Bean	160	2	11%

WEIGHT WATCHERS

	C	F	%fc
Chicken Noodle, 10 1/2 oz	150	2	12%
Chicken & Rice, 10 1/2 oz	110	1.5	12%
Minestrone, 10 1/2 oz	130	2	14%
Vegetable, 10 1/2 oz	130	1	6%
Instant Beef/Chicken Broth, 1 pkg	10	0	0%

Enjoy nutritious soup as part of a meal or snack; or especially to beat the '4.30pm snack syndrome'. Choose lower fat varieties.

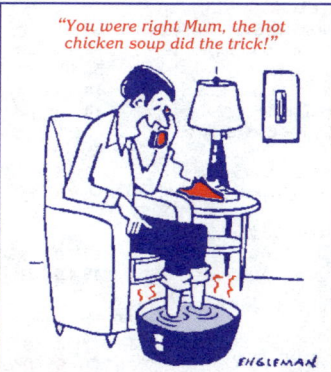

"You were right Mum, the hot chicken soup did the trick!"

HERBS & SPICES
Per 1 teaspoon

	C	F	%fc
Average all types: 1 tsp	5	0	0%
Allspice, ground	5	0	0%
Chili Powder	8	0	0%
Cinnamon, ground	6	0	0%
Curry Powder	6	0	0%
Garlic Powder	9	0	0%
Nutmeg, ground	12	0	0%
Onion Powder	7	0	0%
Parsley, dried	4	0	0%
Pepper, black/red/white, aver.	6	0	0%
Saffron	2	0	0%
Tumeric, ground	8	0	0%
Seeds *(Per 1 tsp):* Fenugreek	12	0	0%
Mustard, yellow	15	1	60%
Poppyseed	15	1	60%
Other types, average	7	0	0%
Parsley Patch, Sesame, 1 tsp	16	1	56%
Salt-free blends, average	10	0	0%
All-purpose, 1 tsp	6	0	0%

SEASONINGS & FLAVORINGS

	C	F	%fc
Accent Flavor Enhancer, 1 tsp	10	0	0%
Angostura Bitters, 1 tsp	12	0	0%
Bacon Bits, average, 1 Tbsp	30	1	30%
Bacon Chips (*Durkee*), 1 Tbsp	45	2	40%
Bac 'N Pieces Chips, 1 Tbsp	25	<1	18%
Best O'Butter, 1 tsp	10	<1	72%
Butter Buds, 1 tsp	8	<1	100%
Garlic Bread Sprinkle, 1 tsp	8	<1	100%
Garlic Salt, 1 tsp	2	0	0%
Italian Seasoning, 1 tsp	4	0	0%
Lemon Pepper Season., 1 tsp	7	0	0%
Meat Tenderizer, aver., 1 tsp	3	0	0%
Molly McButter, 1 tsp	8	0	0%
Perc Salt-free Seasoning, 1 tsp	8	0	0%
Salad Sprinkles (*Lawry's*), 1 tsp	16	<1	45%
Salad Supreme (*McCormick*), 1 tsp	10	<1	45%
Salt: Regular, Sea Salt, Lite Salt	0	0	0%
Seasoning Mixes, aver., 1/4 pkg	25	0	0%
Taco Seasoning, aver., 1/4 pkg	30	<1	6%
Old El Paso			
Taco/Burrito Seasoning Mix, 2 tsp	15	0	0%
Chili Seasoning Mix, 1 Tbsp	25	0.5	18%
Enchilada Seasoning Mix, 2 tsp	10	0	0%
Fajita Seasoning Mix, 1 Tbsp	30	0	0%
Vegit Seasoning Mix, 1 tsp	5	0	0%

SAUCES & CONDIMENTS

	C	F	%fc
Average of Brands & Homemade			
Apple Sce: Swtnd., 1/4 c., 2 1/4 oz	45	0	0%
Unsweetened, 1/4 cup, 2 oz	27	0	0%
Barbecue, average, 1 Tbsp	20	0	0%
Bearnaise Sce, 1/4 cup, 2 1/2 oz	190	19	90%
Catsup (Ketchup): Reg., 1 Tbsp	16	0	0%
Heinz Lite, 1 Tbsp	8	0	0%
Cheese, h/made, 1/4 cup, 2 1/2 oz	150	10	60%
Chili Sauce: *Heinz*, 1 Tbsp	17	0	0%
Del Monte, 1 Tbsp	35	0	0%
Wolf Hot Dog, 1 Tbsp	15	<1	12%
Cranberry Sce, jellied, 1/4 c., 2 1/2 oz	105	0	0%
Escoffier Sauces, 1 Tbsp	20	<1	22%
Horseradish: *Kraft*, 1 Tbsp	10	0	0%
Heinz, 1 Tbsp	70	7	90%
Sauceworks, 1 Tbsp	50	5	90%
Mushroom Sauce, 1/2 cup, 2 oz	50	2	36%
Mustard, average, 1 tsp	5	0	0%
Hot Must. (*Sceworks*), 1 tsp	12	<1	2%
Pizza Sauce, cnd., 1/4 cup, 2 oz	40	2	45%
Salsa, average, 2 Tbsp	15	0	0%
Seafood Cocktail Sce, 1 Tbsp	20	1	45%
Soy Sce, all types, av., 1 Tbsp	10	0	0%
Sour Cream Sce, 1/2 cup	250	15	54%
Spaghetti Sce: 1/2 cup, 4 1/2 oz	135	6	40%
Steak Sauce: A.1., 1 Tbsp	12	<1	2%
Lea & Perrins, 1 Tbsp	20	<1	1%
Heinz - See next page.			
Strawberry Puree Sauce, Unsweet., 2 Tbsp, 1 oz	9	0	0%
Sweet & Sour Sauce:			
Contadina, 1/4 cup, 2 oz	75	<1	6%
Kikkoman, 2 Tbsp, 1 oz	35	<1	6%
La Choy, 2 Tbsp, 1 oz	60	<1	5%
Tabasco Sauce, 1 Tbsp	2	0	0%
Taco Sauce, average, 1/4 cup	20	0	0%
Tartar Sauce, 1 Tbsp	75	7	84%
Teriyaki Sauce, 1 Tbsp	15	0	0%
Tomato Ketchup (*Heinz*), 1 Tbsp	16	0	0%
Weight Watchers, 1 Tbsp	12	0	0%
Tomato Paste, 6 oz pkg, 3/4 cup	150	0	0%
Tomato Puree, 1/2 cup	50	0	0%
Tomato Sauce, 1/2 cup, 4 1/4 oz	40	0	0%
Vinegar: White or wine, 1 fl.oz	4	0	0%
Great Impressions, 1 fl.oz	14	0	0%
White Sauce, 1/2 cup, 5 oz	130	7	48%
Worcestershire Sauce, 1 Tbsp	10	0	0%

BRANDS

	C	F	%fc
BARILLA: *Per 1/2 Cup*			
Marinara; Mushroom & Garlic	80	4	45%
Tomato & Basil	90	2	20%
BOOKBINDERS: *Per 1/2 Cup*			
White Clam Sauce	300	30	90%
CLASSICO: *Per 1/2 Cup*			
Florentine Spinach & Cheese	80	4.5	50%
Garden Zucchini & Parmesan	70	2.5	32%
Italian Sausage & Fennel	90	5	50%
Roasted Peppers & Onions	60	2	30%
Spicy Red Pepper	60	2.5	38%
Sun Dried Tomato; 4 Cheese	80	4	45%
Tomato & Basil; Mushr. & Olives	50	1	18%
Tomato Pesto	90	6	60%
CONTADINA: *Per 1/2 Cup*			
Alfredo Sauce	360	32	80%
Lite	160	10	56%
Creamy Tomato & Pesto	80	9	100%
Garden Vegetable Sauce	40	0	0%
Marinara Sauce	80	4	45%
Pesto with Basil	440	48	98%
Pesto w. Sundried Tomato	400	32	72%
Plum Tomato	70	2.5	32%
DEL MONTE: *Per 1/2 Cup*			
Chunky: Average all varieties	60	1	15%
D'Italia Pasta: Four Cheese	60	2	30%
Other varieties	50	1.5	27%
Picante Sauce, 2 Tbsp	10	0	0%
Salsa, all flavors, 2 Tbsp	10	0	0%
Sloppy Joe Sce, all flavors, 1/4 cup, 2 1/2 oz	55	0	0%
Spaghetti Sauce: Traditional	80	1	11%
Garlic & Herb	60	1.5	23%
ENRICO'S: *Per 1/2 Cup (4 oz)*			
Italian	60	0.5	8%
Peppers & Mushroom	75	1.5	18%
ESTEE			
Barbecue Sauce, 1 Tbsp	18	<1	10%
Spaghetti Sauce, 1/4 cup, 4 oz	60	2	30%
Steak Sauce, 1 Tbsp	14	<1	12%

SAUCES & CONDIMENTS CONT

BRANDS (CONT)

	C	F	%fc
FEATHERWEIGHT			
Barbecue Sauce, 1 Tbsp	14	0	0%
Catsup, Chili Sauce, 1 Tbsp	8	0	0%
Mustard, 1 tsp	5	0	0%
Spaghetti Sce w. Mushr., 4oz	60	2	30%
FIVE BROTHERS: Per 1/2 Cup			
Creamy Alfredo	220	20	82%
Creamy Alfredo w. Mushrooms	160	12	68%
Creamy Tomato Alfredo	140	8	51%
Marinara w. Burgundy Wine	80	3	34%
Mediterranean	80	4	45%
Roasted Garlic & Onion	70	1.5	19%
Romano & Garlic	90	4	40%
Sauteed Mushroom	80	3	34%
Spicy Triple Pepper	80	3	34%
Summer Tomato & Basil	60	1.5	23%
HEINZ			
Per 1 Tbsp - Approx. 1/2 oz			
Barbecue Sauces: All flavors	18	0	0%
Chili Sauce; 57 Sauce	15	0	0%
Horseradish Sauce	70	7	90%
Mustard: Pourable/Mild	8	<1	56%
Spicy Brown	13	1	69%
Seafood Cocktail Sauce	16	0	0%
Steak Sauce (Traditional)	11	0	0%
Tartar Sauce	66	7	95%
Tomato Ketchup	16	0	0%
Worcestershire Sauce	8	0	0%
KRAFT			
Sauceworks: Cocktail, 2 Tbsp	30	0.3	10%
Horseradish, 1 tsp	20	1.5	67%
Sweet 'n Sour, 1 Tbsp	30	0	0%
Tartar: 1 Tbsp	50	5	90%
Lemon & Herb, 1 Tbsp	75	8	96%
Barbecue Sauces:			
Average all types, 2 Tbsp	50	0.5	9%
Other Sauces: Per 1 Tbsp			
Horseradish: Reg./Cream Style	10	0	0%
Mustard	10	0	0%
Sandwich Spread & Burger	50	5	90%
Sweet 'n Sour	80	0.5	6%
Nonfat Tartar	12	0	0%

	C	F	%fc
LAS PALMAS			
Red Chile Sauce, 1/4 cup, 2 oz	15	0.5	30%
Enchilada Sauces: Green Chile	25	1.5	54%
Hot/Original, 1/4 cup, 2 oz	15	0.5	30%
Salsa: Mexicana. Mild, 2 Tbsp, 1oz	5	0	0%
Mexicana Hot/Medium, 2 Tbsp	10	0	0%
OLD EL PASO			
Salsa: Thick 'n Chunky varieties			
2 Tbsp, 1oz	15	0	0%
Homestyle; Green Chili; Verde			
2 Tbsp, 1oz	10	0	0%
Taco Sce: All varieties, 2 Tbsp, 1oz	10	0	0%
Thick 'n Chunky Sauces,			
All varieties, 2 Tbsp, 1oz	10	0	0%
Enchilada Sauces:			
All varieties, 1/4 cup, 2 oz	30	1.5	45%
Tomatoes & Green Chiles,			
1/4 cup, 2 oz	10	0	0%
Tomatoes & Jalapenos,			
1/4 cup, 2 oz	10	0	0%
PRITIKIN			
Mexican Sauce, 1/4 can, 4 oz	50	1	18%
Spaghetti/Mushrooms, 1/4 can	60	0	0%
ROSARITA			
Enchilada Sauce, 1/4 cup, 2 oz	12	0	0%
Nacho Cheese, 1/4 cup, 2 1/4 oz	105	8	69%
Taco Sauce, 1/4 cup, 2 oz	20	0	0%

TOMATO PRODUCTS

	C	F	%fc
Whole/Chopped/Crushed/Diced			
1 cup, 8 1/2 oz	50	1	18%
In Aspic, 1/2 cup	50	0	0%
w. Green Chili, 1 cup, 8 1/2 oz	45	<1	10%
Stewed, 1/2 cup	40	2.5	56%
Wedges in Tom Juice, 1 cup	70	0.5	6%
Salsa, average, 1 Tbsp	15	0	0%
Tomato Ketchup, Paste, Puree ~ See Page 68.			
Tomato Sauce:			
Regular, 1/2 cup	40	0	0%
Spanish Style, 1/2 cup	40	0	0%
w. Mushrooms, 1/2 cup	40	0	0%
w. Onions, 1/2 cup	50	0	0%
Tomato Seasoning, 3 tsp	20	0	0%
Sundried Tomatoes:			
Natural, 5-6 pces, 0.4 oz	22	0	0%
In Oil, drained, 6 pces, 1/2 cup	60	4	60%

SAUCES CONT

PASTA/SPAGHETTI SAUCES

	C	F	%fc
Frank Sinatra: Per 1/4 Cup			
Alfredo	130	14	97%
Marsala Cooking Sauce; Scampi	100	9	81%
Pesto	160	14	79%
Hagerty: Per 1/2 Cup			
Artichoke Pasta Sauce	100	6	54%
Jambalaya Pasta Sauce	70	5	64%
Healthy Choice: Per 1/2 Cup			
Garlic & Herbs; Roasted Garlic	50	0.5	9%
Other varieties, average	45	0	0%
Huxtables: Per 7oz			
Marinara, No Salt	100	1	9%
Tomato, Basil & Garlic	75	<1	3%
Mallard: Per 1/2 Cup			
Creamy: Basil & Parmesan	320	29	82%
Sundried Tomato Pesto	220	17	70%
Lite Alfredo	190	13	62%
Sundried Tomato & Garlic	115	6	47%
Muir Glenn (Organic): Per 1/2 Cup			
Chunky Style	80	2	23%
Roasted Garlic	45	0	0%
Tomato Basil, Garlic & Onion	50	0	0%
Newman's Own: Per 1/2 Cup			
Bombolina	100	4	36%
Sockarooni	60	2	30%
Spaghetti Cheese	90	3	30%
Venetian Spag. Sce w. Mushrooms	60	2	30%
Prego: Per 1/2 Cup			
Four Cheese	80	2	23%
Garlic & Onion; Herb & Garlic	80	2	23%
Mushroom	70	2	26%
Regular: Fresh Mushroom	150	5	30%
Diced Onion Garlic; Tom. & Basil	110	3	25%
Garlic Supreme	130	3	21%
Marinara	110	6	49%
Meat	140	6	39%
Mushroom Parmesan	120	3.5	26%
Mushroom Supreme	130	4.5	31%
Three Cheese	100	2	18%
Tomato Onion Garlic	110	3.5	29%

PASTA SAUCES (CONT)

	C	F	%fc
Prego (Cont)			
Traditional	140	4.5	29%
Vegetable Supreme	90	3	30%
Zesty Garlic & Cheese	130	3.5	24%
Zetsy Mushroom	120	4	30%
Progresso: Per 1/2 Cup, 4 1/4 oz			
Pasta Sauces:			
Alfredo (Authentic)	300	28	84%
Creamy Clam; Lobster, average	105	6.5	56%
Marinara, average	85	5	53%
Meat Flavor; Spaghetti	100	4.5	40%
Chunky Mushroom; Red Clam	80	3	34%
Pizza Sauce	70	2	26%
White Clam (authentic)	90	7	70%
White Clam, regular	130	9	62%
Ragu: Per 1/2 Cup			
Hearty Italian Tomato	120	4	30%
Mushroom; Old World varieties	80	3	34%
Chunky Garden Style:			
Mushroom Green Pepper	110	3.5	29%
Tomato Garlic Onion	120	3.5	26%
Super Mushroom	120	3.5	26%
Super Veg. Primavera	110	3.5	29%
Pasta Toss	120	8	60%
Select: Garlic Basil, 1/2 cup	70	4	51%
Mushroom Onion	60	4	60%
Sutter Home: Per 1/2 Cup			
Italian Style Pasta Sauce	110	4	33%
Sicilian Style	110	3	25%
Spicy Mediterranean	100	3	27%
Marinara Pasta Sauce	80	3	34%

PIZZA SAUCES

	C	F	%fc
Per 1/4 Cup			
Contadina: Pizza Squeeze	35	1.5	39%
Ragu: Pizza Sauce	30	1	30%
Pizza Quick	40	1.5	34%

SALSA

	C	F	%fc
Salsa			
Average all types			
Regular, no oil, 2 Tbsp	15	0	0%
w. Oil, homemade, 2 Tbsp	40	3	68%

SAUCES, GRAVY, PICKLES, RELISHES

SAUCE MIXES

	C	F	%fc
BORDEN (Made Up)			
El Molino: Hot Enchilada, 1/4 c.	32	2	56%
Mild Gr.Chili; Red Taco, 1/4 c.	20	0	0%
Snow's: Newburg, 1/3 cup	120	8	60%
Welsh Rarebit Ch., 1/2 cup	170	11	58%
CAJUN KING			
Seasoning Mix:			
Etoufee, 3 1/2 oz	385	6	14%
Jambalaya, 3 1/2 oz	375	9	22%
HAIN - Pasta & Sauce			
Creamy Parmesan, 1/4 pkg	150	3	18%
Fettucini Alfredo, 1/4 pkg	180	4	20%
Italian Herb, 1/5 pkg	110	2	16%
Marinara, 1/4 pkg	120	1	7%
Primavera, 1/4 pkg	140	4	26%
KNORR (Mix)			
Made As Directed: Per 1/4 Cup, 2oz			
Au Jus	8	0.2	2%
Bearnaise	170	17	90%
Classic Brown Gravy	25	1	36%
Demi-Glace	30	1	30%
Hollandaise	170	18	95%
Hunter; Lyonnaise	25	0.3	10%
Mushroom Sauce	60	3	45%
Napoli Sauce	100	3	27%
Pepper Sauce	20	1	45%
McCORMICK - Per 1/2 Package			
Beef Stew; Beef Stroganoff	65	0.5	7%
Cheese Sauce	70	3	39%
Chili Season; Meat Marinade	55	1	16%
Hamburger	65	2	28%
Hollandaise	100	8	72%
Nacho Cheese	85	3	32%
Sour Cream	90	6	60%
Spaghetti Sce; Taco Seasoning	65	0.5	7%
Pasta Prima:			
Alfredo, 1/2 cup (made up)	255	13	46%
Herb & Garlic, 1/2 cup	325	12	33%
Marinara, 1/2 cup	330	8	22%
Pesto, 1/2 cup	195	6	28%
Pasta Salad, 1/2 cup	390	23	53%

GRAVY

	C	F	%fc
Homemade Gravy:			
Thin, little fat, 2 Tbsp, 1oz	20	1	45%
Thick, 2 Tbsp, 1 1/4 oz	50	2	36%
1/4 cup, 2 1/2 oz	100	4	36%
Franco-American (Canned)			
Au Jus Gravy, 2oz	10	0	0%
Beef/Mushroom Gravy, 2oz	25	1	36%
Chicken Gravy, 2oz	50	4	72%
Pork Gravy, 2oz	40	3	68%
Turkey Gravy, 2oz	30	2	60%
Estee (Gravy Mixes) - Made Up			
Brown Gravy, 1/4 cup, 2oz	14	0	0%
Chicken & Herb, 1/4 cup, 2oz	20	0.3	14%
Pillsbury (Gravy Mixes)			
Brown; Homestyle, 1/4 cup	15	0	0%
Chicken, as prep., 1/4 cup	20	0	0%

PICKLES & RELISH

Average All Brands

	C	F	%fc
Bread & Butter Pickles, 4 sl:1oz	20	0	0%
Chutney, 2 Tbsp, 1 1/4 oz	40	0	0%
Dill Pickle: 1 large,			
(3 3/4"x 1 1/4" diam.), 2 1/4 oz	12	0	0%
Extra large (4"x 1 3/4" diam.), 5oz	30	0	0%
Halves: Small, 1oz	3	0	0%
Large, 2 1/2 oz	8	0	0%
Slices, 4 slices, 1oz	3	0	0%
Sweet, small, 1/2 oz	22	0	0%
Gherkins, sweet, 1 med., 1oz	15	0	0%
Green Chilies, chopped, 2 Tbsp	5	0	0%
Horseradish, 1 Tbsp	10	0	0%
Jalapenos, pickled, 2 whole	5	0	0%
Jalapeno Relish, 1 Tbsp, 1/2 oz	5	0	0%
Mustard, aver. all brands, 1 tsp	5	0	0%
Peppers: Hot/Mild, 1 Tbsp	8	0	0%
Pickled: Beets, 1/2 cup, 4oz	75	0	0%
Onions, 1 medium, 3/4 oz	10	0	0%
Cocktail Onion, 1 onion	2	0	0%
Red Cabbage, 1/2 cup, 3 oz	60	0	0%
Pickles: Sweet, 2 Tbsp, 1oz	35	0	0%
Large (3" x 3/4 dia.), 1 1/4 oz	40	0	0%
Relishes: S/wich Spread, 1 tsp	20	1	45%
Cranberry-Orange, 1 Tbsp	30	0	0%
Hot Dog (*Heinz*), 1 Tbsp	17	0	0%
Sweet Pickle, 1 Tbsp	20	0	0%
Sauerkraut, 1/2 cup, 3 1/2 oz	25	0	0%
Sweet Cauliflower	35	0	0%

SALAD DRESSINGS

MAYONNAISE

QUICK GUIDE	C	F	%fc
REGULAR			
Average All Brands, 1 Tbsp	100	11	98%
(*Bestfoods, Kraft*), 1 Tbsp	100	11	98%
1/2 cup, 4 oz	800	88	98%
LIGHT/REDUCED FAT			
Kraft; Best Foods, 1 Tbsp	50	5	90%
1/2 cup, 4 oz	400	40	90%
Hain, 1 Tbsp	60	6	90%
Hellman's; Estee, 1 Tbsp	50	5	90%
Smart Beat, 1 Tbsp	40	4	90%
Weight Watchers, 1 Tbsp	25	2	72%
FAT FREE			
Kraft; Weight Watchers, 1 Tbsp	10	0	0%
1/2 cup, 4 oz	80	0	0%

MAYONNAISE TYPE DRESSINGS

Per 1 Tbsp (Approx. 1/2oz)

	C	F	%fc
BAMA Dressing, 1 Tbsp	50	4	70%
Miracle Whip Salad Dressing:			
Regular	70	7	90%
Light	40	3	65%
Free	15	0	0%
Nayonaise (Nasoya)			
(Tofu Base/Dairy Free/Eggless)			
Regular, 1 Tbsp	35	3	80%
Fat-Free, 1 Tbsp	10	0	0%
Smart Beat Dressing, 1 Tbsp	12	0	0%
Spin Blend Dressing, 1 Tbsp	60	5	75%

"It's time to curb this inflation."

SALAD DRESSINGS

QUICK GUIDE
Average All Brands
Per 2 Tbsp (Approx 1 oz)

	C	F	%fc
Blue Cheese: Regular	150	16	96%
Light/Reduced Fat	80	8	90%
Caesar: Regular	140	14	90%
Light/Reduced Fat	50	5	90%
French: Regular	130	11	76%
Light/Reduced Fat	50	3	54%
Fat/Oil-Free	40	0	0%
Italian: Regular	130	11	76%
Light/Reduced Fat	70	7	90%
Fat/Oil-Free	10	0	0%
Ranch: Regular	180	18	90%
Light/Reduced Fat	90	8	80%
Fat-Free	50	0	0%
Russian: Regular	130	10	69%
Light/Reduced Fat	50	5	90%
Fat-Free	30	0	0%
Thousand Island: Regular	130	12	83%
Light/Reduced Fat	50	4	72%
Fat-Free	35	0	0%

BRANDS

Per 2 Tbsp (Approx 1 oz)

	C	F	%fc
BERNSTEIN'S			
Cheese - Garlic Italian, 2 Tbsp	110	11	90%
Cheese Fantastico	110	11	90%
Fat Free Blue Cheese	20	0	0%
Fat Free Cheese & Garlic Ital	10	0	0%
Fat Free Italian Parmesan	10	0	0%
Fat Free Peppercorn Ranch	30	0	0%
Italian	140	16	100%
Lt. Fantastic Cheese Fantastico	30	1	30%
Original Italian Parmesan	130	13	90%
Light Parmesan	45	1	20%
Original Mighty Caesar	130	13	90%
Restaurant Recipe Italian	130	13	90%
BEST FOODS			
Chunky Blue Cheese, 2 Tbsp	140	15	96%
Creamy Caesar	170	18	95%
Creamy French	160	16	90%
Creamy Ranch	140	15	96%
Creamy Thousand Island	130	13	90%

SALAD DRESSINGS CONT

Per 2 Tbsp (Approx 1 oz)

	C	F	%fc
BLANCHARD & BLANCHARD			
Caesar, 2 Tbsp	100	10	90%
Garlic	90	9	90%
Honey Dijon	40	3	68%
Lemon Pepper Vinaigrette	110	12	98%
Mustard w. Tarragon	90	9	90%
BRIANNA'S			
Blue Cheese, 2 Tbsp	130	13	90%
Blush Vintage	100	6	54%
French Vinegar	150	17	100%
Honey Mustard	130	12	83%
Poppy Seed	130	13	90%
CARDINI'S			
Caesar, 2 Tbsp	160	17	96%
Italian	120	13	98%
Lemon Herb	130	13	90%
Lowfat Parmesan	20	1	45%
Pesto Pasta	140	14	90%
Zesty Garlic	120	13	98%
FRANKIE'S FAVORITE			
Italian/French/Celery Seed, 2 Tbsp	12	0	0%
Single Serve Packet, 1/2 oz	5	0	0%
(Direct Sales: 1-800-279 4476)			
GIRARDS			
Caesar, 2 Tbsp	150	16	96%
Lite	80	7	79%
Greek Vinegarette	100	11	99%
Honey Dijon	140	13	84%
Italian	130	13	90%
Light Champagne	60	5	75%
Original French	120	13	98%
Raspberry Salad	160	12	68%
Spinach Salad	140	12	77%
Fat Free: Balsamic Vinaigrette	35	0	0%
Caesar; Raspberry Vinaigrette	40	0	0%
Red Wine Vinaigrette	40	0	0%

Per 2 Tbsp

	C	F	%fc
GOOD SEASONS (Mix)			
As Prepared, 2 Tbsp (Approx 1 oz)			
Blue Cheese, Cheese Garlic	145	16	99%
Cheese Italian, Garlic & Herbs	145	16	99%
Classic Dill, 1 pkg	28	0	0%
Italian	145	16	99%
Italian Lite	55	6	98%
Lite Cheese Italian	55	6	98%
Mild Italian; Zesty Italian	145	16	99%
Ranch	115	12	94%
HAIN			
Regular Pourable - Per 2 Tbsp			
Canola: Garden Tomato	120	12	90%
Italian; French Mustard	100	10	90%
Creamy Caesar: French	120	12	90%
Creamy Italian	160	16	90%
Garlic & Sour Cream	140	14	90%
Poppyseed Rancher's	120	14	100%
Savory Herb (No Salt Added)	180	20	100%
Thousand Island	100	10	90%
Traditional Italian	160	16	90%
(No Salt Added)	120	12	90%
Mix (Made Up Per 2 Tbsp)			
No Oil Range			
Bleu Cheese	28	2	64%
Buttermilk	22	tr.	0%
Caesar	12	0	0%
French	24	0	0%
Italian	4	0	0%
HEALTHY SENSATION			
Blue Cheese, French, 2 Tbsp	40	2	45%
Honey Dijon	50	2	36%
Italian	15	0	0%
Ranch	30	0	0%
Thousand Island	40	0	0%
HIDDEN VALLEY			
Blue Cheese (Low Fat), 2 Tbsp	20	0	0%
Creamy Parmesan	140	15	96%
Fat Free: Blue Cheee	20	0	0%
Caesar; Italian Herb & Cheese	30	0	0%
Honey Dijon Ranch	35	0	0%
Ranch			
Red Wine & Herb Vinaigrette	45	0	0%
French	40	0	0%
Light Original French	80	8	90%

Enjoy healthy salads but don't drown your salad in high fat salad dressings.

SALAD DRESSINGS CONT

Per 2 Tbsp (Approx 1 oz)

	C	F	%fc
HIDDEN VALLEY (Cont)			
Honey - Bacon French	150	12	70%
Honey Dijon (Low Fat)	40	2	45%
Italian	32	0	0%
Original Ranch	140	14	90%
Light Original Ranch	80	7	79%
Original Ranch w. Bacon	140	14	90%
Ranch Caesar Creamy	110	11	90%
Ranch Cole Slaw Dressing	150	15	90%
RanchGarlic & Spice	130	13	90%
Thousand Island	40	0	0%
HOLLYWOOD			
Caesar; Creamy French	140	14	90%
Italian; Creamy Italian	180	18	90%
Italian Cheese	160	16	90%
Poppy Seed Rancher's	150	16	96%
Thousand Island	120	12	90%
JOHNNY'S			
Great Caesar; Honey & Mustard	50	2	36%
KNOTTS BERRY FARM			
Honey Dijon, 2 Tbsp	130	13	90%
Roasted Garlic	140	14	90%
Sun Dried Tomato Vinaigrette	100	10	90%
Tropical Fruit Vinaigrette Low Fat	45	1	20%
KOZLOWSKI			
Fat Free: Honey Mustard	20	0	0%
Other varieties	10	0	0%
KRAFT			
Regular Dressings - Per 2 Tbsp			
Bacon & Tomato	140	14	90%
Buttermilk Ranch	150	16	95%
Caesar	130	13	90%
Caesar Ranch	140	15	95%
Catalina	120	10	75%
Free	35	0	0%
Catalina French/ with Honey	140	12	77%
Chunky Blue Cheese	90	7	70%
Coleslaw	150	12	70%
Creamy Caesar; Cucumber Ranch	140	15	95%
Creamy Garlic; Creamy Italian	110	11	90%
French	120	12	90%
Honey Dijon	150	15	90%
House Italian	120	12	90%

Per 2 Tbsp

	C	F	%fc
KRAFT (Cont)			
Peppercorn Ranch	170	18	95%
Pesto Italian	140	15	95%
Ranch	170	18	95%
Free	50	0	0%
Roka Brand Blue Cheese	90	7	70%
Russian	130	10	70%
Salsa Ranch	130	13	90%
Salsa Zesty Garden	70	6	77%
Sour Cream & Onion Ranch	170	18	95%
Thousand Island	110	10	80%
Thousand Island w. Bacon	120	12	90%
Zesty Italian	110	11	90%
Kraft Deliciously Right			
Reduced Calorie Dressings			
Bacon & Tomato; Caesar	60	5	75%
Creamy Italian	50	5	95%
Cucumber Ranch	60	5	75%
French	50	3	55%
Italian	70	7	90%
Ranch	110	11	90%
Thousand Island	40	4	90%
Kraft Free (Fat Free)			
Blue Cheese, Catalina, French	50	0	0%
Honey Dijon, Peppercorn Ranch	50	0	0%
Creamy Italian	50	0	0%
Italian	10	0	0%
Ranch	50	0	0%
Red Wine Vinegar	15	0	0%
Thousand Island; Sr Cream & Onion	45	0	0%
LADY LEE			
Fat Free Thousand Island	30	0	0%
Fat Free Ranch	40	0	0%
Fat Free Italian	5	0	0%
LAWRY'S			
Caesar, 2 Tbsp	130	13	90%
Italian	140	14	90%
MAPLE GROVE			
Fat Free: Caesar, 2 Tbsp	30	0	0%
Poppy Seed	45	0	0%
Raspberry Vinaigrette	35	0	0%

SALAD DRESSINGS CONT

Per 2 Tbsp	C	F	%fc
MARZETTI			
Regular Dressings			
Blue Cheese	160	17	96%
Buttermilk: Bacon Ranch	180	19	95%
Blue Cheese	160	18	100%
Ranch	180	20	100%
Caesar; Chunky Blue Cheese	150	16	96%
California French; Celery Seed	160	13	73%
Classic Caesar Ranch	190	20	95%
Country French	150	13	78%
Creamy Italian	150	16	96%
Dijon Honey Mustard	140	13	84%
Garden Ranch	180	19	95%
Honey French/Blue Cheese	160	13	73%
Italian w. Olive Oil	120	13	98%
Potato Salad Dressing	120	13	98%
Ranch	180	20	100%
Red Wine Vinegar & Oil	130	14	97%
Slaw	170	16	85%
Southern Slaw	100	11	99%
Thousand Island	150	15	90%
Light Dressings: Blue Cheese	60	6	90%
Buttermilk Ranch	90	9	90%
California French	80	6	68%
Chunky Blue Cheese	80	7	79%
French	40	2	45%
Honey French	80	4	45%
Italian	60	5	75%
Ranch	90	8	80%
Red Wine Vinegar & Oil	20	1	45%
Slaw	60	7	100%
Sweet & Sour	100	6	54%
Thousand Island	70	5	64%
Fat Free Dressings			
California French; Honey French	45	0	0%
Honey Dijon	60	0	0%
Italian	15	0	0%
Ranch; Peppercorn Ranch	30	0	0%
Slaw; Sweet & Sour	45	0	0%
Thousand Island	35	0	0%
NEWMAN'S OWN			
Balsamic Vinegar, 2 Tbsp	90	9	90%
Caesar	150	16	96%
Italian Light	20	0	0%
Olive Oil & Vinegar	160	18	100%
Ranch	180	18	90%

Per 2 Tbsp	C	F	%fc
NASOYA			
Vegi-Dressing (Tofu Base/Dairy Free)			
Creamy Dill; Creamy Italian	60	5	75%
Garden Herb; Sesame Garlic	60	5	75%
Thousand Island	60	4	60%
(Nayonaise - See Mayonnaise)			
PFEIFFER			
California French, 2 Tbsp	140	12	77%
French	150	13	78%
Honey Dijon	140	13	84%
Lite Italian	50	5	90%
Ranch	180	20	100%
Savory Italian	110	12	98%
Thousand Island	140	14	90%
RED WING			
Chunky Blue Cheese, 2 Tbsp	130	13	90%
Creamy Ranch	150	15	90%
French Traditional	130	11	76%
Italian Traditional	100	9	81%
"K" Dressing	140	14	90%
Spicy Sweet French	130	11	76%
Thousand Island	110	9	74%
RALPH'S CHEF EXPRESS			
Blue Cheese, 2 Tbsp	170	18	95%
Lite Ranch	90	8	80%

"Take two of these and call me in the morning."

SALAD DRESSINGS cont

Per 2 Tbsp	C	F	%fc
SEVEN SEAS			
Regular Dressings			
Chunky Blue	90	7	70%
Creamy Caesar	140	15	96%
Creamy Italian	110	12	98%
Green Goddess	120	13	98%
Herbs & Spices	120	12	90%
Ranch	150	16	96%
Red Wine Vinegar & Oil	110	11	90%
Two Cheese Italian	70	7	90%
Viva Caesar	120	12	90%
Viva Italian	110	11	90%
Viva Russian	150	16	96%
Free (Fat-Free): Italian	10	0	0%
Ranch	50	0	0%
Red Wine Vinegar	15	0	0%
Reduced Calorie			
Creamy Italian	60	5	75%
Italian w./Olive Oil	50	5	90%
Ranch	100	9	81%
Red Wine Vinegar & Oil	60	5	75%
Viva Italian	45	4	80%
S & W			
Light: Oriental Rice Wine, 2 Tbsp	30	0	0%
Red Wine Vinegar Herb	40	0	0%
Low Calorie Range			
Blue Cheese; Creamy Cucumber	50	4	90%
Creamy Italian	20	2	90%
French	35	0	0%
Italian No-Oil	4	0	0%
Russian	50	2	36%
Thousand Island	50	4	72%
ULTRA SLIM FAST			
French, 2 Tbsp	40	0	0%
Italian, 2 Tbsp	12	0	0%
WALDEN FARMS			
Fat Free Range			
Balsamic Vinegar, 2 Tbsp	15	0	0%
Italian: Sugar Free	0	0	0%
w. Sun Dried Tomato	10	0	0%
Creamy	15	0	0%
Bleu Cheese; Caesar; French	25	0	0%
Honey Dijon; Ranch	25	0	0%
Thousand Island	35	0	0%

Per 2 Tbsp	C	F	%fc
WEIGHT WATCHERS			
Salad Celebrations Dressings			
Fat Free: Caesar (Single), 0.75 oz	5	0	0%
Caesar, 2 Tbsp	10	0	0%
3 Cheese Caesar	40	2	40%
Creamy Italian (8 oz), 2 Tbsp	30	0	0%
French Style, 2 Tbsp	40	0	0%
Honey Dijon, 2 Tbsp	45	0	0%
Italian (8 oz), 2 Tbsp	10	0	0%
Ranch Style, 2 Tbsp	35	0	0%
Ranch (Single), 0.75 oz	25	0	0%
Russian, 2 Tbsp	45	1.5	30%
Thousand Island, 2 Tbsp	45	1.5	30%
WISHBONE			
Chunky Blue Cheese: Regular	170	17	90%
Lite	80	8	90%
Caesar	110	10	82%
Caesar w. Olive Oil (Lite)	55	6	98%
Classic Lite Olive Oil	40	4	90%
Creamy Caesar	180	18	90%
Creamy Italian	110	12	98%
Deluxe French	120	11	83%
Fat Free Honey Dijon	45	0	0%
Fat Free Italian	15	0	0%
Fat Free Parmesan - Onion	45	0	0%
Fat Free Ranch	40	0	0%
Fat Free Red Wine Vinaigrette	35	0	0%
Fat Free Thousand Island	35	0	0%
French: Lite	60	6	90%
Fat-Free	12	0	0%
Sweet 'N Spicy; Red	125	1	86%
Lite	35	0	0%
Italian: Regular	100	9	80%
Lite	15	0.5	30%
Italian Cream Lite	50	4	69%
Olive Oil Vinaigrette	60	6	90%
Parmesan - Onion	110	10	82%
Ranch: Regular	160	17	96%
Lite	85	8	85%
Robutso Italian	100	10	90%
Russian: Regular	110	6	50%
Lite	40	0	0%
Thousand Island: Regular	130	12	82%
Lite	80	5	56%

BREAKFAST CEREALS

COOKED CEREALS

	C	F	%fc
Buckwheat Groats, roasted:			
Dry, 1/2 cup, 3 oz	280	2	4%
Cooked, 1 cup, 7 oz	180	1	4%
Bulgar: Dry, 1/2 cup, 2 1/2 oz	240	1	2%
Cooked, 1 cup, 6 1/2 oz	150	<1	2%
Corn/Hominy Grits:			
Dry, 1/4 cup, 1.4 oz	145	<1	3%
3 Tbsp, 1 oz	110	<1	3%
Cooked, 3/4 cup, 6 1/2 oz	110	<1	3%
Instant, 1 pkt, 0.8 oz	80	<1	3%
w/ Imit. Bacon Bits, 1 oz	100	<1	5%
Cream of Rice, ckd, 3/4 c, 6 oz	90	0	0%
Cream of Wheat:			
Regular, ckd, 3/4 cup, 6 oz	180	<1	3%
Quick, ckd, 3/4 cup, 6 oz	95	<1	3%
Instant, ckd, 3/4 cup, 6 oz	110	<1	3%
Farina: Cooked, 3/4 cup, 6 oz	85	0	0%
Millet, dry, 1/4 cup, 1 oz	100	0	0%
Oat Bran, raw, 1/3 cup, 1 oz	75	2	14%
Cooked, 1/2 cup	45	<1	14%
Oatmeal, dry, 1/3 cup, 1 oz	110	0	0%
Regular, ckd, 3/4 cup, 6 oz	110	2	15%
1 cup, 8 oz	145	3	15%
Instant: Regular, aver., 1 oz	100	2	15%
Flavored, average	150	2	12%
Quaker: See Brands			
Wheat Hearts, 1 oz dry, 3/4 c. ckd	110	1	7%

BRANS & WHEATGERM

	C	F	%fc
Bran: Wheat, unprocessed,			
1 Tbsp, 3g	10	0	0%
Rice Bran, raw, 1 Tbsp, 5g	16	1	6%
1/3 cup, 1 oz	90	6	40%
Oat Bran, 1 Tbsp, 5g	15	<1	14%
1/3 cup, 1 oz	75	2	14%
Wheat Germ, 1 Tbsp, 1/4 oz	25	1	36%
1/4 cup, 1 oz	108	3	25%

CEREAL ADD-ONS

	C	F	%fc
Milk: Per 1/2 Cup, 4 fl. oz			
Whole, 1/2 cup	80	4.5	48%
2%, 1/2 cup	60	2.3	38%
1%, 1/2 cup	50	1	22%
Nonfat, 1/2 cup	43	0	0%
Yogurt: Per 1/2 Cup, 4 fl. oz			
Plain: Whole	90	4	33%
Skim	60	0	0%

CEREAL ADD-ONS (Cont)

	C	F	%fc
Yogurt, fruit: Whole, 1/2 cup	125	2.6	18%
Lowfat, 1/2 cup	120	2	15%
Nonfat, 1/2 cup	60	0	0%
Soy Drink: Regular, 1/2 cup	65	2	27%
Lite, 1/2 cup, 4 fl. oz	50	1	15%
Fruit: Dried, average, 1 oz	80	0	0%
Banana, 1/2 medium	50	0	0%
Prunes in Syrup, 5 (3 oz)	90	0	0%
Honey: 1 Tbsp, 3/4 oz	65	0	0%
Lecithin Granules, 1 Tbsp, 10g	50	5	90%
Nuts: Almonds, 6 (1/4 oz)	40	44	75%
Pollen (Bee) Granules, 1 T., 8g	25	1	35%
Psyllium Husks, 1 Tbsp, 5g	10	0	0%
Seeds: Sunflower, 1 Tbsp	65	6	55%
Soy Grits, 1 Tbsp, 8g	32	1.5	37%
Sugar: 1 heaping tsp	25	0	0%
1 Tbsp, 12g	46	0	0%

COLD CEREALS - QUICK GUIDE

Average All Brands

	C	F	%fc
Bran (processed), 1/3 cup, 1 oz	70	<1	3%
Bran Flakes, 3/4 cup, 1 oz	90	<1	3%
Corn Flakes, 1 cup, 1 oz	110	<1	3%
Granola, 1/4 cup, 1 oz	130	4	30%
Oat Bran Cereal, 1/3 cup, 1 oz	110	1	7%
Puffed Rice, 1 cup, 1/2 oz	55	0	0%
Puffed Wheat, 1 cup, 1/2 oz	55	0	0%
Raisin Bran, 1/2 cup, 1 oz	85	<1	3%
Rice Crisps, 1 cup, 1 oz	110	1	3%
Shredded Wheat, 1 bisc., 3/4 oz	80	<1	3%
Sugar-frosted Flakes, 3/4 cup, 1 oz	110	<1	3%
Wheat Flakes, 1 cup, 1 oz	105	<1	3%

READY-TO-EAT

ARROWHEAD

	C	F	%fc
Amaranth Flakes, 1 cup, 1.2 oz	130	2	14%
Apple Corns, 1 cup, 1.5 oz	150	2	12%
Bran Flakes, 1 cup, 1 oz	100	1	9%
Kamut Flakes, 1 cup, 1.1 oz	120	1	8%
Maple Corns, 1 cup, 1.9 oz	190	3	14%
Multi Grain Flakes, 1 cup, 1.2 oz	140	2	13%
Nature O's, 1 cup, 1.1 oz	130	2	14%
Oat Bran Flakes, 1 cup, 1.2 oz	110	2	16%
Puffed Corn, 1 cup, 0.8 oz	80	0	0%
Puffed Kamut, 1 cup, 0.6 oz	50	0	0%
Puffed Millet/Wheat, 1 cup, 0.9 oz	90	1	10%
Puffed Rice, 1 cup, 0.8 oz	90	0	0%
Spelt Flakes, 1 cup, 1.1 oz	100	1	9%

BREAKFAST CEREALS CONT

	C	F	%fc
BARBARA'S BAKERY			
Breakfast O's, 1 cup, 1 oz	120	2	15%
Brown Rice Crisps, 1 cup, 1 oz	120	1	8%
Corn Flakes, all types, 1 cup, 1 oz	110	0	0%
High 5, 3/4 cup, 1 oz	100	0.5	5%
Puffins, 3/4 cup, 1 oz	90	1	10%
Shredded Oats, 1 1/4 cup, 2 oz	220	2.5	10%
Shredded Spoonfuls, 3/4 cup	120	1.5	11%
Shredded Wheat, 2 bisc.	140	1	6%
Stars: Cocoa Crunch, 1 cup, 1 oz	110	0.5	4%
Honey Crunch, 1 cup, 1 oz	110	0	0%
Toasted O's: Honey Nut, 3/4 cup	120	2	15%
Apple Cinnamon, 3/4 cup	110	1	8%
BETTY CROCKER			
Dutch Apple, 1 cup, 2 oz	220	2	8%
Streusel, 3/4 cup, 1 oz	120	1.5	11%
BREADSHOP			
Granola: Breadshop, aver., 1 oz	120	5	36%
Nectar-Sweet, aver., 1 oz	110	4	33%
Muesli, Rye Date/Oat Bran, 1 oz	100	2	18%
Triple Bran/Oat Bran, 1 oz	100	2	18%
CAP'N CRUNCH			
All varieties, aver., 3/4 cup	110	2	16%
CHEX: Corn, 1 1/4 cup, 1 oz	110	0	0%
Wheat, 3/4 cup, 1.8 oz	190	1	5%
DR McDOUGALL'S: *Per Cup*			
Oatmeal & Wheat, 2.4 oz	220	2	8%
Oatmeal & 4 Grains, 2.3 oz	210	1.5	6%
EREWHON: Aztec, 1 oz	100	0	0%
Crispy Brown Rice, 1 oz	110	1	9%
Fruit 'n Wheat, 1 oz	100	1	9%
Raisin Bran, 1 oz	100	0	0%
Super-O's, 1 oz	110	0	0%
Wheat Flakes, 1 oz	100	0	0%
ESTEE: Corn Flakes, 1 oz pkg	90	0	0%
Raisin Bran, 1 oz pkg	90	1	10%
GENERAL MILLS			
Basic 4, 1 cup, 2oz	200	3	13%
Body Buddies, 1 cup, 1 oz	120	1	8%
Boo Berry, 1 cup, 1 oz	120	0.5	4%
Cheerios: Regular, 1 cup, 1 oz	110	2	16%
Apple Cinnamon, 3/4 c., 1 oz	120	2	15%
Frosted, 1 cup, 1 oz	120	1	8%
Honey Nut, 1 cup, 1 oz	120	1.5	11%
Multi-Grain, 1 cup, 1 oz	110	2	18%
Cinnamon Tst Crunch, 3/4 c., 1 oz	130	3.5	24%
Cocoa Puffs, 1 cup, 1 oz	120	1	8%
Count Chocula, 1 cup, 1 oz	120	1	8%
Country Corn Flakes, 1 cup, 1 oz	120	0.5	4%
Crispy Wheaties 'N Rais., 1 c., 2 oz	190	1	5%
Fiber One, 1/2 cup, 1 oz	60	1	15%
Frankenberry, 1 cup, 1 oz	120	1	8%
French Toast Crunch, 3/4 c., 1 oz	120	1.5	11%
Golden Grahams, 3/4 cup, 1 oz	120	1	8%
Honey Nut Clusters, 1 cup, 2 oz	210	2.5	11%
Kaboom, 1 1/4 cup, 1 oz	120	1.5	11%
Kix, 1 1/3 cup, 1 oz	120	0.5	4%
Berry Berry, 3/4 cup, 1 oz	120	1.5	11%
Lucky Charms, 1 cup, 1 oz	120	1	8%
Oatmeal Crisp Almond, 1 c., 2 oz	220	5	20%
Apple Cinnamon, 1 cup, 2 oz	210	2	9%
Raisin, 1 cup, 2 oz	210	2.5	11%
Raisin Nut Bran, 3/4 cup, 2 oz	200	4	18%
Reece's Peanut Butter Puffs, 3/4 cup, 1 oz	130	3	21%
S'Mores Grahams, 3/4 cup, 1 oz	120	1	8%
Sun Crunchers, 1 cup, 2 oz	220	3	12%
Total, 1 cup, 1 oz	100	1	9%
Total Corn Flakes, 1 1/3 cup, 1 oz	110	0.5	4%
Total Raisin Bran, 1 cup, 2 oz	180	1	5%
Total Whole Grain, 3/4 cup, 1 oz	110	1	8%
Triples, 1 cup, 1 oz	120	1	8%
Trix, 1 cup, 1 oz	120	1.5	11%
Wheaties, 1 cup, 1 oz	110	1	8%
Honey Frosted, 3/4 cup, 1 oz	110	0	0%
GLENNY'S			
Maple Frosted Corn, 1 oz	110	0	0%
Oat/Rice Mini Puffs, 1 oz	110	0	0%
GOOD SHEPHERD			
Millet Rice Flakes, 1 oz	95	1	9%
Spelt Flakes, 1 oz	100	6	54%

Start the day right with a high fiber breakfast of cereals, milk/soy and fruit.

BREAKFAST CEREALS CONT

	C	F	%fc
GRIST MILL			
Apple Cinn. Nat., 1/2 c., 1.9 oz	260	10	35%
Bran, 1/2 cup, 1.9 oz	250	8	29%
Oat & Honey Nat., 1/2 c., 1.9 oz	270	12	40%
Oat Honey & Rais., 1/2 c., 1.9 oz	260	10	35%
HEALTHY CHOICE			
Multigrain Raisins & Almonds,			
1 1/4 cup, 2 oz	200	2	9%
Flakes, 1 cup, 1.1 oz	100	0	0%
HEARTLAND			
Granola: Lowfat, 1/2 cup, 2 oz	210	3	13%
Original; Raisin, 1/2 cup, 2 1/4 oz	300	11	33%
HEALTH VALLEY			
Per Serving			
Amaranth Flakes, 3/4 cup	100	0	0%
Bran Cereal (w. Fruit), 3/4 cup	160	0	0%
Corn Bran Flakes, 3/4 cup	100	0	0%
Fiber 7 Flakes (100% Orig.), 3/4 c.	100	0	0%
Golden Flax, 1/4 cup	190	3	14%
Granola O's, all types, 3/4 cup	120	0	0%
Healthy Crunches & Flakes, 3/4 c.	130	0	0%
Healthy Fiber Flakes, 3/4 cup	100	0	0%
Honey Sweetened: Corn, 1 cup	80	0	0%
Crisp Brown Rice, 1 cup	110	0	0%
98% Fat Free Granola 2/3 cup	180	1	5%
Oat Bran Flakes, all types, 3/4 c.	100	0	0%
Oat Bran O's, 3/4 cup	100	0	0%
Raisin Bran Flakes, 1 1/4 cup	190	0	0%
Real Oat Bran, 1/2 cup	200	3	14%
10 Bran O's, 3/4 cup	100	0	0%
HOT CEREALS			
Wheat Hearts, 1/4 cup, dry	130	1	7%
KASHI			
Brittles Sesame/Maple, 3 1/2 oz	473	19	36%
Puffed, 3/4 oz	74	1	12%
KELLOGGS			
Per 1 oz Serving (unless indicated)			
All-Bran, 1/2 cup	80	1	11%
with Extra Fiber, 1/2 cup	50	0.5	9%
Apple Cinn. Rice Crispies, 3/4 c.	110	0	0%
Apple Cinn. Squares, 3/4 c., 2 oz	180	1	5%
Apple Jacks, 1 cup, 1 oz	120	0	0%
KELLOGGS (Cont)			
Apple Raisin Crisp, 1/2 cup	90	0	0%
Blueberry Squares, 3/4 cup, 2 oz	180	1	5%
Bran Buds, 1/3 cup, 1 oz	80	0.5	0%
Cinnamon Mini Buns, 3/4 cup	120	0.5	4%
Complete Bran Flakes, 3/4 cup	90	0.5	5%
Cocoa Krispies, 3/4 cup	120	1	7%
Common Sense O/Bran, 3/4 cup	110	1	8%
Corn Flakes, 1 cup	110	0	0%
Honey Crunch, 3/4 cup	110	1	8%
Corn Pops, 1 cup	120	0	0%
Cracklin Oat Bran, 3/4 cup, 2 oz	190	6	28%
Crispix, 1 cup	110	0	0%
Double Dip Crunch, 3 3/4 cup	110	0	0%
Froot Loops, 1 cup	120	1	8%
Frosted: Bran, 3/4 cup	100	0	0%
Flakes, 3/4 cup	120	0	0%
Krispies, 3/4 cup	100	0	0%
Mini-Wheats, 1/2 cup	85	0.7	5%
Bite Size, 1 cup	200	1	5%
Fruity Marshmallow Crispies, 3/4 c.	110	0	0%
Healthy Choice:			
Almond Crunch, w. Raisins, 1 c.	210	2	9%
Golden Multi-Grn Flakes, 3/4 c.	110	0	0%
Tst Brown Sugar Sq., 1 cup	210	2	9%
Just Right, 1 cup, 2 oz	210	1.5	6%
Low Fat Granola: 1/2 cup, 2 oz	190	3	14%
w. Raisins, 3/4 cup, 2 oz	220	3	12%
Müeslix: Apple & Almond, 3/4 c.	200	5	23%
Raisin & Almond, 2/3 cup	200	3	14%
Nut & Honey Crunch, 1 1/4 c., 2 oz	220	2.5	10%
Nutri-Grain: Almond, 1 1/4 c., 2 oz	180	3	15%
Golden Wheat, 3/4 cup, 1 oz	100	1	9%
Pop Tarts Crunch, 1 cup	130	1	7%
Product 19, 1 cup, 1 oz	100	0	0%
Raisin Bran, 1 cup	200	1.5	7%
Raisin Squares, 3/4 cup, 2 oz	180	1.5	8%
Rice Krispies, 1 1/4 cup	120	0	0%
Treats, 3/4 cup	120	1.5	11%
Smacks, 3/4 cup	100	0.5	5%
Special K, 1 cup	110	0	0%
Strawberry Squares, 3/4 c., 2 oz	170	2	15%
Temptations:			
French Vanilla Almond, 3/4 c.	100	1.5	14%
Honey/Rst. Pecan, 2/3 c., 1 oz	120	1.5	11%
LA LOMA			
Ruskets Biscuits, 2 bisc., 1 oz	110	0	0%

BREAKFAST CEREALS CONT

Item	C	F	%fc
MUESLIX			
Crispy Blend, 2/3 cup, 1.9 oz	200	2	9%
NABISCO			
100% Bran, 1/3 cup, 1 oz	70	1	13%
Fruit Wheats, 1/2 cup, 1 oz	90	0	0%
Shredded Wheat: 1 biscuit	80	<1	5%
Spoon size, 2/3 cup	90	1	5%
Shredd. Wheat'n Bran, 2/3 cup	90	0	0%
Shredd. Wheat w. Oatbran, 1 oz	100	1	8%
Team Flakes, 1 cup, 1 oz	110	1	7%
NATURE VALLEY			
Cinnamon & Raisin, 3/4 cup	240	8	30%
Fruit & Nut, 2/3 cup	250	11	40%
Lowfat Fruit Granola, 2/3 c., 2 oz	210	2.5	11%
NUTRI-GRAIN			
Almond Raisin, 1 1/4 cup, 1.9 oz	200	2	9%
Golden Wheat, 3/4 cup, 1 oz	100	1	9%
POST			
Per 1 oz: Alpha Bits, 1 cup	110	1	8%
Banana Nut Crunch, 1 cup	250	6	22%
Cocoa Pebbles, 7/8 cup	115	1	8%
Cranberry Apple Crunch, 1 cup	220	3.5	14%
Great Grains, 2/3 cup	210	5	21%
Fruit & Fiber, 2/3 cup	120	2	20%
Fruit & Fibre Peach, 1 cup	210	3	13%
Grape Nuts; Raisin, 1/4 cup	105	0	0%
Honey Bunches of Oats, 3/4 cup	120	5	38%
w. Almonds, 3/4 cup	130	3	21%
Natural Bran Flakes, 2/3 cup	90	0	0%
Oat Flakes, 2/3 cup	105	1	8%
Raisin Bran, 2/3 cup, 1.4 oz	120	1	7%
Toasties Corn Flakes, 1 1/4 cup	110	0	0%
QUAKER			
Ready to Eat			
Crunchy Corn Oatmeal Bran, 3/4 c.	90	1	10%
100% Natural, 1/2 cup	220	9	37%
Lowfat, 2/3 cup	210	3	13%
w. Raisins, 1/2 cup	230	9	35%
Oat Bran, 1 1/4 cup	210	3	13%
Oat Life, all types, 3/4 cup	120	1.5	11%
Oatmeal Squares, 1 cup	220	1	4%
Puffed Rice; Wheat, 1 cup, 1/2 oz	50	0	0%
Quisp, 1 cup	110	1.5	12%

Item	C	F	%fc
QUAKER (Cont)			
Toasted Oatmeal, 1 cup	190	2.5	12%
Shredded Wheat, 3 bisc.	220	1.5	6%
Instant Grits: Per Pkt, all types, aver.	100	1	9%
Regular Grits			
All types, average, 1/4 cup	130	0.5	3%
Instant Quaker Oatmeal: Per Pkt			
Oatmeal: Regular, 1 oz	100	2	18%
Apples & Cinn.; Cinn. Toast	130	1.5	10%
Blueberries & Cream, 1 1/4 oz	130	2.5	17%
Cinnamon & Spice, 1 1/2 oz	170	2	11%
Maple/Br.Sug; Rais./Spice	160	2	11%
Strawb./Peaches & Cream	130	2.5	17%
Raisin/Date/W'lnut, 1 1/4 oz	140	2	13%
Kid's Choice			
All types, 1 pkt, aver., 1 1/2 oz	160	2.5	14%
Quaker by the Bag			
Apple Zaps; Fruitany O's, 1 cup	120	1	8%
Cocoa Blasts, 1 cup	130	1	6%
Corn Quakes;			
Marshmallow Safari, 3/4 cup	120	1.5	11%
Frosted Flakers, 3/4 cup	120	0	0%
Frosted/Honey Nut Oats, 1 cup	110	1	8%
Popeye Puffed Rice/Wheat, 1 cup	50	0	0%
Sweet Crunch, 1 cup	110	1.5	12%
Sweet Puffs, 1 cup	130	0.5	3%
Microwave Oatmeal: Per Packet			
Regular, 1 oz	110	2	16%
App.Spice; Cinnamon Dble Raisin	170	2	11%
Br.Sugar Cinnamon; Honey Bran	150	2	12%
Quaker/Hot: Multigrain, 1/2 cup	130	1.5	10%
Oat Bran, 1/2 cup	150	3	18%
Whole Wheat Hot Nat. 1/2 cup	130	1	7%
Oats Quick; Old Fash., 1/2 cup	150	3	18%
Unproc. Wheat Bran, 1/3 cup	30	0	0%
OTHER QUAKER BRANDS			
Honey Graham Oh's, 3/4 cup	110	2	16%
King Vitaman, 1 1/2 cup	120	1	8%
Kretschmer Wh/Germ, 2 Tbsp	50	1	18%
Honey Crunch Wh/Germ, 2 T.	50	1	18%
Toasted Wheat Bran, 1/4 cup	30	1	30%
Mother's: Hot Cereals, 1/2 cup	130	1.5	10%
Oatbran; Oatmeal, 1/2 cup	150	3	18%
Popeye: Puffed Rice/Wheat, 1 c.	50	0	0%
Sun Country			
Granola w. Rais. & Dates, 1/2 c.	260	8	28%
Granola w. Almonds, 1/2 cup	270	9	30%

CEREALS • GRAINS & FLOURS

CEREALS (Cont)	C	F	%fc
RALSTON			
Bran Flakes, 3/4 c., 1 oz	110	1	7%
Chex Multi Bran, 1 1/4 cup, 2 oz	220	2	8%
Cocoa Crispy Rice, 1 c., 1 3/4 oz	200	1	4%
Cookie Crisp, 1 cup, 1 oz	120	2	16%
Frosted Flakes, 3/4 cup, 1 oz	120	0	0%
Muesli: Blueberry, 1 cup, 2 oz	200	3	13%
Cranberry, 3/4 cup, 2 oz	200	3	13%
Strawberry, 1 cup, 2 oz	210	3	12%
Raisin Bran, 3/4 cup, 2 oz	190	1	4%
Tasteeos, 1 1/4 cup, 1 oz	130	3	20%
SMACKS: Cereal, 3/4 cup, 1 oz	110	1	8%
STONE-BUHR			
7 Grain, 1/3 cup, 1 1/2 oz	140	2	13%
Bran Flakes, 1/4 cup, 0.5 oz	65	0	0%
SUNBELT: Muesli, 2 oz	210	2	8%
TEAM: 1 cup	110	1	8%
US MILLS			
All varieties, 1 oz	110	1	8%
WEETABIX: 2 bisc., 1.3 oz	140	1	6%

GRAINS & FLOURS

Per 1/2 Cup (8 level Tbsp)

Item	C	F	%fc
Amaranth, 1/2 cup, 3 1/2 oz	365	6	10%
Arrowroot, 1/2cup, 2 1/4 oz	230	0	0%
Barley:			
Regular, 1/2 cup, 3 1/4 oz	325	2	5%
Pearled, raw, 3 1/2 oz	350	1	3%
Flakes, 1/2 cup, 1 1/2 oz	150	<1	3%
Buckwheat: Regular, 1/2 cup, 3 oz	290	3	6%
Groats, roasted, dry, 3 oz	285	2	6%
Roasted, cooked, 3 1/2 oz	90	<1	6%
Flour, whole-goat	200	2	6%
Bulgur: Dry, 1/2 cup, 2 1/2 oz	240	1	3%
Cooked, 1/2 cup, 3 1/2 oz	75	<1	3%
Carob Flour, 1/2 cup, 1.8 oz	95	<1	3%
Corn, kernels (blue/yellow), 3 oz	300	4	10%
Corn Bran, 1/2 cup, 1.4 oz	85	<1	3%
Corn Flour/Masa, 2 oz	210	2	6%
Corn Grits: Dry, 1/2 cup, 2 3/4 oz	290	1	3%
Cooked, 1/2 cup, 4 1/4 oz	75	<1	3%
Corn Germ, toasted	245	13	47%

GRAINS/FLOURS (Cont)	C	F	%fc
Cornmeal: Whole-grain, 2.2 oz	220	2	7%
Self-rising, bolted, 2.2 oz	205	2	7%
w.Wheat Flour added, 3 oz	250	2	7%
Cornstarch, 1/2 cup, 2 1/4 oz	245	0	0%
Couscous: Dry, 3 1/4 oz	345	0	0%
Cooked, 4.1 oz	60	0	0%
Farina: Dry, 3 oz	325	0	0%
Cooked, 4.1 oz	60	0	0%
Flax Seeds, 2 oz	280	20	60%
Garbanzo (Chick Pea), 1/2 cup, 2oz	200	3	13%
Matzo Meal, 1/2 cup	260	1	2%
Milet: raw, 1/2 cup, 3 1/2 oz	380	4	6%
Cooked, 1/2 cup, 4 1/4 oz	145	1	6%
Oats, 1/2 cup, 2 3/4 oz	305	5	13%
Oat Bran: Raw, 1/2 cup, 1.7 oz	115	2	15%
Cooked, 1/2 cup, 4 oz	115	1	7%
Oats, rolled/oatmeal: Dry	155	2	10%
Cooked, 1/2 cup, 4.2 oz	75	1	10%
Polenta, 1/2 cup	220	2	6%
Potato flour, 1/2 cup, 3.2 oz	315	0	0%
Psyllium Husks, 1 Tbsp (5g)	10	0	0%
Quinoa, 1/2 cup, 3 oz	320	5	13%
Rye: Grains, 1/2 cup, 3 oz	280	2	5%
Flakes, 1/2 cup, 1 1/2 oz	150	<1	5%
Flour, dark, 2 1/4 oz	210	2	7%
Medium light, 1.8 oz	185	1	4%
Semolina, 1/2 cup, 3 oz	305	1	2%
Sorghum, 1/2 cup, 3.4 oz	325	3	8%
Soybean Flakes, 1/2 cup, 1 1/2 oz	190	8	38%
Soy Flour, 1/2 cup, 2 oz	250	11	38%
Tapioca, pearl, Dry: 1/2 cup, 2.7oz	260	0	0%
3 Tbsp, 1 oz	100	0	0%
Teff (Seed) Flour, 2 oz	200	<1	2%
Tortilla Flour Mix, 1/2 cup, 2 oz	225	12	48%
Triticale, 1/2 cup, 3.4 oz	325	2	4%
flour, whole-grain, 1/2 cup	220	1	4%
Wheat: Average, 1/2 cup, 3 1/2 oz	320	2	6%
Wheat Bran, unproc., 1/2 cup, 1oz	65	1	14%
Wheat Flakes, 1/2 cup, 1 1/2 oz	160	<1	3%
Wheat Germ: Crude, 1/2 cup, 2 oz	200	8	36%
toasted, 1/2 cup, 2 oz	215	12	50%
Wheat Flour: Whole grain, 2.1oz	205	1	4%
White, all types, 1/2 c., 2.2 oz	220	<1	2%

Also See Arrowhead Mills Cereals ~ Page 77

Rice, Pasta & Noodles

Rice

	C	F	%fc
BROWN RICE			
Raw: Short Grain, 1 cup, 7 oz	700	3	3%
Long Grain, 1 cup, 6 1/2 oz	650	3	3%
Cooked:			
Short Grain; Hot, 1/2 c., 3 3/4 oz	125	<1	3%
Cold, 1/2 cup, 2 3/4 oz	95	<1	3%
Long Grain: Hot, 1/2 cup, 3 1/2 oz	120	<1	3%
Cold, 1/2 cup, 2 1/2 oz	90	<1	3%
WHITE RICE (Polished)			
Raw: Short/Med. Grain, 1 c., 7 oz	720	<1	3%
Long Grain, 1 cup, 6 1/2 oz	670	<1	2%
Cooked (Boiled/Steamed):			
Short/Medium Grain:			
Hot, 1/2 cup, 3 3/4 oz	15	0	2%
1 cup, 7 1/2 oz	230	0	2%
Cold, 1/2 cup, 2 3/4 oz	90	0	2%
Long Grain:			
Hot, 1/2 cup, 3 1/2 oz	110	0	2%
Cold, 1/2 cup, 2 1/2 oz	80	0	2%
Parboiled, ckd, hot, 1/2 c., 3 oz	90	0	2%
Precook./Instant: Dry, 1/2 c., 3 1/2 oz	370	<1	2%
Cooked, Hot, 1/2 cup, 3 oz	90	0	2%
Fried, Chinese (egg/veg/pork), 1 cup, 5 oz	320	13	36%
Wild Rice: Raw, 1 cup, 5 1/2 oz	570	13	36%
cooked, hot, 1 cup, 5 3/4 oz	165	<1	3%
1/2 cup, 3 oz	85	<1	3%
RICE BRAN/FLOUR			
Rice Bran, 1/3 cup, 1 oz	90	6	60%
Rice Flour, 1/2 cup, 2 3/4 oz	290	2	5%
Rice Polish, 1/2 cup	220	7	30%

RICE CAKES ~ See Page 84.
Rice-A-Roni ~ See Page 58.

Macaroni, Spaghetti

- Macaroni includes all shapes and sizes; e.g. elbows, shells, tubes, twists, sheets, cannelloni, manicotti, spaghetti, ziti.
- All regular macaroni products have the same calories/fat on a weight basis.
- 1 oz Dry = approx. 2 1/2 -3 oz cooked.

	C	F	%fc
Dry Macaroni/Spagh.: 1 oz	105	<1	4%
1lb box/pkg., 16 oz	1680	7	4%
Elbows, 1 cup, 3 3/4 oz	395	2	4%
Shells, small, 1 cup, 3 1/4 oz	340	2	4%
Spirals, 1 cup, 3 oz	315	2	4%
MACARONI/SPAGHETTI (Cont)			
Cooked, Plain (no added fat):			
Firm/Al Dente (8-10 mins.), 1 oz	42	<1	4%
Medium (11-13mins.), 1 oz	37	<1	4%
Tender (14-20mins.), 1 oz	32	<1	4%
(Longer cooking increases water absorbed)			
Elbows/Spirals, 1 cup, 5 oz	185	1	4%
Small Shells, 1 cup, 4 oz	150	<1	4%
Spaghetti, 1/2 cup, 2 1/2 oz	90	<1	4%
Med. serving, 1 cup, 5 oz	185	1	4%
Large (restaurant), 2 c., 10 oz	370	2	4%
Corn: Cooked, 1 cup, 5 oz	175	1	3%
Protein-fortified: Dry, 1 oz	107	<1	3%
Cooked, 1 cup, 5 oz	230	<1	3%
Spinach/Vegetable: Dry, 1 oz	105	<1	3%
Cooked, 1 cup, 5 oz	180	<1	3%
Whole-wheat: Dry, 1 oz	100	<1	3%
Cooked, 1 cup, 5 oz	175	<1	3%
FRESH PASTA (Refrigerated)			
Plain/Spinach/Tomato, average:			
As purchased, 4 oz	325	2.5	4%
Cooked, 1 cup, 5 oz	190	1	4%
Home-made, without egg:			
Cooked, 1 cup, 5 oz	175	1	4%

Other Spaghetti/Pasta Listings:

Froz. Foods, Pp. 49; Canned, Pp. 57.
Restaurant Dishes - Italian, Pp. 135.
Spaghetti Sauces - Sauces, Pp. 70.

Noodles

	C	F	%fc
Plain/Egg:			
Dry, 1 oz	108	1	7%
1 cup, 1 1/3 oz	145	1.5	7%
Cooked, 1 oz	38	<1	7%
1/2 cup, 2 3/4 oz	105	1	7%
1 cup, 5 1/2 oz	210	2	7%
'No Yolks' (*Foulds*), ckd, 1 cup	210	2	7%
Chinese:			
Celloph./Rice, dry, 1 oz	100	0	0%
Chow Mein/hard, dry, 1 oz	150	5	30%
Japanese:			
Soba, dry, 1 oz	95	<1	3%
cooked, 1 cup, 4 oz	110	<1	3%
Somen, dry, 1 oz	100	<1	3%
cooked, 1 cup, 6 oz	225	<1	3%

BREADS

Note: All breads have similar calories on a weight basis. However, volume may vary. For example, 1 oz of bread may equal 1 slice regular bread or 2 slices of a lighter bread. It is best to weigh bread used and calculate on 1 oz bread = 70 calories.

Average All Varieties:
(White/Brown/Wheat/French/Italian Oat/Buttermilk/Sourdough)

	C	F	%fc
Thin slice (1/4") 1 oz	70	1	12%
Extra thin slice 3/4 oz	55	<1	12%
Light thin slice, 0.6 oz	40	<1	12%
Toasting slice, 1.2 oz	85	1	12%
Thick slice (3/8"), 1.5 oz	105	1.5	12%
Large thick (1/2"), 2 oz	140	2	12%
1-lb Loaf, 16 oz	1120	6	12%

Toast has same calories as bread used.

	C	F	%fc
1 thin slice + 1 tsp of fat	105	5	43%
1 thick slice (3/8") +2 tsp fat	175	10	51%
Bran style, 1 oz slice	70	1	12%
Buttermilk, average, 1 oz slice	80	2	22%
Challah, 1 oz slice	85	2	21%
Corn Bread, aver., 1 pce., 3 oz	180	7	35%
Dark Bread, 1 oz slice	70	1	12%
Date & Nut, 1 oz slice	90	1	10%
'Enriched' Breads, aver., 1 oz sl.	75	1	12%
French Bread, 1 oz slice	70	1	12%
French Toast, 1 slice, 2 1/4 oz	160	7	39%
Garlic Bread, 1 pce. w. fat, 1 oz	125	6	43%
Italian Bread, 1 oz slice	75	1	12%
Light Bread, aver., 0.8 oz slice	40	<1	11%
1 oz slice	70	1	12%
Nut/Health Nut, 1 oz slice	85	2	21%
Oatmeal Bread, 1 oz slice	70	1	12%
Party Breads: (Pepperidge Farm):			
Dijon; Pumpernickel, 1 sl.	18	<1	25%
Rye Slices, 1 slice	15	<1	30%
Pita Bread, aver. all types, 2 oz	150	2	12%
Mini/Pocket, 1 oz	75	1	12%
Poppyseed (Vienna), 0.8 oz sl.	55	1	16%
Pumpernickel, 1 oz slice	75	1	12%
Cocktail size, 0.4 oz	30	<1	15%
Raisin Bread, 1 oz slice	80	1	1%
Roman Meal, 1 oz slice	70	1	12%
Rye, average., 1 thin slice, 1 oz	75	1	12%
1 thick slice, 2 oz	150	2	12%
Cocktail size, 0.4 oz	25	<1	18%
Sandwich Bread, 1 oz slice	70	1	12%
Sourdough, 1 oz slice	70	1	12%
Wheat/Cracked Wheat, 1 oz sl.	75	1	17%

BAGELS

Average All Types:

	C	F	%fc
1 small/bagelette, 1 oz	80	<1	5%
1 medium bagel, 2 oz	160	1.5	8%
1 large bagel, 3 oz	240	2	7.5%
Sara Lee: Egg	200	2	9%
Other types, 3 oz	250	1	3%
Amy's Kitchen, aver., 3 1/2 oz	235	2	8%
Bagel Chips (New York Style), 4 slices, 3/4 oz	90	2	20%
Bagel Crisps (Burns Ricker), 1 oz	150	9	54%

BREAD ROLLS & BUNS

	C	F	%fc
Brown 'n Serve, average, 1 oz	80	2	22%
Challah Roll, 2 oz	150	2	12%
Dinner Rolls: 1 medium (2 1/2" diam. x 2" high), 1 oz	85	2	21%
1 extra med. (3" diam),1 1/2 oz	130	3	20%
Frankfurter/Hot Dog: 1 1/4 oz	100	2	18%
1 1/2 oz size	120	2	15%
French: 1 medium, 1.3 oz	110	1	8%
1 large, 3 oz	240	2	7.5%
Hamburger: Regular, 1 1/2 oz	120	2	15%
Large, 3 oz	240	4	15%
Hoagie/Submarine, average (11 1/2" x 3" x 2 1/2" high), 4 3/4 oz	400	8	18%
Kaiser Roll, 2 oz size	170	3	16%
Onion Roll, 2 oz size	170	2	10%
Parker House Roll, 0.7 oz size	65	1	13%
Party Roll, 0.6 oz	55	1	16%
Sandwich Roll, 1.6 oz size	120	2	15%
Soft Pretzel Bun (J & J), 3 oz	235	3	11%
Sweet Rolls, 1 oz	100	2	18%
w. Icing, average	160	6	23%
Wheat Roll: Small, 1 oz	75	<1	6%
Medium, 1 1/2 oz	110	1	8%

PEPPERIDGE FARM - *Per Roll/Bun*

	C	F	%fc
Brown 'n Serve: Club	100	1	9%
French (3 per pkg), 1 roll	240	2	7.5%
French (2 per pkg), 1 roll	360	4	10%
Dinner Rolls: Dinner/Finger	60	2	30%
Old Fashioned	50	2	36%
Fancy Rolls: Crescent/Twist	110	6	49%
Frankfurter Roll	140	3	19%
French: 9 per pkg, 1 roll	110	1	8%
4 per pkg, 1 roll	240	4	15%

Rolls/Buns - Continued Next Page.

BREADS (CONT) • CRISPBREADS

ROLLS, BUNS (Cont)

	C	F	%fc
Sandwich Rolls: Onion	150	3	18%
Buns with Sesame	160	3	16%
Sliced Hamburger	130	2	27%
Soft Family Rolls	110	2	16%
Sourdough (French style)	100	1	9%

BREAD PRODUCTS

	C	F	%fc
Bread Crumbs, dry:			
Plain or seasoned, 1 oz	110	1	8%
1 rounded Tbsp, 10g	35	<1	12%
1 cup, 3 1/2 oz	390	5	11%
Corn Flake Crumbs, 1 oz	110	1	8%
Graham Cracker Crumbs, 1oz	115	1	7%
Keebler, 1cup, 4 1/4 oz	520	14	24%
Bread Dough: Frozen, 1 slice	75	<1	6%
Refrigerated, French, 1" sl.	60	1	15%
Wheat/White, 1" sl.	80	2	22%
Breadsticks:			
Stella D'oro: Sesame, (1)	50	2	36%
Plain/Onion/Wheat, 1pce.	40	1	22%
Keebler/Lance, 2 sticks	30	<1	15%
Salt Sticks, plain, 1 oz	110	1	8%
Croutons: Aver. all brands, 1 oz	130	6	41%
1/4 cup, 11g	50	2	36%
Coating Mixes:			
Seasoned, average, 1oz	110	3	24%
Featherweight, 1.4oz pkg	72	<1	6%
English Muffins, aver., 2 oz	140	2	12%
Pretzels: See Snacks ~ Page 106.			
Stuffing: Average, dry miz, 1 oz	110	1	8%
Made-up, 1/2 cup, 4 oz	180	9	45%

CROISSANTS

Average All Brands

	C	F	%fc
Plain/All Butter, petite, 1 oz	120	7	52%
1 medium, 1 1/2 oz	180	10	50%
1 Large, 2 1/2 oz	300	18	54%
Au Bon Pain: See Page 108.			
Burger King: Croissan'wich-See Page 117.			
Dunkin' Donuts: Coconut	320	20	56%
Chocolate Kreme Filled	320	16	45%
Old Fashioned	280	19	61%
Pepperidge Farm: All Butter	240	14	52%
All Butter Petite	140	3	19%
Sara Lee: All Butter, 1 1/2 oz	180	9	45%
All Butter Petite, 1oz	120	6	45%

RICE CAKES

Average All Types/Brands:

	C	F	%fc
Regular size, 1 cake, 9g	35	0	0%
Lundberg, all types, 15g each	60	<1	7%
Hain, Mini, average, 3g each	12	<1	37%

TACO SHELLS

	C	F	%fc
Regular size, all types	55	3	49%
Super Size	100	6	54%
Mini Size, 1 taco	25	1.5	54%
Salad shell, flour (*Azteca*)	200	5	22%
Tortilla (Soft Taco), each	85	2	21%
Flour Tortilla: each	140	3	19%
Lowfat	110	1.5	12%
Tostada Shells, each	55	3	49%

CRISPBREADS

Per Crispbread/Cracker

	C	F	%fc
Finn Crisp: Original, rye	35	<1	12%
Other types	19	<1	23%
Kavli Norwegian: Thin	17	<1	26%
Thick	20	<1	22%
Malsovit, Meal Wafers	75	4	48%
Rykrisp: Natural, 1 crispbread	20	0	0%
Seasoned	23	<1	19%
Sesame	25	1	36%
Ryvita: Dark/Light, 1 piece	26	<1	17%
High Fiber	23	<1	19%
Wasa: Breakfast; Sesame	50	<1	9%
Extra Crisp; Rye (Light)	25	<1	18%
Fiber Plus	35	<1	12%
Rye (Hearty)	45	<1	10%

MATZOS

MANISCHEWITZ

	C	F	%fc
American Matzos, 1 board, 1 oz	115	2	15%
Passover Matzos, 1 board, 1.1oz	130	<1	3%
Passover Egg Matzos, 1.1oz	130	2	13%
Egg 'n Onion Matzo, 1oz	112	1	8%
Thin Salted Tea Matzos, 0.9oz	100	<1	4%
Unsalted; Whole Wheat, 1oz	110	<1	4%
Dietetic Matzo Thins, 0.83oz	90	<1	5%
Crackers: Miniatures, 1 cr.	9	<1	50%
Passover Egg Matzo, 1 cr	11	<1	40%
Matzo Meal, 1 cup, 4 3/4 oz	515	2	3%
Matzo Farfel, 1 cup, 2.7oz	180	<1	2%

CRACKERS • COOKIES

CRACKERS QUICK GUIDE

Average All Brands: | C | F | %fc |

Cheese Crackers: Per Cracker
	C	F	%fc
Plain, 1" square	5	<1	90%
Small, octagonal	10	<1	45%
Round (2" diam.)	15	<1	30%
Sandwich (Peanut Butter)	35	1	25%
Graham, 2½" square, 1 cracker	30	0.5	15%
Melba Toast, plain, 1 piece	20	0	0%
Oyster & Soup crackers, ¼ oz	60	2	30%
(40 small oysters/20 lge hexagons)			
Rice Crackers: 1 small	9	<1	50%
Rice Snax (*Amsnack*), ½ oz	60	1	15%
Saltines, 2 crackers	25	1	36%
Snack-type, 1 round cracker	15	<1	30%
Soda, 1 cracker, ½ oz	60	2	30%
Uneeda, 1 cracker	30	1	30%
Water (*Carr's*), regular, 1 cr.	32	<1	14%
Bite-size, 1 cracker	13	<1	34%
Wheat, thin, 1 cracker	9	<1	50%
Zweiback Toast, 1 piece	30	<1	15%

COOKIES • CRACKERS

Per Cookie/Cracker Unless Indicated

BARBARA'S BAKERY
	C	F	%fc
Animal Cookies, each	16	0.6	33%
Bites, all types, 26 crackers	120	1.5	11%
Choc Choc Chip, each	75	3.5	42%
Chocolate Chip	85	3.5	37%
Cookies & Creme, all types	60	2.5	38%
Crisp Cookies, all types	80	4	45%
Homestyle Cookies, all types	40	0	0%
Rite Lite Rounds, 5 crackers	55	0.5	8%
Small Indulgence, all types	23	1.5	50%
Snackimals	15	0.5	30%
Wheetines, all types, 1 large sq.	50	1.5	27%
Fat Free:			
Mini, all types, each	18	0	0%
Wheat Free Bars, each	60	0	0%

BREMNER
	C	F	%fc
Wafers: All varieties, 1 wafer	10	0.3	27%

DELICIOUS
	C	F	%fc
Butter Finger, each	45	2	40%
Skippy, each	50	3.5	63%

ESTEE
	C	F	%fc
Chocolate Chip	38	2	47%
Coconut Cookies, Oatmeal Raisin	35	1.5	38%
Fig Bars, each	50	0.5	9%
Fudge Cookies	38	2	47%
Sandwich Cookies	55	2	33%
Shortbread	35	1	26%
Vanilla; Lemon	35	1.5	39%

FAMOUS AMOS
	C	F	%fc
Chocolate Chip, each	35	1.5	38%
w. Pecans, each	35	2	51%
Chocolate Sandwich Cookies, each	50	2.5	45%

FEATHERWEIGHT
	C	F	%fc
Choc. Chip Cookies, each	45	2	40%
Other varieties, average	45	2	40%
Creme Wafers, each	20	1	45%

FRANKIE'S
	C	F	%fc
Oatmeal Choc Chip	40	2	45%
Oatmeal Raisin	40	1	23%

FROOKIE
	C	F	%fc
Cookies: Average all types	45	2	40%
Animal Frackers	10	0.3	27%
Apple Cinnamon Oatbran, each	45	2	40%
Fruitins: Apple; Fig	60	1	15%
Large Frooks: All types	120	4	30%

GRANDMA'S
	C	F	%fc
Choc Chip; Nutty Fudge	190	9	43%
Fudge Choc; Oatmeal Apple	170	6	32%
Old Time Molasses	160	4	23%
Peanut Butter varieties, aver.	190	9	43%
Snack Bars: Granola; Oatmeal Ap.	180	6	30%
Fudge Choc Chip	190	7	33%
Peanut Butter Choc Chip	210	10	43%
Sandwich: Fudge Vanilla (3)	150	4	24%
Fudge; Vanilla (3)	180	5	25%
Wafer, 4 cookies	160	6	34%

HEALTH VALLEY
	C	F	%fc
Graham: Amaranth; Oat Bran	15	0	0%
Original Amaranth/Oat Bran	20	0.5	23%
Healthy Pizza, all flavors	8	0	0%
Lowfat, all flavors	10	0.3	27%
Original Rice Bran	18	0.5	25%
Whole Wheat, all flavors	10	0	0%

CRACKERS • COOKIES CONT

HEALTH VALLEY (Cont)

Cookies (each):

	C	F	%fc
Apple Spice; Hawaiian Fruit	35	0	0%
Apricot Delight; Date Delight	35	0	0%
Healthy Biscotti, all flavors	60	1.5	23%
Healthy Chips, all flavors	35	0	0%
Healthy Choc, all flavors	35	0	0%
Jumbo, all flavors	80	0	0%
Raisin Oatmeal	35	0	0%
Raspberry Fruit Center	70	0	0%
Tarts: All types, 1 tart	150	0	0%

KEEBLER

Crackers:

	C	F	%fc
Town House, Reg (5)	80	4.5	50%
Reduced Fat (6)	70	2	26%
Club: Original, 50% Red. Sod. (4)	70	3	39%
33% Red. Fat (5)	70	2	26%
Cracker Paks S'wiches, aver (1)	190	11	52%
Graham Selects: Honey (8)	150	6	36%
Original Cinnamon Crisps, av (8)	140	4	25%
Low-fat varieties, aver. (8)	115	1.5	12%
Munch'ems: Regular, aver. (30)	130	4	28%
55% Reduced Fat (35)	130	4	28%
Toasteds: Reduced Fat (10)	120	3	23%
Regular varieties (9)	140	6	39%
Wheatables: Reduced Fat (29)	130	4	28%
Regular varieties (25)	150	7	42%
Zesta: Soup & Oyster (42)	70	2.5	32%
Fat Free (5)	50	0	0%
Other varieties, aver, (5)	60	2	30%

Cookies:

	C	F	%fc
Chips Deluxe: Reg, P'nut Butter (1)	90	4.5	45%
Chewy; Rainbow, 1 cookie	80	4	45%
25% Reduced Fat, 1 cookie	70	3	38%
Chocolate Lovers, 1 cookie	90	5	50%
Choc/Vanilla Wafers (8)	130	3.5	24%
Classic Collection: Per 2 Cookies			
Plentiful Peanut Butter	150	9	54%
Sparkling Sugar	140	7	45%
Hearty Oatmeal	150	8	48%
Sandwich Cookies, each	80	3.5	39%
Danish Wedding (4)	120	5	38%
E.L. Fudge S'wich, 2 cookies	120	6	45%
Golden Vanilla Wafers (8)	150	7	42%
Iced Animal, (6)	150	5	30%
Krisp Kreem, (5)	140	7	45%
Soft Batch, all types (1)	80	3.5	39%
Wafers (8)	130	3.5	24%

LANCE

	C	F	%fc
Soft Fudge/Chocolate Chip, each	65	3	42%
Oatmeal, each	65	3	42%
Apple-Cinn; Strawb./Blueberry	60	2	30%
Coated Graham, 1 pkt	200	10	45%
Peanut Butter Creme Wafer, 1 pkt	240	10	38%

Cracker Sandwiches: See Snacks Page 106.

Crackers (Food Service):

	C	F	%fc
Saltines, 2 pak	25	1	36%
Other Crackers, average, 2	30	1	30%
Melba Toast, aver., 2 slices	25	0	0%
Bread Sticks, 2	30	0	0%

LITTLE DEBBIE

	C	F	%fc
Oatmeal Creme Pies: each	170	7	37%
Light Pies, each	130	2.5	17%
Peanut Clusters, each	190	11	52%
Figaroos, each	150	3.5	21%
Peanut Butter & Jelly Sandwich	130	5	35%

LU MARIE LU

	C	F	%fc
Butter Twist; Marie Lu (3)	170	6	32%
Crokine	18	0	0%
Chocolatiers (4), 1 oz	170	8	42%
Creme Wafer	37	2	49%
Dipped Chocolatiers	52	3	52%
Little Schoolboy (2), 1 oz	130	7	48%
Mini Marie Lu	10	0.3	27%
Petit Beurre	40	1	23%
Pims	48	1	19%
Prince	67	3	40%
Truffle Lu (4)	180	11	55%
Wheat & Cinnamon	45	1	20%

MRS FIELDS COOKIES

Estimates Only — Per Cookie

	C	F	%fc
Chocolate (Semi-Sweet/Milk), aver.	240	13	49%
with Walnuts/Pecans, aver.	270	14	47%
Chewy Fudge	240	13	49%
Cocomac (Coconut/Macadamia)	250	14	50%
Debra's Special (Oatm/Raisin/Nut)	240	11	41%
Double Fudge Brownie	420	25	54%
Milk Chocolate w. Macadamia	260	14	48%
Peanut Butter Dream Bar, 4 oz	570	34	54%
Pecan Whites	250	13	47%
Triple Chocolate	270	15	50%
White Chunk with Macadamia	260	15	50%

Frozen (Supermarkets):

	C	F	%fc
Chocolate Chip w. Walnuts	270	14	47%
Oatmeal & Raisin Nut	240	11	41%

CRACKERS • COOKIES CONT

MANISCHEWITZ	C	F	%fc
Matzo Boards ~ See Page 84.			
Matzo Cracker, Miniatures	9	0	0%
Whole Wheat Crackers	9	0	0%
Tam Tams, all types	15	1	60%
Chocolate Macaroons, each	45	2	40%

MOTHER'S BRAND			
Almond Shortbread	60	4	60%
Butter Flav.; Vanilla Wafers	24	1	38%
Checkerboard Wafers	20	1	45%
Chocolate Chip: Cookies	80	4	45%
Cookies (bag)	30	2	60%
Cookie Parade Assortment, each	35	1.5	38%
Chocolate Chip Parade	35	1.5	38%
Angel Cookies	60	4	60%
Chocolate Creme Sandwich	55	4	65%
Circus Animal Cookies	25	1	36%
Cocodas Coconut Cookies	30	2	60%
Dinosaur Grrrahams: Average	75	3	36%
Double Chips, all flavors	80	3.5	39%
Double Fudge	90	4.5	45%
Duplex S/wich	50	2	36%
English Tea Sandwich	90	3.5	35%
Fig Bars: Regular; Wheat	57	1	16%
Flaky Flix Fudge/Vanilla	70	3.5	45%
Fudge 'n Chip Cookies	30	2	60%
Fudge Swirl Cookies	74	6	73%
Gaucho Peanut Butter S'wich	95	5	47%
Iced Raisin; Macaroon	80	4	45%
Mini Dinosaurs: Average, each	10	0	0%
Mint Patties	60	2	30%
Oatmeal Cookies: Regular	55	2.5	40%
Iced; Chocolate Chip	65	2	28%
Oatmeal Raisin Cookies	30	2	60%
Oatmeal Walnut Choc. Chip	65	3	42%
Royal Grahams; Walnut Fudge	70	4	51%
Striped Shortbread Cookies	55	2.5	40%
Sugar Cookies	70	3	39%
Taffy Sandwich	90	4	40%
Triplets	65	3	42%

NABISCO	C	F	%fc
Crackers - Per Cracker			
Bacon Flavored Thins, each	10	0.5	45%
Better Cheddars: Reg; Low Salt	7	0.3	38%
Toasted Bran Thins, each	9	0.5	50%
Cheddar Wedges, 1/2 oz (31)	70	3	39%
Chicken in a Basket, 1/2 oz (7)	80	5	56%
Crown Pilot	70	2	26%
Dandy: Soup & Oyster, 1/2 oz (20)	60	2	30%
Escort	23	1	39%
Garden Crisps	10	0.3	27%
Meal Mates: Ses. Bread Wafers	23	1	39%
Nips Cheese, 1/2 oz, (13)	70	3	39%
Oysterettes, 1/2 oz (18)	60	1	15%
Premium: Saltines, all types	12	0.5	38%
Fat Free Saltine	10	0	0%
Premium Bits, 1/2 oz (16)	70	3	39%
Ritz: Regular; Low Salt	17	1	53%
Ritz Bits: All types, 1/2 oz, (22)	70	4	51%
S/wiches: Chse./P'nut But., (1)	13	1	69%
Royal Lunch	50	2	36%
Sociables; Swiss Cheese	12	0.5	38%
Tid Bits, cheese, 1/2 oz (16)	70	4	51%
Triscuit Wafers: All types	20	1	45%
Triscuit Bits Wafers	7	0.3	39%
Twigs Snack Sticks	14	1	64%
Uneeda, Unsalted Tops	30	1	30%
Vegetable Thins	10	0.5	45%
Waverly: Reg; Low Salt	17	1	53%
Wheat/Oat Thins: All types	9	0.5	50%
Wheatsworth; Stone Ground	17	1	51%
Zings! 1 pkg, 1.8 oz	240	11	41%
Zwieback Toast	30	0.5	15%
Cookies - Per Cookie/Wafer			
Almost Home: All types, average	65	3	41%
Baker's Bonus: Oatmeal	80	3	34%
Banana Bar, 1 bar	130	2	14%
Barnum's Animal Crackers	12	0.5	38%
Biscos: Sugar Wafers	17	1	53%
Waffle Cremes	35	2	51%
Brown Edge Wafers	28	1	32%
Bugs Bunny Graham Cookies	12	0.5	38%
Cameo Creme Sandwich	70	3	38%
Chips Ahoy: Chewy	60	3	45%
Choc. Chip; Sprinkled	50	2	36%
Mini	12	0.5	38%
Reduced Fat	50	2	36%
Other types, average	95	5	47%
Choc Cherry Bar, 1 bar	130	2	14%

'*Be sure to stay healthy.*
You can kill yourself later! '
(Yiddish Proverb)

CRACKERS • COOKIES CONT

NABISCO (Cont): Per Cookie	C	F	%fc
Chocolate Chip Bite Size	10	0.3	27%
Chocolate Grahams	60	3	45%
Chocolate Snaps	17	0.5	26%
Cookie Break; Van. Crm. S'wich	50	2	36%
Cookies 'n Fudge: Party Grahams	45	2	40%
Striped Shortbread	60	3	45%
Striped Wafers	70	4	45%
Devil's Food Cakes	50	0.5	9%
Famous Chocolate Wafers	28	1	32%
Fig Newtons, 2	110	2.5	20%
Fat Free, 2	100	0	0%
Fudge Brownie Bar, 1 bar	130	2	14%
Fudge Cakes	90	4	40%
Giggles Sandwich Cookies	60	3	45%
Golden Snack Bar, 1 bar	130	2	14%
Grahams	15	0.5	30%
Heyday Bars: All types	110	6	49%
Honey Maid: Grahams	30	0.5	15%
Graham Bites: All types	5	0.1	18%
Ideal Bars: Chocolate & Peanut	90	5	50%
Lorna Doone: Shortbread	35	2	51%
Mallomars: Chocolate Cakes	60	3	45%
Marshmallow Puffs	90	4	40%
Marshmallow Twirls	140	6	38%
Mystic Mint Sandwich	90	5	50%
Old Fash. Ginger Snaps	30	0.6	18%
Pure Chocolate Middles	80	5	56%
National Arrowroot Biscuit	20	1	45%
Newtons: Cobblers, all varieties	50	0	0%
Variety Pack, each	120	3	23%
Nilla Wafers: Regular; Cinnamon	15	0.3	18%
Nutter Butter: P'nut Butter S/wich	70	3	39%
Peanut Creme Patties, 1	40	2	45%
Oreo: Chocolate Sandwich	50	2	36%
Reduced Fat	45	1.5	32%
Fudge Chocolate Sandwich	110	6	49%
Big Stuf Choc. Sandwich	250	12	43%
Brownie Bars, 1 bar	160	7	39%
Cheese	55	2.5	40%
Double Stuf Choc. S/wich	70	4	51%
Pantry: Molasses Cookies	80	3	34%
Pecan Shortbread	80	5	56%
Pinwheels: Choc./Marshmallow	130	5	35%
Social Tea Biscuits	20	1	45%
Suddenlys' Mores	100	4	36%
Teddy Grahams Bearwich's	17	1	53%
Teddy Grahams Snacks: All types	5	0.1	18%

PEPPERIDGE FARM	C	F	%fc
Cookies: Per Cookie			
Brussels	50	2.5	45%
Mint Brussels	65	3.5	48%
Chesapeake Choc Chunk Pecan	140	8	51%
Chessman	40	1.5	34%
Chocolate	60	3.5	53%
Chocolate Mousse	100	5	45%
Creme de Menthe	90	5	50%
Delica au Chocolat	55	2	33%
Double Chocolate Milano	75	4	48%
Fruitful: Apricot	45	2	40%
Raspberry Tart	60	1.5	23%
Strawberry Cup	45	2	40%
Geneva	55	3	49%
Gingerbread Man	30	1	30%
Hazelnut	55	2.5	40%
Lemon Nut Crunch	60	3	45%
Mint Milano; Orange Choc	70	4	51%
Nantucket Choc Chunk	130	7	48%
Sante Fe Oatmeal Raisin	100	4	36%
Sausalito Milk Choc. Macadamia	140	7	45%
Selection de Choix	30	1.5	45%
Shortbread	70	3.5	45%
Soft Baked: Choc Chunk	130	6	55%
Reduced Fat	120	4.5	34%
Oatmeal Raisin	110	4	33%
Reduced Fat	110	3	25%
Tahoe White Choc. Macadamia	130	7	48%

SALERNO	C	F	%fc
Crackers: Graham	17	0.5	26%
Oyster Crackers, 1/4 cup, (20)	30	1	30%
Royal Graham: Small	47	2	38%
Large	70	4	51%
Saltines: All varieties	12	0.5	38%
Cookies: Almond Crescent	20	1	45%
Animal Cookies	8	0.3	33%
Bonnie Shortbread	32	1	28%
Butter Cookies: Regular	28	1	32%
Mini, each	6	0.3	45%
Dinosaurs: Large	70	2	26%
Mini, each	8	0.3	33%
Gingerbread; Gingles	23	1	39%
Iced Oatmeal	65	2	28%
Patties: Peanut; Mint Creams	75	4	48%
Royal Stripes	70	3	39%
Vanilla Wafer	19	0.5	23%
WWF Superstars; Super Mario	13	0.5	35%

CRACKERS • COOKIES CONT

	C	F	%fc
SNACKWELL'S			
Chocolate Chip, 2	20	0.5	25%
Choc/Creme Sandwich	55	1.3	21%
Oatmeal Raisin, each	55	1	22%
STELLA D'ORO			
Per Cookie			
Almond Toast (Mandel)	60	1	15%
Angel Bars	80	5	56%
Anisette Sponge/Toast	50	1	18%
Apple Pastry	80	3	34%
Castelets, regular/chocolate	70	3	39%
Coconut Cookies	50	2	36%
Dutch Apple Bars	110	3	25%
Egg Biscuits, Low Sodium	40	1	23%
Egg Jumbo	50	1	18%
Fruit Delight Apple Cinnamon	70	0	0%
Golden Bars; Love Cookies	110	4	33%
Hostess/Lady Stella Assorted	40	2	45%
Kichel, low sodium	7	0.4	51%
Margherite, chocolate/vanilla	70	3	39%
Peach Apricot/Prune Pastry	90	4	40%
Swiss Fudge	70	3	39%
SUNSHINE			
Crackers: Krispy Saltine	12	0.5	38%
Cheez-It Crackers	6	0.3	45%
Wheats Snack Crackers	9	0.3	30%
Animal Crackers	10	0.3	27%
Oyster & Soup, 16 crackers	60	1	15%
Honey Graham, 1 whole	60	2	30%
Cinnamon Graham, each	70	3	39%
Cookies: Grahamy Bears	14	0.5	32%
Ginger Snaps	20	1	45%
Hydrox (Reduced Fat)	45	1.5	26%
Oatmeal Cookies	55	3	49%
Grahams Fudge/Honey, each	50	2	36%
Choc. Chip w. Pecans, each	110	7	57%
Vienna Fingers, each	70	3	39%
Vanilla Wafers, each	20	1	45%
WEIGHT WATCHERS			
Apple Raisin Bars (1)	70	2	26%
Chocolate Chip (2)	140	5	32%
Choc. S'wich Cookies (2)	140	3.5	23%
Fruit Filled, 1 bar	70	0	0%
Oatmeal Raisin (2)	120	2	15%
Vanilla Sandwich Cookies	140	3	19%

COOKIES, BISCUITS-REFRIGERATED

	C	F	%fc
THAW/BAKE & SERVE			
COOKIETREE: *Per Cookie*			
Chocolate varieties, average	130	7	48%
Buttersugar; Cinn. Apple Oatmeal	120	5	38%
Cookie w. *M&M's*; Dble Fudge	120	6	45%
Peanut Butter/Chocolate	130	7	48%
Raisin Oatmeal	110	3.5	29%
White Chocolate Pecan/Macad.	130	7	48%
GUILTLESS INDULGENCE (1.3 oz Cookie)			
Fat Free varieties, aver.	120	0	0%
Lowfat Fudge/Choc., aver.	130	2	14%
GRANDS!: *Per Biscuit*			
Butter Tastin'; Buttermilk	200	10	45%
Reduced Fat	190	7	33%
Cinnamon Raisin; Extra Fluffy	200	8	36%
Extra Rich	220	12	49%
Flaky; Homestyle	190	9	43%
Southern Style	200	10	45%
PILLSBURY COOKIES: *Per 1 oz*			
Bunny (2), 1 oz	130	7	48%
Chocolate Chip/Chunk	130	6	42%
Choc. Chip. Reduced Fat	110	4	33%
Chocolate Chip w. Walnuts	140	7	45%
Flag; Halloween (2), 1 oz	130	7	48%
Heath	140	7	45%
Holiday (2), 1 oz	130	7	48%
M&M's	130	6	42%
Oatmeal Choc. Chip; Reeses	130	6	42%
Peanut Butter	110	5	41%
SnackWells, Choc. Chip, Red. Fat	110	3	25%
SnackWells, Chocolate Fudge	90	1.5	15%
Snowman; Valentine (2), 1 oz	130	7	48%
Sugar (2), 1 oz	130	5	35%
MRS FIELD'S: *Per 1.9 oz (53g)*			
Chocolate Chip w. Walnuts	270	14	47%
Oatmeal & Raisin Nut	240	11	41%

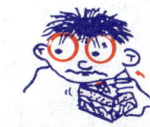

89

CAKES, PASTRIES, MUFFINS

CAKES, PASTRIES

	C	F	%fc
Angel Food: Plain, 2 oz	160	0	0%
w. Cream Icing	230	7	27%
Banana w. Butter Cream, 3 oz	300	13	39%
Black Forest, 3 oz	230	10	39%
Carrot Cake: Plain, 3 oz	230	8	31%
w. Cream Cheese Icing	380	21	50%
Cheesecake: Small serving, 3 oz	260	18	62%
Large serving, 5 oz	430	30	63%
w. Lowfat Cheese/fruit, 3 oz	150	8	48%
Cheesecake Factory: 1 sl., 7 oz	700	48	62%
Lite, 1 slice, 7 oz	570	28	44%
Denny's Cheesecake, 1 slice	580	33	49%
Chocolate Cake: Plain, 2 oz	220	11	45%
w. Chocolate Icing, 3 oz	320	15	40%
& Cream Filling, $3^{1}/_{2}$ oz	360	21	53%
Cinnamon Roll (*Denny's*)	670	30	40%
Coffee Cake, $2^{1}/_{2}$ oz	230	7	27%
Cream Puff (custard fill), $4^{1}/_{2}$ oz	300	18	54%
Croissants: Plain ~ See Page 84.			
Almond	420	25	54%
Apple	250	10	36%
Chocolate	400	24	54%
Au Bon Pain ~ See Page 108.			
Cupcake: Plain, $1^{1}/_{2}$ oz	140	6	38%
w. Icing	170	7	37%
Danish Pastry: Small, 2 oz	220	10	41%
Large, 4 oz	440	20	41%
Date Nut Roll, $^{1}/_{2}$" slice	80	2	23%
Eclair, Choc., Cust. fill, $3^{1}/_{2}$ oz	240	14	52%
Fig Bars, average, each	150	3	20%
Fruit Cake, Dark/Light, $1^{1}/_{2}$ oz	165	7	38%
Gingerbread: From mix, 3" sq.	200	6	27%
Homemade, $2^{1}/_{2}$ oz	270	4	13%
Lemon Cake, $2^{1}/_{2}$ oz	220	9	37%
Mud Cake, 1 piece, $3^{1}/_{2}$ oz	350	16	41%
Pineapple Upside Down, $2^{1}/_{2}$ oz	230	9	35%
Peach Melba, $3^{1}/_{2}$ oz	300	8	24%
Pecan Roll (*Au Bon Pain*)	800	45	50%
Pound Cake, 1 oz	130	7	48%
Sponge: Plain, $2^{1}/_{2}$ oz	190	3	14%
w. Cream & Strawberry	325	8	22%
w. Chocolate Icing	300	12	36%
Raisin Bun, 1 bun, $2^{1}/_{4}$ oz	180	2	10%
Strudel, fruit, average, 3 oz	280	8	26%
Sweet Roll, average, $1^{1}/_{2}$ oz	155	7	40%
Tiramisu, 1 piece, 5 oz	400	29	65%
Turnovers, fruit, aver., 3 oz	270	12	40%

MUFFINS

	C	F	%fc
READY-TO-EAT			
Average All Types:			
Small, 1 oz	80	3	34%
Medium, 2 oz	160	6	34%
Large, 3 oz	240	9	34%
Jumbo/Extra Large, 4 oz	320	12	34%
English: Average, 1 muffin	150	2	12%
Carl's: Blueberry Muffin	340	14	37%
Bran Muffin	370	13	32%
Dunkin' Donuts: Per Muffin	340	14	37%
Apple 'n Spice	330	10	27%
Banana Nut	340	12	32%
Blueberry; Cranberry Orange	310	10	29%
Corn	350	14	36%
Hostess: Oat Bran, each, $1^{1}/_{2}$ oz	160	7.5	42%
Blueberry; Raspberry, 1, 4 oz	440	19	39%
McDonald's: Apple Bran	300	3	9%
Pepperidge Farm: Multigrain	200	8	36%
Other types, average	175	6	30%
Sara Lee: Apple Oat Bran	190	6	28%
Golden Corn	240	13	49%
Other types	210	8	34%
Weight Watchers: Per Muffin			
Chocolate Chocolate Chip	190	2	9%
Harvest Honey Bran	220	4.5	18%
Fat Free: Banana; Blueberry	170	0	0%
MUFFIN MIXES: *Prepared - Per Muffin*			
Betty Crocker: Banana Nut	150	5	30%
Cinnamon Streusel	170	7	37%
Lemon Poppyseed	190	7	33%
Twice the Blueberry	140	4	26%
Fat Free, all flavors	120	0	0%
Duncan Hines: Blueberry, reg.	120	3	23%
Bakery Style Blueberry	190	6	28%
Oat Bran Blueberry	110	4	33%
Cinnamon Topp. Oatbran Honey	140	5	32%
Bakery Style: Cinnamon Swirl	200	7	32%
Cranberry Orange Nut	200	8	36%
Pecan Crunch	220	11	45%
Oatmeal & Apples/Walnuts	210	9	39%
Robin Hood:			
Blueberry; Corn	160	6	34%
Other flavors	170	8	42%
Snackwell's:			
Blueberry, $^{1}/_{6}$ pkt, 1 oz	120	0	0%
Sweet Rewards: Fat Free	120	0	0%

90

DONUTS

QUICK GUIDE

	C	F	%fc
DONUTS *Average All Brands:*			
Plain, 1 3/4 oz	210	12	51%
Sugared, 1 3/4 oz	220	11	45%
Glazed, 2 oz	250	12	43%
Chocolate Iced, 2 oz	260	14	48%

BRANDS

	C	F	%fc
AWREY'S DONUTS			
Plain, 2 oz	240	14	53%
Chocolate Iced, 1 3/4 oz	200	13	58%
Crunch, 2 1/2 oz	280	16	51%
Glazed, honey, devil's food, 1 pce	310	16	46%
Powdered sugar, 1 1/2 oz	170	10	53%
DOLLY MADISON DONUTS			
Regular, 1 3/4 oz	270	12	40%
Gem varieties, 1/2 oz each	65	3	41%
Powdered Mini, 1/2 oz each	60	3	45%
DRAKE'S: Old Fashioned Donuts	180	8	40%
Powd. Sugar Delites, each	45	2	40%
DUNKIN' DONUTS			
See Fast-Foods Section ~ Page 133.			
DUTCH MILL: Plain, 1 3/4 oz	210	12	51%
Sugared, 1 3/4 oz	220	11	45%
Glazed, 2 oz	250	12	43%
Double-Dipped Chocolate, 2 oz	280	17	55%
ENTENMANN'S DONUTS			
Softee Variety, 2 oz	230	13	51%
Country Powdered, 1 3/4 oz	240	15	56%
Rich, Frosted, 2 oz	290	19	59%
Light Fantastic Fudge, 2oz	210	9	39%
Light, 2oz	220	9	37%
Glazed Buttermilk, 2 1/4 oz	270	13	43%
Poppettes, all varieties, 2oz (3)	240	15	56%
HOSTESS DONUTS			
Regular: Assorted, 1 1/2 oz	200	11	50%
Cinnamon, Family Pack, 1 oz	110	5	41%
Cinnamon Swirl, 1 1/2 oz	180	7	35%
Frosted, 1 1/2 oz	180	11	55%
Jumbo, frosted, 2 oz	260	16	55%
Old Fashioned; Glazed, 2 oz	250	12	43%
Plain, 1 1/2 oz	170	9	37%

	C	F	%fc
HOSTESS (Cont)			
Regular (Cont):			
Powdered Family Pack, 1 oz	110	6	50%
Raspberry Filled, 2 1/4 oz	230	10	39%
Gem Donettes: Frosted, 1/2 oz	65	4	55%
Crumb; Powdered, 1/2 oz	60	2.5	38%
Frosted Chocolate Donettes, 2 1/2 oz each	75	4.5	54%
LIGHTEN UP DONUTS			
Powdered, 1 3/4 oz	160	1.5	8%
Double Chocolate, 2 1/4 oz	200	2.5	11%
Choc. Buttermilk; B'milk Maple, 2 1/4 oz	210	2	9%
LITTLE DEBBIE DONUTS			
Donut Sticks, 1.6 oz pkg	210	13	56%
3 oz pkg	390	23	53%
RICH'S (Frozen) DONUTS			
Ever Fresh: Glazed, 1 1/4 oz	140	7	45%
Jelly, 2 1/4 oz	210	9.5	40%
SARA LEE DONUTS			
Plain; Powdered, 2 1/4 oz	200	7	32%
Old Fashioned Glazed, 2 1/4 oz	280	14	45%
Reduced Fat Chocolate, 2oz	220	9	37%
Choc. Frosted Mini, 3/4 oz each	75	2.5	30%
Powdered Mini, 1/2 oz each	85	4.5	48%
Reduced Fat, 1/2 oz each	55	2.5	40%
TASTY KAKE DONUTS			
Cinnamon, 1 1/2 oz	180	8	40%
Frosted Rich, 2 oz	260	16	55%
Honey Wheat, 2 oz	210	8	34%
Orange Glazed, 2 oz	210	9	39%
Plain, 1 1/2oz	190	10	47%
Powdered Sugar, 1 1/2 oz	180	9	45%
VAN DE KAMPS DONUTS			
Plain, 1 1/4 oz	180	8	40%
Choc; Powd; Cinn; Crumb, 1 1/2 oz	180	9	45%
Old Fashioned: Chocolate, 2.4oz	340	22	58%
Powdered, 2 oz	240	11	41%
Assorted, 2 1/4 oz	280	13	42%

PIES & TARTS

PIES & TARTS

	C	F	%fc
Average All Brands			
1/8 of 9" Pie, 4 oz Serving			
Apple; Blueberry; Cherry	290	13	40%
Boston Cream Pie	330	14	38%
Chocolate Pie	300	18	54%
Custard; Coconut Custard	250	13	47%
Lemon Chiffon Pie	360	14	35%
Lemon Meringue	270	11	37%
Mince Pie	300	13	39%
Pecan Pie	470	24	46%
Pumpkin Pie	240	13	49%
Strawberry Pie	230	9	35%

BRAND NAMES (Frozen)
See ~ Cakes & Desserts (Frozen)

SNACK PIES

	C	F	%fc
Hostess, fruit, average, 4 1/2 oz	440	21	43%
Pudding Pies, average, 5 oz	480	18	34%
TastyKake, Fruit, average	310	10	29%
French Apple	350	11	28%
Coconut Creme	380	20	47%

DENNY'S

Pies - *Per Serving*

	C	F	%fc
Apple Pie	430	20	42%
with Equal	370	20	49%
Cherry Pie	540	21	35%
Chocolate Pecan Pie	790	37	42%
Coconut Cream Pie	480	36	49%
Dutch Apple Pie	440	19	39%
French Silk	650	43	59%
German Chocolate	580	33	51%
Key Lime	600	27	41%
Lemon Meringue	460	17	33%
Pecan Pie	600	28	42%

McDONALD'S

	C	F	%fc
Baked Apple Pie, 2 3/4 oz	260	13	45%

LONG JOHN SILVER

	C	F	%fc
Chocolate Cream Pie	280	17	55%
Double Lemon Pie	350	18	46%
Key Lime Cream Cheesecake	310	19	55%

PASTRY & PIECRUSTS

	C	F	%fc
Pie Crust:			
Baked, 9" diameter shell			
1 Pie Shell, 6 1/2 oz	900	60	60%
2-crust Pie, 9", 11 1/4 oz	1500	93	56%
Betty Crocker, 9", 1/8 shell	110	8	65%
Pet-Ritz, all types, 1/8, 3/4 oz	90	5	50%
Pillsbury (All Ready), 1/8 pie, 1 oz	120	7	53%
Piecrust Sticks, 8 oz	960	64	60%
Choux Pastry, raw, 1 oz	60	4	60%
Filo Pastry, 4 sheets, 2 1/2 oz	210	2.5	10%
Flaky Pastry, 1 sheet, 6 oz	780	72	83%
Puff *(Pepp.Farm),* 1/2 sheet	520	34	59%
Shell	210	15	64%
Pizza Crust, 1/8 whole	90	1	10%
Bisquick Baking Mix: 1/3 c., 1 1/2 oz	170	6	32%
Reduced Fat, 1/3 cup, 1 1/2 oz	150	2.5	15%

PIE FILLING

Canned - *Average All Brands*

	C	F	%fc
Apple, 4 oz	120	0	0%
1 Can, 21 oz	600	0	0%
Apricot, 4 oz	150	0	0%
Blackberry, Blueberry, 4 oz	120	0	0%
Bosenberry, Cherry, 4 oz	120	0	0%
Chocolate, Coconut, 4 oz	140	3	20%
Lemon, 4 oz	200	2	9%
Mincemeat, 4 oz	190	1	4%
Peach, 4 oz	120	0	0%
Pumpkin, 4 oz	170	0	0%
Libby, 1/2 cup	100	0	0%
Raisin, 4 oz	130	1	6%
Raspberrry, Black/Red, 4 oz	190	0	0%
Strawberry, 4 oz	120	0	0%

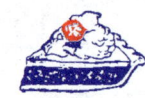
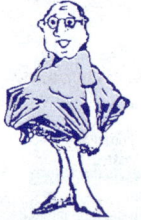

EAT IT TODAY ... WEAR IT TOMORROW !!

CAKES & DESSERTS - FROZEN

AMY'S

	C	F	%fc
Apple Pie, 8 oz	280	12	39%
Chocolate Fudge Cake, 3 1/4 oz	320	9	25%
Strawberry Cheesecake, 4 oz	290	13	40%

SARA LEE

All Butter Pound:

	C	F	%fc
Original, 1/10 whole	130	7	48%
Family Size Original, 1/15	130	7	48%

All Butter Coffee: *Per 1/8 Whole*

	C	F	%fc
Butter Streusel, Pecan	160	7	39%
Cheese, 2 oz	210	11	47%

Single Layer Iced: *Per 1/8 Whole*

	C	F	%fc
Banana, 1.7 oz	170	6	32%
Carrot, 2.4 oz	250	13	47%

Two Layer: *Per 1/8 Whole*

	C	F	%fc
Black Forrest; Strawb. Shortcake	190	8	38%

Three Layer: *Per 1/8 Whole*

	C	F	%fc
Double Chocolate	220	11	45%

Lights: *Per Whole Cake*

	C	F	%fc
Carrot; Lemon Cream, average	180	6	30%
Double Chocolate	150	5	30%

Indiv. Wrapped Coffee: *Per Whole*

	C	F	%fc
Apple Cinnamon	290	13	40%
Butter Streusel	230	12	47%
Pecan	280	16	51%

Original Cheesecake: *Per 1/6 Whole*

	C	F	%fc
Cherry/Strawberry Cream, aver.	245	8	30%
Plain Cream, 2.8 oz	230	11	43%

Classics: *Per 1/8 Whole*

	C	F	%fc
Choc. Mousse; French Cheesecake	260	17	59%
Strawb.French Ch/Cake, 3.2 oz	240	13	49%

Classic Lights: *Per Whole Cake*

	C	F	%fc
Chocolate Mousse	170	8	42%
French Cheesecake	150	4	24%
Strawberry French Cheesecake	150	2	12%

Snacks: *Per Cake*

	C	F	%fc
All Butter Pound; Carrot	200	11	50%
Chocolate Fudge Cake	190	10	47%
Classic Cheesecake	200	14	63%
Country Apple Pie	230	9	35%
Fudge Brownie; Pecan	270	14	47%

Danish Twist: *Per 1/8 Whole*

	C	F	%fc
Apple; Raspberry	190	10	47%
Cheese	200	12	54%

Individual Danish: *Per 1 Roll*

	C	F	%fc
Apple	120	6	45%
Cheese; Cinnamon; Raisin	140	8	51%

SARA LEE (Cont)

Homestyle Pies (9"):
Per 4 oz Serving (1/10 of Pie)

	C	F	%fc
Apple; Cherry; Peach; Raspberry	280	12	38%
Pumpkin	240	10	38%
Blueberry; Dutch Apple; Mince	300	13	39%
Pecan	400	18	40%

HOSTESS

Per Cake:

	C	F	%fc
Snoballs	175	5.5	28%
Suzy Q's	225	9	36%
Twinkies	150	4.5	27%
Dessert Cups, each	90	1.5	15%
Light: Brownie	140	2.5	16%
Cupcakes; Twinkies	135	1.5	10%
Crumb Cakes	85	0.5	5%
Crumb Coffee	120	4.5	34%
Chocolate/Orange Cupcake, aver.	170	6	31%
Ding Dongs; King Dongs	180	9.5	48%
Ho Ho's, each	130	6	42%
Honey Bun: Glazed	320	19	25%
Iced/Frosted	390	20	21%

MARIE CALLENDER

	C	F	%fc
Berry/Peach Cobbler, 1/4 pie, 4 1/4 oz	390	19	44%

PEPPERIDGE FARM

Cakes Supreme: *Per 3 oz Slice*

	C	F	%fc
Boston Cream, Lemon Coconut	290	14	43%
Chocolate	310	17	49%
Peach Melba	270	7	23%
Raspberry Mocha	310	14	40%

Cream Cakes Supreme:

	C	F	%fc
Pineap./Strawb. Cr., 2 oz sl.	190	7	33%

Layer Cakes: *Per 1 1/2 oz Slice*

	C	F	%fc
Butterscotch Pecan	160	7	39%
Choc. Fudge/Mint; German Choc.	180	10	50%
Devil's Food; Coconut; Golden	180	9	45%
Vanilla	190	8	38%

Old Fashioned Cakes: *Per 1 oz Sl.*

	C	F	%fc
Butter Pound	130	7	48%
Carrot w. Cream Cheese Icing	140	8	51%
Cholesterol Free Pound Cake	110	6	49%

Fruit Squares: Single

	C	F	%fc
Apple; Blueberry; Cherry	220	12	49%
Turnovers: All types, aver., 3 oz	290	15	47%

WEIGHT WATCHERS ~ Next Page.

CAKE & DESSERT MIXES

FROZEN DESSERTS (CONT)

WEIGHT WATCHERS

	C	F	%fc
Apple Crisp; Chocolate Mousse	190	5	24%
Brownie a la Mode	190	4	19%
Chocolate Frosted Brownie	100	2.5	23%
Chocolate Eclair	150	4	24%
Choc. Chip Cookie Dough Sundae	180	4	20%
Chocolate Mocha Pie	170	4	21%
Choc. Rapsberry Royale	190	3	19%
Double Fudge Brownie Parfait	190	2.5	12%
Double Fudge Cake	190	4.5	21%
French Style Cheesecake	180	5	25%
Mississippi Mud Pie	160	5	28%
New York Style Cheesecake	150	5	30%
Peanut Butter Fudge Brownie	110	2.5	20%
Praline Toffee Crunch Parfait	190	3	14%
Strawberry Parfait Royale	180	2	10%
Triple Choc Caramel Mousse	200	4	18%
Triple Chocolate Cheesecake	200	5	23%
Triple Chocolate Eclair	160	5	28%

CAKE & DESSERT MIXES

Made As Directed

	C	F	%fc
AUNT JEMIMA: Coffee, 1/8 cake	170	5	26%

BETTY CROCKER
Cakes: Super Moist - *Per 1/12 Cake*

	C	F	%fc
Chocolate Chip; Butter Chocolate	280	14	45%
Peanut Butter Choc; White	240	10	38%
Other flavors, average	250	11	40%
Per 1/10 Cake: Carrot	300	13	39%
Cherry; Sour Cream; Strawberry	280	12	39%
Light: White	210	3.5	15%
Devil's Food; Yellow	230	4.5	18%

If using No Cholesterol Recipe, deduct 40 calories; and 4 grams fat.

	C	F	%fc
Angel Food Cakes: 1/12 mix	140	0	0%
Brownie Mixes: Caramel	190	9	43%
Choc Chip;Cookies. & Cr; Walnut	200	11	50%
German Chocolate	220	9	37%
Fudge, all types, average	190	9	43%
Frosted	230	10	39%
Original: P'Nut Butter Candies; White Choc.	210	10	43%
Classic Dessert Mixes:			
Boston Cream Pie (1/10)	200	4.5	20%
Choc. Pudding Cake (1/8)	170	3.5	19%
Date Bar, 1/12 mix, dry	160	7	39%

BETTY CROCKER (Cont)
Classic Dessert Mixes: (Cont)

	C	F	%fc
Gingerbread:			
Cake & Cookie (1/8)	230	7	27%
Fun Kit, 2 cookies	150	4.5	27%
Golden Pound (1/8)	290	13	40%
Lemon Chiffon (1/16)	140	3	19%
Lemon Pudding (1/8)	180	4	20%
Pineapple Upside Down (1/6)	400	15	34%
Creamy Chilled: Banana Crm (1/9)	250	11	40%
Choc. French Silk (1/8)	270	11	37%
Coconut Cream (1/9)	290	13	40%
Cookies & Cream (1/6)	380	16	38%
Sunkist Lemon Supreme (1/9)	320	13	36%
Supreme Dessert Bars: *Per Bar*			
Caramel Oatmeal; Choc. Chunk	180	9	45%
Strawberry Swirl Cheesecake	180	10	50%
Sunkist Lemon	140	4	26%
Other varieties,	170	8	42%

DUNCAN HINES

	C	F	%fc
Angel Food, 1/12 whole	140	0	0%
Other flavors, average, 1/12	190	5	24%
Cookies: All flavors, 1 cookie	65	3	42%

ESTEE

	C	F	%fc
Brownie, 1 pce, 2"x 2"	50	2	36%
All cakes, 1/5 cake	200	4	18%
Choc. Chip Cookie, 1 cookie	45	2.5	50%

PILLSBURY
Moist Supreme: *Per 1/12 Cake (Prepared)*

	C	F	%fc
Angel Food Cake	140	0	0%
French Vanilla; Lemon (1/10)	300	13	39%
Other flavors, average (1/12)	260	12	42%
Streusel Swirl: 1/16 Cake	260	11	38%
Bundt: Hot Fudge, 1/12	350	20	51%
Chocolate Caramel Nut, 1/16	290	18	56%
Strawberry Cream Cheese, 1/16	300	17	51%
Brownies: *Per 2" Square*			
Thick'n Fudgy Walnut	190	10	47%
Hot Fudge; Fudge; Dble Choc.	150	6	36%
Other flavors	180	8	40%
Bar Mixes: *Per Serving*			
Lemon Cheesecake	190	10	47%
Other flavors, average	170	7	37%
Toaster Strudel pastry, all types	190	7	23%
Yellow, 1/5 cake	280	13	42%

CAKE FROSTINGS & INGREDIENTS

CAKE & DESSERT MIXES

	C	F	%fc
ROBIN HOOD			
Devil's Food, (1/5)	310	17	49%
Yellow 1/5 cake	280	13	42%
SWEET REWARDS			
Fat Free Snack, all flavors (1/8)	170	0	0%
Reduced Fat, all flavors (1/12)	220	7	29%
Brownie Mix: Supreme, 1 pce	150	4	24%
Lowfat Fudge, 1/18 pkg	130	2.5	17%
SNACKWELL'S			
Brownie: Devil's Food, (1/12)	150	2.5	15%
Fudge (1/12)	150	2.5	15%
Cookies: Choc. Chip, 1 oz (1/18)	110	3	25%
Chocolate Fudge, 1 oz (1/18)	90	1.5	15%
Cakes: Devil's Food, 1/6 cake	200	4	18%
White; Yellow, 1/6 cake	210	4.5	19%

CAKE FROSTINGS

	C	F	%fc
BETTY CROCKER			
Creamy Deluxe (Ready-to-Spread)			
All flavors, average, 2 Tbsp	150	6	36%
Light, 2 Tbsp	120	1	7%
Creamy Frosting Mix: Made as directed, 2 Tbsp			
Coconut Pecan	160	8	45%
Other flavors, average	140	4	26%
Fluffy Frosting Mix:			
White, 3 Tbsp mix (dry)	100	0	0%
Whipped Deluxe: All flav., 2 T.	110	5	40%
DUNCAN HINES			
Lemon, 1/12 tub	120	6	45%
Other flavors, average, 1/12 tub	160	7	39%
ESTEE: Frosting Mix, 1/5 pkg	100	2.5	23%
Whipped Topping, 3/4 tsp	10	0.5	45%
PILLSBURY - Per 1/12 Tub, 2 Tbsp			
Caramel Pecan	150	8	48%
Cream Cheese; Lemon	150	6	36%
Milk Chocolate; Fudge	140	6	38%
Coconut Pecan	160	10	56%
Dark Choc	130	6	41%
All other flavors	150	6	36%
Decorators, Choc, 1 Tbsp	70	2	26%
SWEET REWARDS			
All flavors, 1 Tbsp	130	2.5	17%

BAKING INGREDIENTS

	C	F	%fc
Almond Paste:			
(Marzipan), 1 oz	125	7	50%
Baking Powder: Regular, 1 tsp	3	0	0%
Cream of Tartar, 1 tsp	2	0	0%
Butter/Margarine: 1/2 cup, 4 oz	820	91	100%
Carob Flour, 1/2 cup	90	<1	5%
Chocolate Baking Bars: *Average All Brands*			
Unsweetened, 1oz	150	15	90%
Grated, 1 cup, 4 1/2 oz	680	68	90%
Semi-sweet, 1oz	160	8	45%
Bitter-sweet/White Baking 1oz	160	9	50%
Baker's German Sweet, 4 sq., 1oz	120	7	40%
Chocolate Baking Chips: *Average All Brands*			
Milk Choc./Semi Sweet 1 oz	140	8	50%
1/4 cup, 1 1/2 oz	210	12	50%
1 cup, 6 oz	840	48	50%
Cocoa Powder, Baking:			
Hershey's, 1 Tbsp	20	0.5	28%
1/3 cup, 1 oz	115	3.5	28%
Nestle, 1 Tbsp	15	1	45%
1/3 cup, 1 oz	80	4	45%
Coconut, dried: Unsweet., 1 oz	190	18	85%
Sweetened/flaked, 1 oz	135	9	60%
1/2 cup, 1.3 oz	175	12	60%
Toasted (*Baker's*), 1 oz	170	13	70%
Creamed,1 oz	195	19	90%
Coconut Cream (*Coco Lopez*), 2 T	120	5	37%
Cornstarch, 1 Tbsp	30	0	0%
Flour: All Purpose, 1 cup, 5 oz	400	0	0%
Flavor Extracts, average all brands			
Imitation, 1 tsp	15	0	0%
Pure Extract, 1 tsp	20	0	0%
Almond, Vanilla, 1 tsp	10	0	0%
Fruit Pectin: Swtnd, 1 Tbsp, 1/2 oz	35	0	0%
Unsweetened, 1 Tbsp	2	0	0%
Gelatin, dry, 1/4 oz pkg	30	0	0%
Herbs & Spices ~ Page 67.			
Lemon/Orange Peel, 1/4 cup	30	0	0%
Nuts & Seeds ~ Pages 107 - 108.			
Pie Crusts & Fillings ~ Page 92.			
Rennin, 1 pkg (11g)	12	0	0%
Sugar/Syrups ~ Pages 98 - 99.			
Vinegar, aver. all types, 1 oz	4	0	0%
Whey, sweet, dry, 1 oz	90	<1	5%
Yeast: Active, dry, 1/4 oz pkg	15	0	0%
Fleischmann's, 0.6 oz pkg	15	0	0%
Bakers, compressed, 1 oz	25	0	0%
Brewers; Torula, 1 oz	80	<1	5%

PUDDINGS, DESSERTS, GELATIN

PUDDINGS

	C	F	%fc
INSTANT PUDDING & PIE MIXES			
Per 1/2 Cup			
Regular, average all flavors	170	4	21%
Reduced Calorie: D-Zerta	70	<1	6%
Estee	70	<1	6%
Featherweight	80	0	8%
Jell-O, sugar-free	80	2	23%
Royal, sugar-free	100	2	18%

READY-TO-SERVE

Per Serving

	C	F	%fc
Del Monte: Pudding Snacks			
Chocolate; Chocolate Fudge	130	4	28%
Butterscotch; Tapioca; Vanilla	120	3	23%
Fat Free Vanilla	90	0	0%
Dr McDougall's			
Rice Pudding, 3 oz	310	1.5	4%
Hunts: Pudding Snacks			
Chocolate	140	5	32%
Mild Chocolate; Vanilla	130	4	28%
Light Choc.; Fat Free Tapioca	90	0	0%
Jell-O: Americana Rice Pudding	90	0	0%
Cooked/Instant Pudding, aver.	95	0	0%
Fat Free Puddings	90	0	0%
Sugar Free varieties	25	0	0%
Refrigerated varieties, aver.	160	5	28%
Fat Free, average	100	0	0%
Kozy Shack: Rice Pudding	130	3	21%
Creme Caramel Flan, 1 cup, 4 oz	150	4	24%
Tapioca Pudding, 4 oz	140	3	21%
Swiss Miss: Choc. varieties, aver.	165	6	33%
Tapioca	140	4	26%
Fat Free varieties	100	0	0%
Weight Watchers (Frozen)			
Chocolate Mousse, 2 3/4 oz	190	5	24%
Triple Choc. Caramel Mousse	200	4	18%
Other Desserts ~ See Page 94.			

PUDDING BARS (FROZEN)

	C	F	%fc
Bullwinkle Pudd. Stix, 2 1/2 fl.oz:			
All flavors	120	2	15%
Good Humour Pudding Stix	90	2	20%
Jell-O Pudding Pops: Regular	80	2	23%
Deluxe Chocolate covered	210	10	43%

HOMEMADE PUDDINGS

	C	F	%fc
Apple Tapioca, 1/2 cup	150	<1	3%
Bread Pudding, 1/2 cup	250	8	29%
Blancmange, 1/2 cup	140	5	32%
Chocolate, 1/2 cup	190	6	28%
Corn Pudding, 1/2 cup	135	7	47%
Plum Pudding, 2 oz	170	3	16%
Rennin Dessert, 1/2 cup	115	5	39%
Rice with Raisins, 1/2 cup	200	4	18%
Sponge Pudding, 3 1/2 oz	340	16	42%
Tapioca Cream, 1/2 cup	110	4	33%
Trifle, 1/2 cup	180	7	35%

MERINGUES

	C	F	%fc
Meringue Swirl, 1/2 oz	50	0	0%
Meringue Shell, 1 oz Shell	100	0	0%
(Add extra calories/fat for fillings)			

CUSTARDS

	C	F	%fc
CUSTARD MIX			
Jell-O (Americana) Golden Egg:			
Prep. w. whole milk, 1/2 cup	160	5	28%
Prep. w. skim milk, 1/2 cup	125	1	7%
Royal, 1/2 cup	150	5	30%
HOMEMADE CUSTARD			
Baked, plain, 1/2 cup, 4 1/3 oz	150	7	42%
w. skim milk, artif. sweetened	70	3	38%
Boiled, 1/2 cup	165	7	38%

GELATIN/JELL-O

	C	F	%fc
Gelatin Mix: *Average, (Jell-O, Royal)*			
Regular, all flavors, 1/2 cup	80	8	0%
Sugar Free/Low Cal., 1/2 cup	8	0	0%
Snack Cups (Del Monte/Jell-O):	70	0	0%

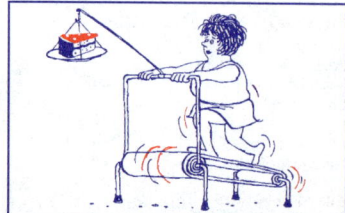

PANCAKES & WAFFLES

PANCAKES

QUICK GUIDE

	C	F	%fc
PLAIN: *Average All Types:*			
Small (3" diam.), 3/4 oz	50	1	18%
Medium (4" diam.), 1 1/4 oz	80	2	23%
Large (5" diam.), 2 1/2 oz	160	4	23%
Add Extra for Syrups/Butter			
Pancake Syrup: Regular, 1 Tbsp	50	0	0%
1/4 cup	200	0	0%
Lite, 1 Tbsp	25	0	0%
1/4 cup	100	0	0%
Butter/Margarine: Regular, 1 T.	100	11	100%
Whipped, 1 Tbsp	70	7.5	100%

RESTAURANT STYLE PANCAKES

	C	F	%fc
Denny's Pancakes: Plain, 3	490	7	13%
w. Syrup & Butter	725	17	21%
Grand Slam Breakfast	800	50	57%
w. Syrup & Margarine	1030	60	52%
Hardees: 3 Pancakes (no fat)	280	2	6%
w. Sausage Pattie	430	16	33%
w. 2 Bacon Strips	350	9	23%
Syrup, 1 serving	120	0	0%
Margarine/Butter Blend, 1 pkg	35	4	100%
Jack in the Box:			
Pancake Platter	400	12	27%
Pancake Syrup	120	0	0%
McDonalds: Hotcakes, Plain	310	7	20%
w. Marg. & Syrup	580	16	23%
IHOP (International House of Pancakes)			
Pancakes (Syrup/Butter extra):			
Buttermilk, 1 (2 oz)	105	3	25%
Short Stack, 3	315	9	25%
Full Stack, 5	525	15	25%
Buckwheat, 1 (2 1/2 oz)	135	5	33%
Country Griddle, 1 (2 1/4 oz)	135	4	26%
Harvest Grain 'N Nut, 1	160	8	45%
Crepes (Pancake Type), 1 (2 oz)	100	5	45%
Syrup: 1 Tbsp	50	0	0%
Whipped Butter, 1 Tbsp	70	7	90%
Waffles (Plain): Regular, 1 (4 oz)	300	15	45%
Belgian: Regular, 1 (6 oz)	410	20	44%
Harvest Grain 'N Nut, 1	450	28	56%
Perkins			
Pancakes: Buttermilk, 3, plain	440	12	25%
Harvest Grain: Plain, 3	270	2	6%
w. lowcal Syrup	295	2	6%
5-Stack w. lowcal Syrup	475	3.5	6%

BRANDS

	C	F	%fc
Aunt Jemima:			
Frozen: Blueberry (3)	210	4	17%
Buttermilk	180	3	15%
Lowfat	130	2	14%
Original	200	3	14%
Pancake & Waffle Mix:			
Original, 1/3 cup	150	1	6%
Regular, 1/3 cup	190	2	9%
Buckwheat, 1/4 cup	120	1	8%
Buttermilk Complete, 1/3 cup	190	2	9%
Reduced Calorie, 1/3 cup	140	1.5	10%
Wholewheat, 1/4 cup	130	1	7%
Betty Crocker Pancake Mixes:			
Complete Original, 3	200	3	14%
Complete Buttermilk, 3	200	2.5	11%
Bisquick (Shake 'N Pour)			
Pancake & Waffle Mixes:			
Average, all types, 3	210	4	17%
Estee: 3 x 4" pancakes	180	0	0%
Featherweight: 3 x 4" pancakes	140	2	13%
Hungry Jack			
Mixes: *Per 1/3 Cup (prep.)*			
Buttermilk: Original,			
w. 2% Milk, Oil, Egg	290	13	40%
w. Skim Milk, Oil, Egg Whites	230	6	23%
Buttermilk: Complete, 1/3 cup	160	1.5	8%
Complete Packets, 1/2 pkt	200	3	14%
Extra Lights: w. 2% Milk, Oil, Egg	240	8	30%
w. Skim Milk, Oil, Egg Whites	230	6	23%
Complete	150	2	12%
Microwave: *Per 3 Pancakes, 4 oz*			
Blueberry	230	3.5	14%
Buttermilk; Original	280	8	26%
Buttermilk Minis, (11)	260	7	24%
Robin Hood (Mix): Buttermilk, 3	230	6	23%

WAFFLES

	C	F	%fc
Homemade: 7" waffle, 2 1/2 oz	245	13	48%
From Mix: 7" waffle, 2 1/2 oz	205	8	35%
Aunt Jemima (Frozen):			
Blueberry, 1 Waffle, 2 1/2 oz	175	5	26%
Wholegrain Wheat/Oat	155	3	17%
Other varieties, 1 waffle	175	6	31%
Eggo (Frozen): Aver. all types, 1	120	5	38%
Downyflake (Frozen):			
Average, 2 waffles, 2 1/2 oz	180	6	30%
Homestyle Lowfat, (2), 2 1/2 oz	170	2	11%

SUGAR, SWEETENERS, JAMS

SUGAR

	C	F	%fc
White Sugar, granulated:			
1 level teaspoon, 4g	15	0	0%
1 heaping teaspoon, 6g	25	0	0%
1 cube, 1/2"	24	0	0%
Single portion, 1 packet	25	0	0%
1 Tablespoon, 12g	46	0	0%
1 ounce, 1oz	110	0	0%
1 cup, 7 oz	770	0	0%
1 pound	1760	0	0%
Brown Sugar:			
1 Tbsp, 13g	50	0	0%
1 ounce, 1oz	109	0	0%
1 cup, not packed, 5 oz	540	0	0%
1 cup, packed, 7 3/4 oz	845	0	0%
Powdered/Confectioners:			
Sifted, 1 cup, 3 1/2 oz	385	0	0%
Unsifted, 1 cup, 4 1/4 oz	460	0	0%
OTHER SUGARS			
Glucose, 1 oz	110	0	0%
Tablets (*Dex 4*), 1	15	0	0%
Cinnamon Sugar, 1tsp	15	0	0%
Dextrose, 1 oz	110	0	0%
Fructose: 1 tsp	15	0	0%
3 Tbsp, 1 oz	110	0	0%
Estee, 1 pkg	10	0	0%
FruitSource, 1oz	110	0	0%
Sorbitol, 1oz	110	0	0%
Turbinado Sugar, 2 Tbsp, 1oz	110	0	0%
Unrefined Cane Sugar, 1oz	110	0	0%

SUGAR ALTERNATIVES

	C	F	%fc
Equal: Tablet/Liquid	0	0	0%
Granulated, 1 pkg	4	0	0%
NutraSweet Spoonful, 1 tsp	2	0	0%
Nutra Taste, 1 pkt	0	0	0%
Sprinkle Sweet, 1 tsp	2	0	0%
Sugar Delight: 1 pkt	8	0	0%
Sugar Like (Bateman's), 1 tsp	4	0	0%
Sugar Twin: 1 pkt	3	0	0%
Sugar Substitute, 1 tsp	2	0	0%
Sweet 'N Low, 1 pkt	0	0	0%
Sweet One, 1 pkt	0	0	0%
Weight Watchers Sweetener, 1 tsp	4	0	0%

HONEY, JAM, PRESERVES

	C	F	%fc
HONEY			
1 tsp, 1/4 oz	22	0	0%
1 Tbsp, 3/4 oz	65	0	0%
1 ounce, 1 oz	86	0	0%
1 cup, 12 oz	1030	0	0%
Single Portion, 1/2 oz pkg	43	0	0%
JAMS/JELLIES/PRESERVES			
Regular, 1 tsp, 1/4 oz	18	0	0%
1 Tbsp, 3/4 oz	55	0	0%
1 ounce	75	0	0%
Single Portion, 1/2 oz pkg	38	0	0%
Fruit Spreads:			
Regular, 1 tsp	16	0	0%
Low Sugar, 1 tsp	8	0	0%
Low Cal. *(Featherweight)*, 1 tsp	4	0	0%
Jelly: Regular, average, 1 tsp	18	0	0%
Imitation, Low Calorie, 1 tsp	4	0	0%
Marmalade, citrus, 1 tsp	18	0	0%
Apple/Fruit Butters, 1 tsp	12	0	0%

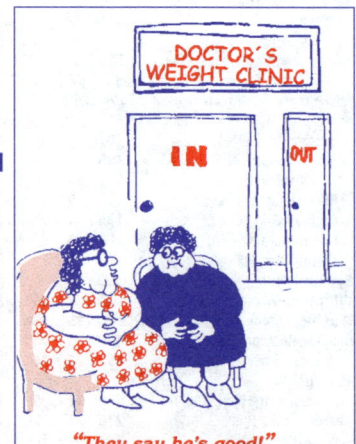

"They say he's good!"

SYRUPS

QUICK GUIDE

SYRUPS	C	F	%fc
Average All Types (Corn/Rice/Maple/Pancake/Waffle)			
Regular/Dark/Light Color:			
1 Tbsp: 3/4 oz	55	0	0%
2 Tbsp: 1 1/2 oz	110	0	0%
1/4 cup: 3 oz	220	0	0%
1 cup: 12 oz	880	0	0%
Single Portion: 1oz pkg	115	0	0%
1 1/2 oz: pkg	170	0	0%
Lite (e.g *Weight Watchers*),			
1 Tbsp: 0.6 oz	25	0	0%
2 Tbsp	50	0	0%
1/4 cup: 2 1/2 oz	100	0	0%

BRANDS

Per 2 Tbsp (1 fl.oz Serving)
(For 1/4 cup serving, double the figures.)

	C	F	%fc
Aunt Jemima:			
Original; Butter Rich	105	0	0%
Lite; Butterlite	50	0	0%
Br'er Rabbit, dark/light	120	0	0%
Country Kitchen: Regular	100	0	0%
Lite	6	0	0%
Eden, Barley Malt Syrup	120	0	0%
Estee, Maple/Blueberry	40	0	0%
Featherweight	30	0	0%
Golden Griddle	100	0	0%
Grocer's Pride	105	0	0%
Hungry Jack: Regular	100	0	0%
Lite	50	0	0%
Karo, all types	120	0	0%
Knott's Berry Farm: All types	105	0	0%
Log Cabin: Regular	100	0	0%
Lite	50	0	0%
MacDonalds Premium	105	0	0%
Maple House	105	0	0%
McIlhenny, Cane Syrup	130	0	0%
Mrs. Butterworth's, Lite	60	0	0%
Original; Country Best Recipe	115	0	0%
Mrs. Richardson's: Original	105	0	0%
Lite	50	0	0%
Quik, strawberry	120	0	0%
Ralph's: Regular	105	0	0%
Lite	50	0	0%
S & W: Calorie Reduced	8	0	0%
Smucker's Fruit Syrup; Regular	105	0	0%
Light	65	0	0%

BRANDS (Cont)

	C	F	%fc
Tree of Life: Maple	100	0	0%
Rice Syrup	120	0	0%
Tropical Pancake	110	0	0%
Vons: Regular	105	0	0%
Lite	50	0	0%
Weight Watchers Syrup	50	0	0%

MOLASSES

	C	F	%fc
Dark/Light: 1 Tbsp	55	0	0%
1 cup, 11 1/2 oz	880	0	0%
Blackstrap: 1 Tbsp, 3/4 oz	47	0	0%
1 cup, 11 1/2 oz	750	0	0%

ICECREAM TOPPINGS

Per 2 Tbsp

	C	F	%fc
Hershey: Choc. Fudge	100	4	36%
Kraft: Butterscotch	130	2	14%
Caramel	120	0	0%
Chocolate	110	0	0%
Hot Fudge	140	4	26%
Pineapple; Strawberry	110	0	0%
Marzetti: Caramel Apple	60	7	100%
Car. Apple Reduced Fat	30	3	90%
Smuckers: Butterscotch	130	1	7%
Chocolate Fudge	130	1	7%
Fat Free Choc. Fruit Dip	130	0	0%
Hot Caramel	120	3	23%
Hot Fudge	140	4	26%
Lite Hot Fudge	90	0	0%
Marshmallow	120	0	0%
Magic Shell Toppings	220	16	65%
Peanut Butter Caramel	150	4.5	27%
Pecans in Syrup	190	11	52%
Pineapple; Strawberry	110	0	0%
Sundae Syrups, all flavors	110	0	0%

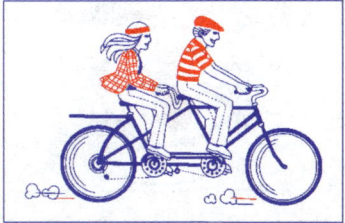

CANDY, CHOCOLATE

QUICK GUIDE

	C	F	%fc
Average all Brands			
Milk Chocolate, regular:			
Plain/Nuts/Fruit, aver., 1 oz	150	10	60%
1 1/2 oz Bar	225	15	60%
2 oz Bar	300	20	60%
4 oz Block	600	40	60%
8 oz Block	1200	80	60%
1 Pound, 16 oz	2400	160	60%
Dark/White Chocolate, 1 oz	150	10	60%
Chocolate-coated:			
Almonds, 5-6, 1 oz	160	11	61%
Macadamias, 2-3 pces., 1 oz	180	13	65%
Peanuts, 12 med., 1 oz	160	11	61%
Clusters, nut, 2, 1 oz	160	11	61%
Raisins, 30 med., 1 oz	120	4	30%
Mints, 1 med., 11g	45	1	20%
Fudge, 1 oz	125	5	36%
Nougat & Caramel, 1 oz	120	4	30%
Creme/Cordial Centres, 1 oz	120	4	30%
Cooking Chocolate:			
Sweet/Semi-sweet, 1 oz	160	8	45%
Chips, 1/4 cup, 2 1/2 oz	210	12	51%
Unsweetened, 1 oz	150	15	90%
Also See Baking Ingredients - Page 95			
Carob Candy — See Page 104			
Carob, plain, 1 oz	160	11	61%

BRANDS & GENERIC

	C	F	%fc
Per Piece/Serving			
Abba Zabba, 2 oz bar	250	5	18%
Aero Bar, 1.45 oz bar	210	13	56%
After Dinner Mints, 1 small	45	1	20%
After Eight Mint, each	35	1.2	31%
Almond Joy, 1.76 oz bar	240	13	49%
Almond Roca, each	65	3	42%
Almonds, sugar-coated (7), 1 oz	130	5	34%
Altoids (C & B), each	3	0	0%
Amazin' Fruit, 1 bag	180	0	0%
Andes: Creme de Menthe,			
8 pces, 1.3 oz	210	13	56%
Toffee Crunch, 8 pces, 1.3 oz	210	12	51%
Anthon Berg: Cognac, each	180	8	40%
Marcipan Brod, each	120	7	52%
After Dinner Sweet:			
Marzipan w. Madeira, 1.4 oz	175	7.5	39%
Baby Ruth, 3.7 oz bar	495	21	38%
2.1 oz bar	280	12	39%
Fun size, each	95	4.5	43%
Baci *(Perugino)*, each	85	5	53%
Bar None, 1.5 oz bar	240	14	52%
Barley Sugar, 1 pce., 0.2 oz	23	0	0%
Bit-O-Honey, 1.7 oz	200	4	18%
Bonus Bar, 2.1 oz bar	290	16	50%
Brach's: Butterscotch Disks,			
3 pces, 0.6 oz	70	0	0%
Choc Bridge Mix, (16), 1.4 oz	190	9	43%
Dlbe Dip Choc Peanuts, 15 pce	220	14	57%
International Toffee, each	25	0.6	22%
Jordan Almonds (10), 1.4 oz	180	6	30%
Lemon Drops, (4), 0.6 oz	70	0	0%
Malted Milk Balls, each	12	0.6	45%
Milk Maid Caramel, each	35	1	26%
Orange Slices Hi-C, each	50	0	0%
Breath Savers, all types, each	10	0	0%
Brock: Candy Corn, (10) 0.7 oz	75	0	0%
Gummy Bears, each	26	0	0%
Lemon Drops, each	20	0	0%
Orange Slices, each	35	0	0%
Sour Balls, each	25	0	0%
Spice Drops, each	12	0	0%
Starlight Mints, each	20	0	0%
Toffee, each	25	0.8	29%
Buncha Crunch, 1/2 cup, 1.3 oz	190	9	43%

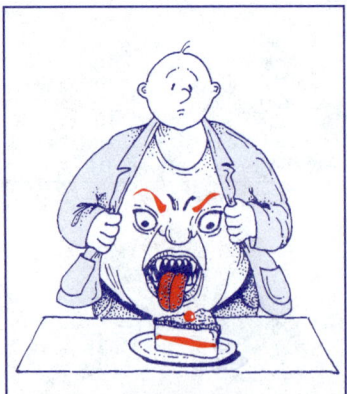

CANDY, CHOCOLATE CONT

Per Piece/Serving	C	F	%fc
Butterfinger, 3.7 oz bar	510	21	37%
2.1 oz bar	270	11	37%
Fun size, each	110	4	33%
Mini, each	20	1	45%
Butterfinger B.B.'s, 1/4 cup, 1.4 oz	200	9	40%
Butterscotch, 6 pces	115	5	39%
Chips, 1 oz	150	7	42%
Candy Corn, 1 oz	105	0	0%
Caramels, each	30	1	30%
Chocolate, each	25	0.3	1%
Caramel Nips, each	30	1	30%
Caramel Truffles (Godiva), 1 pce	110	6.5	53%
Caramello (Hershey's) 1.6 oz bar	220	10	41%
Cellas Choc Cherries, .5 oz pce	55	2	33%
Certs: Breath Mints, 1 pce	6	0	0%
Sugar-free, 1 piece	7	0	0%
Chews, all types, 1 oz	110	1	8%
Chocolate Mints, each	55	4	65%
Chocolate Parfait Nips, each	30	1	30%
Chuckles, each	35	0	0%
Chunky Bar, 1.4 oz	200	11	49%
Coffee Go Coffee/Cappuccino, each	18	0.4	20%
Coffee Rio-Gold, each	15	0.5	30%
Cote d'Or: Bouchee, each	130	8	55%
Chokotoff, each	210	9	39%
Nougatti	150	8	48%
Bar & Nuts, 35g	220	18	74%
Crisped Rice: Almond, 1 bar	130	6	42%
Choc Chip, 1 bar	115	4	31%
Crunch, 5 oz bar	725	38	47%
2.75 oz bar	400	21	47%
1.55 oz bar	230	12	47%
Fun size, each	50	2.5	45%
Double Dip Stick, 1 stick	16	0.5	28%
Dove: Dark/Milk, 1.3 oz bar	200	12	54%
Truffles, each, 0.4 oz	67	4.5	60%
English Toffee, 1 pce	48	3	56%
Estee:			
Caramels, all flavors, 1 pce.	30	1	30%
Chocolate, Dark, Mint, 1/2 bar	200	14	63%
Milk Chocolate, 1/2 bar	230	17	67%
Gummy Bears; Gum Drops, 1 pce.	7	0	0%
Lollipops, 1 pop	25	0	0%
Peanut Butter Cups, 1 cup	40	3	67%
Fructose Sweetened, 1 cup	40	2	45%
Peanut Brittle, 1/4 box, 1.1 oz	150	6.5	40%
5th Avenue, 2.1 oz bar	290	13	40%
Featherweight:			
Candy (Fruit Blends), 1 pce.	12	0	0%
Chocolate Bars:			
Almonds, 1 section	90	6	60%
Milk/Crunch, 1 section	80	7	78%
Peppermint Swirls, 1 pce.	20	0.2	9%
Cool Blue Mints: Butterscotch	25	0.3	11%
Caramels, 1 piece	30	1	30%
Fruit Drops, all flavors, 1 pce.	30	0	0%
Ferrero Rocher, each	75	5	60%
Fondant: Choc-coated,			
1 piece, 1.2 oz	130	3	21%
Mint, 1 oz	105	0	0%
Franklin Crunch 'N Munch:			
All varieties, aver. 1.25 oz	170	7	37%
Fruit Drops, each	6	0.1	15%
Fruit Leathers, average, 1/2 oz	40	0	0%
Fruit Pastilles, 1 roll, 1.4 oz	100	0	0%
Fruit Rolls, 1 roll	80	0	0%
Fruit Roll-Ups, 1/2 oz	50	<1	9%
Fruit Waves, 0.5 oz	50	0	0%
Fudge: Chocolate/Vanilla, 1 oz	115	3	23%
with Nuts, 1 oz	120	4	30%
Choco. Marshmallow, 1 oz	120	5	38%
w. Nuts, 1 oz	125	5.5	40%
Peanut Butter, 1 oz	105	2	17%
Ghiradelli: Milk/Dark Chocolate,			
1.5 oz piece	220	14	57%
Choc Nuts & Chews, 1 pce	55	3.5	57%
Go Lightly: Sugar-free, each	12	0	0%
Godiva: Hearts, each	45	2	40%
Almond Butter Dome, 1 pce	80	6	67%
Bouchee au Chocolate, 1 pce	210	11	47%
Gold Ballotin, 1 pce	70	3.5	45%
Truffle Amaretto, 1 pce	105	6	51%
Golden Almond Bar, 1 bar	520	34	59%
Golden 111 Bar, 1 bar	500	30	54%
Goobers Peanuts, 1 pkg, 1.4 oz	210	13	56%
Good & Fruity, 1 box, 1.8 oz	140	1	6%
Good & Plenty: Box, 1/5 bar, 1.4 oz	130	0	0%
Candy Bar, 1/5 bar, 1.4 oz	130	0	0%

Continued Next Page

CANDY, CHOCOLATE CONT

Per Piece/Serving	C	F	%fc
Gum (Per Piece):			
Bazooka, each	30	0	0%
Beechies	6	0	0%
Big League Chew	10	0	0%
Bubble Yum; Bubblicious	25	0	0%
Candilicious	30	0	0%
Carefree: Bubble Gum	10	0	0%
Wild Cherry	10	0	0%
Cinnamon; P'mint; Spearmint	5	0	0%
Clorets, stick	10	0	0%
Dentyne; Chiclets	6	0	0%
Estee, bubble/regular	5	0	0%
Extra Plen-T-Pak	8	0	0%
Featherweight	4	0	0%
Freshen-Up	13	0	0%
Hubba Bubba, regular	23	0	0%
Sugar-free, average	14	0	0%
Sticklets	7	0	0%
Trident: Slab	5	0	0%
Soft Bubble Gum	9	0	0%
Wrigley's, all types	10	0	0%
Gum Drops, 1 small	15	0	0%
1 large, 0.4 oz	40	0	0%
Gummi Bears, each	7	0	0%
Gummi Worms, each	25	0	0%
Halvah: Plain or w/Nuts, 1 oz	160	7	39%
Chocolate-covered, 1 oz	160	8	45%
Hard Candy, all flavors, 1 oz	110	0	0%
1 regular piece	18	0	0%
Heath: Original, 1.4 oz bar	210	13	56%
Sensations Singles, 1.4 oz	210	12	51%
Hershey's: Bar, 1.55 oz bar	240	14	52%
w. Almonds, 1.45 oz bar	230	14	55%
Almond: 7 oz (1/5 bar)	210	13	56%
Almond Chocolate, 2.6 oz bar	410	25	5%
Almond Nuggets (4), 1.4 oz	210	13	56%
Cookies 'N Mint, 1.55 oz bar	230	12	47%
2.6 oz bar	390	20	46%
7 oz bar, 1/5 bar	190	10	47%
Cookies 'N Mint Nuggets, (4) 1.4 oz	200	10	45%
Cookies & Creme, (4) 1.4 oz	200	11	49%
Milk Chocolate, 1.35 oz bar	230	13	51%
2.6 oz bar	400	23	52%
7 oz bar, 1/5 bar	200	12	54%
Milk Choc. Nuggets, (4) 1.4 oz	210	12	51%
Miniatures, 5 pces, 1.5 oz	230	13	51%

Per Piece/Serving	C	F	%fc
Honeycomb: Plain, 1 oz	113	<1	4%
Choc-coated, 1 oz	125	5	36%
Hugs, 8 pces, 1.3 oz	210	12	51%
w. Almonds, 9 pces, 1.4 oz	230	13	51%
Jellies, 3 medium, 1 oz	120	3	22%
Jelly Beans: Small, each	6	0	0%
24 pces, 1.4 oz	150	0	0%
Jelly Bellys, each	4	0	0%
35 pces, 1.4 oz	140	0	0%
Jells Raspberry *(Joyva)*, each	70	1	13%
Jolly Rancher Candy (3), 0.6 oz	70	0	0%
Jr Mints, 1.6 oz box	180	3	15%
16 pces, 1.4 oz	160	2.5	14%
Juicefuls: Red Raspb., (3), 0.6 oz	60	0	0%
Assorted Fruits, 1 pce	20	0	0%
Jujifruits, each	10	0	0%
Jujubes, each	3	0	0%
Kisses, All types, (8) 1.4 oz	210	12	51%
Kit Kat, 2.6 oz bar	405	21	47%
1.6 oz bar	250	13	47%
Multipack, each	80	4	45%
Krackel, 1.55 oz bar	230	13	50%
Snack size, 0.35 oz	55	3	50%
Lance: Popscotch, 1.2 oz pkg	160	6	34%
Chocolaty Peanut Bar, 2 oz bar	320	18	51%
Peanut Bar, 1.8 oz pkg	260	14	48%
Licorice: Average all types, 1 oz	100	0	0%
Bites *(Switzer)*, each	4	0	0%
Chews *(Panda)*, each	10	0	0%
Tid Bits, each	5	0	0%
Twists: Black/Red, aver. 1 pce	30	0	0%
Amer. Lic. Co: Stick, (1) 0.5 oz	45	0	0%
Choco Sticks, (4) 1.4 oz	145	0	0%
Red Bites, 1.4 oz	140	0	0%
Red Ropes, 1 rope	220	0	0%
Laces, 1 pce	35	0	0%
Vines, 1 pce	70	0	0%
Lifesavers: Regular, all types, ea.	20	0	0%
Sugar-free Delites:			
Orchard Fruits; Summer Blend	5	0	0%
Butter Toffee; European Collect.	9	0.4	40%
Gummi Savers, 1.4 oz roll	130	0	0%
Lollipops Fruit, 1 pce, 0.4 oz	45	0	0%
Lindt: Dark Choc Truffles, each	70	6	77%
Lindor, Balls, average	73	4	49%
Lollipops, each, 0.2 oz	20	0	0%
Lollipops C Pops *(Glenny's)*, each	35	0.2	5%

CANDY, CHOCOLATE CONT

Per Piece/Serving	C	F	%fc
M & M's:			
Almond Choc., 1.3 oz pkg	200	11	49%
1.5 oz pkg	230	13	51%
Mint/Plain, 1.7 oz pkg	230	10	39%
Peanut, 1.7 oz pkg	250	13	47%
Peanut Butter/Choc, 1.5 oz	220	12	49%
Peanut Candy, 1.5 oz	220	11	45%
Peanut Choc, 3.2 oz bar	480	24	45%
Plain Chocolate, 3.2 oz bar	440	18	37%
Mr Goodbar, 2.6 oz bar	410	25	55%
1.75 oz bar	290	19	59%
Mars Bar, all varieties, 1.8 oz	240	13	49%
Marshmallows: Firm/Soft, 1 oz	90	0	0%
Regular size, 1 pce	25	0	0%
Miniature, 1 pce	2	0	0%
Choc-coat. Twists (Joyva), ea.	95	2	19%
Kraft: Mini, 1/2 cup	80	0	0%
Creme, 2 Tbsp	40	0	0%
Jet Puff, 4 pces	90	0	0%
Funmallows, each	25	0	0%
Miniature, 1/2 cup	50	0	0%
Teddy Bear, 1/2 cup	50	0	0%
Marshmallow Egg, 1 egg	110	0	0%
Mauna Loa: Choc., 2.5 oz bar	420	29	62%
Mega Fruit Gummi, each	10	0	0%
Milk Chocolate, 1.55oz bar	225	14	56%
with Almonds, 1.45 oz bar	215	14	59%
Milk Choc. Crisp, 1.45 oz bar	205	11	48%
Milk Duds, 13 pces, 1.4 oz	180	6	30%
Milk Shake Bar, 1.8 oz bar	220	7	29%
Milky Way, 2.15 oz bar	270	10	33%
Snack size, each	90	3.5	35%
Mini, each	38	1.4	33%
Dark, 1.8 oz bar	220	8	33%
Milky Way Lite, 1.57 oz	170	5	26%
Mints: uncoated, 1 oz	100	<1	5%
1 small mint (3/4 " diam)	7	0	0%
1 large mint 1 1/2" diam.)	30	0	0%
Mounds, 1.9 oz bar	250	13	47%
Neuhaus, average all types	80	5	56%
Nougat, 2 pces, 1 oz	115	1	7%
Chocolate Covered, 1 oz	120	4	30%
Nougat Nut Cream, 3.5 oz	340	31	82%
Now & Later: Radberry, 2.9 oz pkg	270	2.5	8%
Nutrageous Bar, 2.8 oz	460	28	55%
1.6 oz bar	240	15	56%

Per Piece/Serving	C	F	%fc
Oh Henry! 1.8 oz bar	230	9	35%
100 Grand, 1.5 oz bar	180	12	60%
PayDay Bar, 1.85 oz bar	240	12	45%
Peanut Bar, 1.4 oz bar	210	14	60%
Peanut Brittle, 1 pce	25	1	36%
Peanut Chews (Goldenberg's), ea.	60	3	45%
Peanuts, choc-covered, each	25	1.5	54%
Peppermints, 7 small, 1/2 oz	50	<1	9%
Pez, 1 roll	30	0	0%
Planters Orig. Peanut Bar, 1.6 oz	230	14	55%
Popcorn - See Snacks Page 105			
Pralines, average, 1 pce	35	2	51%
Pretzels, choc-covered, (1) 0.4 oz	50	2	36%
Quik (Nestle), 1.65 oz bar	180	3.5	18%
Raisinets, 1 pkg, 1.6 oz	200	8	36%
Raspberry Cream, each	80	2.5	28%
Reese's: Chocolate Bar, 2.8 oz	420	24	51%
Candy (Multipack), each	95	5.5	52%
Candy (miniatures), each	40	2.5	56%
Peanut Butter Cups, 1.8 oz cup	280	17	55%
Pieces, 1 pce	42	2.5	54%
Snack Size Candy, 1 pce	95	5.5	52%
Riesen Choc. Chew, (5) 1.4 oz	180	7	35%
Rolo, each	32	1.5	42%
Seashells (Guylian) 1 shell	65	4	55%
Sesame Crunch, 10 pces, 0.6 oz	90	6	60%
Skittles, 1.5 oz	170	1	5%
Bite Size, 1 bag	250	2.5	9%
Skor Toffee Bar, 1.4 oz	220	13	53%
Simply Lite:			
Li'l Bits Chocolatey, 1/2 ctn, 36 pieces	130	5	35%
Li'l Bits Peanut Buttery, 1/2 ctn, 36 pieces	140	5	32%
Patteez, 1/2 ctn, 5 pieces	110	2.5	20%
Sweet 'N Low:			
Sugar-Free Hard Candy, each	8	0	0%
Sugar-Free Chews, each	11	0.2	16%
Smarties Candy Rolls, 1 roll	30	0	0%
Snickers Bar: 2.1 oz	280	14	45%
Munch Bar, 1.4 oz bar	230	15	59%
Fun size, each	95	5	47%
Miniatures, each	40	2.3	52%
Sno Caps, 2.3 oz box	300	13	39%
Soft 'N Chewy Butter Toffee, ea.	32	1.2	34%
Solitaires, 1/2 bag	260	17	59%

103

CANDY CONT

CANDY (CONT)
Per Piece/Serving

	C	F	%fc
Sour Punch, all types, 6 pces	130	0.5	3%
Spearmint Leaves, 1 oz	110	0	0%
Starburst: Fruit Chews, each	20	0.4	18%
Fruit Twist, each	190	1	5%
Jellybeans, 1.5 oz	150	0	0%
Original Candy, 2.7 oz pack	240	5	19%
Trop. Fruit Chews, 2.7 oz pack	240	5	19%
Sweet Escapes: Choc Toffee	80	3.5	39%
Other varieties, average	75	2.5	30%
Sweet Success Bars, 1 bar	120	4	30%
Sweetarts. 0.5 oz	60	0	0%
Symphony: All types, 7 oz (1/5 bar)	220	14	57%
3 Musketeers, 2.28 oz	260	8	28%
Mini, 2 bars, 1.4 oz	140	4	26%
Tastetations: Peppermint, each	20	0	0%
Butterscotch; Caramel; Choc	20	0.5	22%
Terry's Orange Milk Choc, 1 pce	50	3	54%
Tic Tac, all varieties, each	1.5	0	0%
Toblerone, 1 bar, 3.5 oz	540	30	50%
Toffees: Regular, 1 oz	150	9	54%
Tootsie Roll Pops, 1/2 oz pop	60	0	0%
Turtles *(Nestle),* each	85	4.5	48%
Twix Caramel/Cookie, 2 oz pkg	280	14	45%
Twizzlers Strawberry, 1.3 oz pce	120	0.5	4%
Ultra Slim Bars, 1 bar	120	4	30%
Werther's: Original Butter, 3 pce	60	1	15%
Whatchamacallit Bar, 1.8 oz	260	13	45%
Whitman's Pecan Roll, 2 oz roll	300	20	60%
Yogurt Candy: Plain, 1 oz	20	6	45%
Coated Raisins, 1 oz	120	4	30%
York Mints: 1.5 oz patty	170	3	16%
Snack size, 0.5 oz	55	1	16%
Zero Bar, 1 pce, 0.7 oz	85	3	32%

COUGH DROPS & LOZENGES

	C	F	%fc
Beech Nut, 1 tablet	10	0	0%
Halls, 1 tablet	15	0	0%
Hall's Plus, 1	78	0	0%
Helps Cough, all flavors, 1	14	0	0%
Listerine Loz. (Amer.Chicle)	9	0	0%
Luden Throat, all flavors, 1	8	0	0%
Pine Bros, 1 cough drop	10	0	0%
Rolaids/Sodium Free (1)	4	0	0%
Squibb Cough/Throat Loz.'s, 1	16	0	0%
Sucrets (Beecham) Lozenges, 1	10	0	0%
Cough Medications - Page 109			

CAROB CANDY

	C	F	%fc
Carob: Plain/Natural, 1oz	160	11	61%
Carob coated: Raisins, 1 oz	130	8	55%
Almonds/Peanuts, 1 oz	150	10	60%
Malt Balls, 1 oz	135	8	53%
Caramels, 1 oz	110	4	32%
Dates, 1 oz	125	5	36%
Soybeans	145	9	55%
Trail; Party Mix, 1 oz	140	9	57%
Carob Chips, unsweetened, 1 oz	140	7	45%
Carob Bars, average all brands:			
Plain/Nut, 1 oz	160	11	61%
Fruit & Nut, 1 oz	155	10	58%
Mint/Orange, 1 oz	160	11	61%
Caroby Natural Touch, 3 oz	450	27	54%
Joan's Natural Bars, 3 oz:			
Coconut; Peanut, average	520	35	60%
Fruit & Nut	560	38	61%
Honey Bran	490	33	60%
Nature Snacks (Sun Maid):			
Carob Crunch, 1 oz	145	8	49%
Carob Peanuts, 1 1/4 oz	190	12	56%
Carob/Yogurt Raisins, 1 1/4 oz	160	10	56%
Tahitian Treat; Yogurt Cr., 1 oz	125	7	50%
Queen Bee: Carob Turtles, 1 pce.	230	15	58%
Fantasy Truffles, 1 piece	225	12	48%
Tiger's Milk, carob-coated bar	160	6	33%
with Peanut Butter	160	7	39%

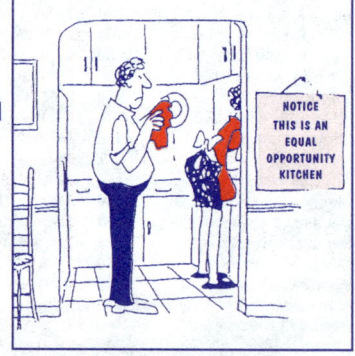

SNACKS

Per 1 oz (Unless Indicated)

	C	F	%fc
Bacon Cheese Crackers	140	6	39%
Beef Jerky: Average, 1 oz	70	1	12%
(Brands - See Page 42)			
Beef Sticks *(Frito-Lay's)* 0.3 oz	50	4	32%
Bugles: Original, 1 1/3 cup, 1 oz	160	9	50%
Baked Bugles, 1 1/2 cup, 1.1 oz	130	3.5	23%
Carrot Chips *(Hain)*	160	9	50%
Cheddar Sticks/Lites	140	5	32%
Chee•ta Cheesy Crackers, 1 oz	150	10	60%
Cheese Balls, 1 1/8 oz pkg.	190	13	62%
Cheese Crackers, 1 oz	130	6	42%
Cheese Filled *(Frito-Lay's)*	210	11	47%
Cheese Curls, 1 oz	160	9	51%
Reduced Fat *(Utz)*, 1 oz	140	6	39%
Cheese Puffs, average, 1 oz	150	10	60%
Lowfat, 1 oz	140	5	32%
Health Valley, 1 1/2 cup	110	0	0%
Cheese Straws, 4 pieces	110	1	8%
Cheese Twists, 1 1/2 oz pkg.	260	13	45%
Cheetos: Regular all flavors	160	10	56%
Light, cheese flavored	140	6	39%
Chex *(Ralston)* 2/3 cup, 1 oz	130	5	35%
Cheez Balls/Curls/Doodles	160	10	56%
Cheez Waffies	140	8	51%
Churros *(Mex. Pastry)* 10" stick,1.2 oz	140	9	58%
Corn Chips: Average all varieties			
1/2 oz bag	80	5	56%
1 oz bag	160	10	56%
8 oz bag	1280	80	56%
Corn Crunchies/Spirals, 1 oz	160	10	56%
Corn Crisps *(Pringle)*, 1 oz	140	7	45%
Corn Nuggets *(Fr. Lay's)*, 1.38 oz	170	5	26%
Corn Puffs *(Health Valley)* 2 cup	120	1.5	11%
Dunkeroos, 1 tray, 1 oz	130	5	35%
Funyun's Onion flavor., 1 oz	140	7	45%
Frankie's (1-800-279 4476):			
Apple D'Lites	100	0	0%
Fudge Brownie (Fat Free)	94	0	0%
Pound Cake Snacks, 2 oz	90	0	0%
Goldfish *(Pepperidge Farm)* 1 oz	140	7	45%
Gold-N-Chee *(Lance)*, 1 3/8 oz pkg.	180	9	45%
Hot Sausage *(Frito-Lay's)*	80	7	79%
Lance Sandwich: Fig, 1 pkg	150	2	12%
Captain's Wafers w. Crm. Chse	170	9	48%
Other varieties, average, 1 pkg	190	10	47%
Munchos, 16 pieces, 1 oz	160	10	56%
Party Mix *(Flavor Tree)* 1/4 cup	160	11	62%

POPCORN

	C	F	%fc
Popping Corn Kernels: 2 Tbsp, 1oz	100	1	9%
(makes approx. 3 1/2 cups)			
Air-popped (no oil), plain, 1oz	100	<1	10%
1 cup (6g)	20	0	0%
Oil-popped, plain, 1 oz	220	13	53%
1 cup (11g)	55	3	49%
Popcorn Oil, 1 Tbsp	120	14	100%
Popcorn (Popped) *Per 1 Cup:*			
Microwave: *(Average All Brands)*			
Regular: Plain	30	1.5	45%
Butter/Cheddar	35	2.5	64%
Caramel, 1 cup	90	5.5	55%
Movie Theater (Brands)	35	2	51%
Light: Plain/Natural	20	0.5	23%
Butter	25	1	36%
Fat-Free: Plain/Butter	20	0	0%
Bagged: Reg./flav'd., 1/2 oz	80	5	56%
1 oz pkg.	160	10	56%
Light, 1/2 oz pkg.	60	3	45%
Caramel: Regular, 1 c., 1 1/4oz	150	4.5	27%
Fat-Free, 1 cup	110	0	0%
Cracker Jack: Original, 1 cup	165	3	16%
Butter Toffee, 1/2 cup	130	4.5	31%
Crunch'N Munch: P'nut, 2/3c.	140	4	26%
Fiddle Faddle: Peanut, 3/4 cup	150	7	42%
Fat Free Snacks, 1 cup	110	0	0%
Frankie's: Caramel/Cinnamon/			
Vanilla, 1.6 oz bag	100	0	0%
Mini Popcorn Cakes, 0.8 oz	97	0	0%
Weight Watchers: Caramel,1oz	100	1	9%
Butter Toffee, 1 cup	110	2.5	20%
Butter Flavor, 2/3 oz	90	2.5	25%
White Cheddar Cheese	90	4	40%
Movie Theater Popcorn: (Oil Popped)			
Small (7 cups): Plain	400	27	60%
with Butter	580	47	73%
Medium (16 cups): Plain	900	60	60%
with Butter	1170	90	73%
Large (20 cups): Plain	1150	76	60%
with Butter	1500	116	73%
Pork Skins/Rind: Baken-ets,1 oz	160	10	56%
2/3 cup *(Grande)*	80	5	56%

Continued Next Page

SNACKS (CONT) • SPORTS BARS

	C	F	%fc
Potato Chips, aver. all brands:			
Reg or flavored, 1 oz bag	150	10	60%
4 oz bag	600	60	90%
Pringle, all flavors, 1 oz	150	10	60%
Crunch Tators, 1 oz	140	7	45%
Kettle Fry (Eagle), 1 oz	150	8	48%
Reduced Fat: *Ruffles,* 1 oz	140	7	45%
Pringles, 1 oz	140	7	45%
Lowfat/Baked varieties, 1 oz	110	1.5	12%
Fat Free (*Childer's/Louise's*), 1oz	100	0	0%
Pretzels: Hard, aver., 1 oz	110	2	16%
Sticks, thin, 2 1/4" (9/oz), 1	1	0	0%
Twisted, thin, 1/4" (5/oz), 1	25	0	0%
Dutch, 2 3/4" x 2 5/8" (2/oz), 1	55	1	16%
Wheels/Nuggets (*Utz*), 1 oz	100	0	0%
Soft Pretzels (Twists) average:			
Plain: Regular, 2 1/2 oz	190	0	0%
King Size, 5 oz	390	0	0%
Super Pretzel: Jalapeno, 5 oz	360	0	0%
Bavarian Twist, 3 oz	210	3	13%
Cinnamon Raisin w/Icing, 5oz	420	4	8%
Sweet Dough Twist, 3.7 oz	300	3	10%
Auntie Anne's: Original	190	1	5%
with Butter	220	4	16%
Rice Chips: Bar-B-Q/Onion, 1/2 oz	70	3	39%
Santitas (*Frito Lay*), 1 oz	140	6	39%
Sesame Sticks, 1 oz	155	8	46%
Spicers Wheat Snacks, 1 1/2 oz	150	7.5	45%
Sunchips (*Frito Lay*), 1 oz	140	7	45%
Toast/Cheese Crackers, 1 pkg.	140	7	45%
Tortilla Chips: Average, 1 oz	150	8	48%
(3 oz = approx. 11 chips or 12 strips)			
Utz: Lowfat Baked, 8/1 oz	120	1.5	11%
Doritos: 18 chips, 1 oz	140	6	39%
Light, 13 chips, 1 oz	130	5	35%
Keebler Suncheros Light	150	8	48%
Padrino Reduced Fat, 1 oz	130	4	28%
Tostitos, 1 oz	140	8	51%
Turkey Jerky Teriyaki (*Oberto*)	80	0.5	6%
Vegetable Snacks/Chips, 1 oz	150	7	42%
***Weight Watchers* Snacks:**			
Apple Chips: 3/4 oz pkg.	70	0	0%
BBQ Flav. Curls, 1/2 oz	60	1.5	23%
Cheese Curls, 1/2 oz	70	2.5	32%
Fruit Snacks, 1/2 oz pkg.	50	0	0%
Oatbran Pretzel Nuggets, 1 1/2 oz	170	2.5	13%
Pizza/Ranch Curls, 1/2 oz	60	2	30%
Yogurt Raisins, 1 oz	120	4	30%

GRANOLA & SPORTS BARS

Per Bar	C	F	%fc
Balance Bar, 50g	180	6	30%
Barbara's Bakery: Real Fruit	50	0	0%
Cereal Bars	110	0	0%
Granola Bars	80	2	23%
Bariatrix: Nutra Bars, 47g	170	5	26%
Proti Bars (15g Protein), 41g	130	5	35%
Right Choice Bars, 40g	140	3	19%
Bear Valley Food Bars, average	420	13	28%
Breakbar (IDN), 2 oz bar	180	4	20%
Calcium Diamond Bar	150	2.5	15%
Cap'N Crunch, all types, 0.8 oz	90	2	20%
Campfire Marshmallow Munchie			
Crisp Rice Treat: Regular, 1oz	100	2	18%
w. Choc. Chip, 0.8 oz	90	2.5	25%
Carnation Breakfast Bars	145	5	31%
Clif Bar, 2.4 oz bar	250	2	7%
Croma Slim, 43g	180	3	15%
Custom Fit, 45g	170	3.5	18%
Diet Fat Burner, 36.4g	130	1.5	10%
Diet Max Hunger Curb, 1.2 oz	120	0.5	4%
Diet Pure Energy, 50g	130	0	0%
Edgebar, 2.5 oz bar	235	2	8%
Energig, 65g	230	2.5	10%
Exceed Sports Bar, 2.8 oz	280	2	6%
Extreme, 2.25 oz	230	3	18%
Fi-Bar: AM 1.5 oz	150	4	24%
Original Fruit, 1 oz bar	100	3	27%
Chewy & Nutty, 1.2 oz bar	130	4	28%
Figurines, average, 1 bar	110	6	49%
Finttalsa Energy Bar	170	2	11%
Frankie's Bars (Hi Protein):			
Chocolate Bar, all flavors	160	4	20%
Peanut Butter Bar	180	7	33%
Future Fix: Pounds Off, 60g	220	4	16%
Weight Loss, 70g	260	4.5	16%
Gatorbar, 2.25 oz	220	2	8%
Glenny's Snack Bars (Fat Free)	120	0	0%
Moist & Chewy Bars:			
Coconut Almondine	190	10	47%
Oatmeal Raisin	160	3	17%
Peanut; Sunflower	180	7	35%
Govindas: Cosmic Combo	240	12	45%
Brazil Pine Divine	230	16	63%
Omega; Peanut; Walnut Date	200	12	54%
Grandma's Snack Bars, all types	180	6	30%
HMR Benefit Bar, 2.1 oz	240	8	30%

GRANOLA, SPORTS & DIET BARS

Per Bar	C	F	%fc
Hardbody, 2 1/2 oz (71g)	290	8	25%
High Carbohydrate Energy	300	9	27%
Health Valley: Fruit Bars	140	0	0%
Bakes: Breakfast, all types	110	0	0%
Apple; Date; Raisin	70	0	0%
Brownie Bar w.Fudge Filling	110	0	0%
Granola Bars, all types	140	0	0%
Fat Free: Cereal, all types	110	0	0%
Choc. Flavored Sandwich	150	0	0%
Crisp Rice, all types	110	0	0%
Marshmallow, all types	90	0	0%
Tarts, all types	150	0	0%
Healthy: Cheesecake, all types	160	1.5	8%
Energy, all types	180	1.5	8%
Oatbran Fruit Bar	160	1	6%
Healthy Lifestyle Bar	180	5	25%
Hot Stuff, 65g	220	2	8%
Kellogg's: Nutri Grain, all types	140	3	19%
Kudos: Peaches/Strawb. & Cream	150	6	36%
Peanut Butter & Choc Chip	170	9	48%
Met-Rx, Fudge Brownie, 100g	310	2.5	7%
Vanilla, 100g	320	2.5	7%
MetaForm, 4.3 oz	400	4	9%
Nabisco: Oreo, 1.3 oz	160	7	39%
Chips Ahoy, 1.3 oz	150	5	30%
Natrol Citrimax, 43g	180	3	15%
Nature Valley Crunchy Granola:			
Cinnamon; Oats 'n Honey	100	3	27%
Peanut Butter	100	3	27%
Lowfat varieties	110	2	16%
Nite Bite Snack Bar, 25g	100	3.5	30%
Nutra Blast: Vanilla, 47g	160	2	11%
Honey & Nougat, 47g	170	3	16%
Apple Cranberry, 47g	160	3.5	20%
Phos Pha Gain, 68g	230	4	16%
Planters: Peanut Bar, 1.6 oz	230	11	43%
Honey Roasted Bar	230	13	51%
Sweet 'n Crunchy Bar	250	15	54%
Old Fashioned Bar, 1 oz	140	9	58%
Crackers (4 S'wiches), 1 oz	140	7	45%
Power Bars, 65g	230	2.5	9%
Pro-Amino, 788g	296	7	21%
Pro Gain Weight Gain, 113.4g	463	8	16%
Pro-Sports Performance, 2 oz	210	2	9%

Per Bar	C	F	%fc
PR Bar Ironman	230	8	31%
Pure Energy, Nectar & Honey	180	0	0%
Quaker Granola Bars:			
Chewy: Average	120	4.5	34%
Lowfat, all flavors	110	2	16%
Re-Create, 71g	260	6	21%
Sandoz Nutritional Bars:			
Nutra Recipe Bars	150	4	24%
Healthy Recipe Bars	150	4	24%
Snackwell's: Cereal varieties	120	0	0%
Fudge-Dipped varieties	110	3	25%
Snack Bars, 1.3 oz	130	2	14%
Steel Bar, 3 oz	380	5	19%
Sweet Rewards: Brownie	120	2	15%
Choc. Chip	110	2	16%
Fat Free Bars	120	0	0%
Sweet Success (*Nestle*)	120	4	30%
Thunder Bar, all flavors	220	2	8%
Tiger's Milk, Regular, 35.4g	145	3	31%
Peanut Butter, 35.4g	140	5	32%
Peanut & Honey, 35.4g	150	6	36%
Tiger Sport, 65g	210	2	8%
Twin Lab: Amino Fuel, 78g	285	3	9%
Ultra Fuel, 2 1/2 oz (72g)	230	0	0%
Diet Fuel, 2 1/2 oz (72g)	180	0	0%
Ultra Fuel, 2.6 oz	230	0	0%
Ultra Slim-Fast Crunch Bars	120	4	30%
Universal Muscle, 56.7g	280	5	16%
Weider Sportsfood: Protein	160	4	23%

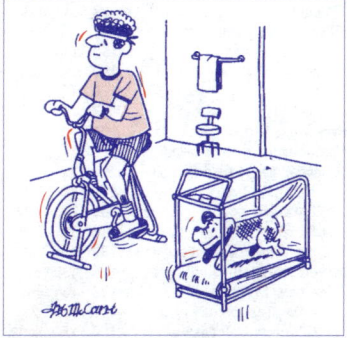

NUTS

Shelled, Per 1 oz (unless shown)	C	F	%fc
Acorns, raw 1 oz	105	7	60%
Almonds, Dried/Dry roasted:			
Whole, 24-28 med., 1 oz	170	15	80%
1/2 cup, 2 1/2 oz	420	37	80%
Chopped, 1/2 cup, 2 1/4 oz	380	34	80%
Sliced, 1/2 cup, 1 2/3 oz	280	25	80%
Choc. coated (5-6), 1 oz	160	11	62%
Oil rstd. (Blue Diamond), 1 oz	175	17	85%
Almond Meal (partially defattened)			
1 cup (not packed), 2 1/4 oz	260	11	36%
Honey roasted, 1 oz	170	13	69%
Brazil Nuts, 8 medium, 1 oz	185	19	92%
Cashews, Dry or Oil roasted:			
14 large/18 med./26 small, 1 oz	165	14	76%
1/2 cup, 2.4 oz	400	33	74%
Honey roasted, 1 oz	170	12	64%
Chestnuts, average all types:			
Raw/Fresh, 5-6 nuts, 1 oz	60	<1	8%
Dried, 1 oz	105	1	9%
Canned, water chestnuts			
sliced/whole/drained, 1 oz	23	<1	8%
Coconut: Flesh (no shell), 1 oz	100	10	90%
Raw: 1 pce. (2" x 2" x 1/2"), 1.6 oz	160	15	84%
1/2 medium (4 1/2" diam.)	650	62	86%
Dried (Desiccated):			
Unsweetened, 1 oz	187	18	87%
Sweetened, shredd., 1 oz	140	9	58%
Grated, 1/2 cup, 1.3 oz	185	12	58%
Cream (can.), 1/2 c., 5.2 oz	285	26	82%
Milk (canned), 1/2 c., 4 oz	225	24	96%
Water (center liq.), 1/2 cup, 4 1/4 oz	23	<1	19%
Filberts or Hazelnuts:			
Shelled, 18-20 nuts	180	18	90%
Chopped, 1/4 cup	180	18	90%
Ground, 1/4 cup	120	12	90%
Ginko Nuts, can., 14 med., 1 oz	32	<1	14%
Hickory, 30 small nuts	190	18	85%
Macadamia Nuts, shelled:			
Raw, 7 med./14 small, 1 oz	200	21	94%
1/2 cup, 2.3 oz	460	48	94%
Oil roasted, 1 oz	205	22	97%
1/2 cup, 2.4 oz	490	52	95%
Choc. coated, 2-3 pces, 1 oz	180	13	65%
Mixed Nuts: 18-22 nuts, 1 oz	175	13	67%
Planters: Dry roasted	170	15	79%
Honey roasted (dry rst'd)	170	13	69%
Oil roasted, all types	180	16	80%

	C	F	%fc
Nut Toppings:			
Chopped, 1Tbsp, 1/4 oz	40	4	90%
Peanuts:			
Raw/Dried, in shell, 1 oz	117	10	77%
Shelled, 1 oz	160	14	79%
Boiled, 1/2 cup, 1.1 oz	102	7	62%
Roasted, 30 lge./60 sml., 1 oz	165	14	76%
1 cup, 5.1 oz	840	71	76%
Chopped, 3 Tbsp, 1 oz	165	14	76%
Planters: Oil Roasted, 1 oz	170	15	76%
Dry Roasted, 1 oz	160	14	76%
Honey roasted, 1 oz	170	13	69%
Honey/Dry rst'd, 1 oz	160	14	73%
Cocktail, oil rst'd, 1 oz	170	14	74%
Sweet 'n Crunchy, 1 oz	140	8	51%
Pecans:			
kernel halves, 1 oz	190	19	90%
(20 Jumbo or 31 large havles)			
1 cup halves, 3.8 oz	720	73	91%
Chopped, 1/2 cup, 2 oz	380	30	71%
Oil roasted, 1 oz	195	20	97%
Honey roasted, 1 oz	200	18	81%
Pilinuts, dried, 1/4 cup, 1 oz	205	23	100%
Pinenuts, dried, 1 Tbsp, 10g	50	5	90%
Pistachios:			
Unshelled, 1/2 cup, 2 oz	165	14	76%
Shelled, 1/4 c., 45 nuts, 1 oz	165	14	76%
Lance, 1 1/8 oz package	180	14	70%
Planters: Dry Roasted, 1 oz	170	15	79%
Fruit 'n Nut Mix, 1 oz	150	9	54%
Nut Topping, 1 oz	180	16	80%
Tavern Nuts, 1 oz	170	15	79%
Sesame Nut Mix:			
(Planters), 1 oz	160	12	67%
Soybean Nuts:			
Dry roasted, 1 oz	130	6	42%
1/2 cup, 3 oz	390	18	42%
Oil roasted, 1 oz	140	7	45%
Walnuts:			
Black, 15-20 halves, 1 oz	175	16	82%
Chopped, 1/4 cup	190	18	85%
Ground, 1/4 cup	120	12	90%
English/Persian:			
14 halves, 1 oz	185	18	88%
Chopped, 1/4 cup	195	19	88%

SEEDS • VITAMINS • COUGH

SEEDS

	C	F	%fc
Caraway, Fennell, 1 tsp	10	<1	45%
Cottonseed Kernels, rst., 1 Tbsp	50	4	72%
Lotus Seeds, dried, 1/2 c., 1/2 oz	50	<1	9%
Pumpkin & Squash Seeds, whole:			
Roasted, 1 oz	125	5.5	40%
1/2 cup (32g)	140	6	39%
Dried, 1 oz	155	13	75%
Safflower Kernels, dried, 1 oz	150	11	66%
Sesame Seeds: Dried, 1 Tbsp, 9g	50	4.5	81%
Roasted/Toasted, 1 oz	160	14	79%
Sunflower Kernels/Seed:			
Dry roasted, 1 Tbsp, 8g	45	4	80%
1/4 cup, 1 oz	160	14	79%
Oil roasted, 1/4 cup, 1 oz	180	17	85%
Watermelon, dried, 1/4 cup, 1 oz	160	14	76%

NUT & SEED BUTTERS

	C	F	%fc
Almond Butter, 1 Tbsp, 1/2 oz	105	9	77%
Beanut Butter, 1 Tbsp, 1/2 oz	88	5.5	56%
Cashew Butter, 1 Tbsp	92	7	68%
Hazelnut Butter, 1 Tbsp	100	10	90%
Peanut Butter: Average, 1 oz	170	14	74%
Chunky/Creamy, 1 Tbsp, 16g	95	8	76%
Smucker's Honey Swtnd., 1 Tbsp	100	8	72%
Goober Grape/Strbry, 1 Tbsp	90	5	50%
Skippy, honeynut, 1 Tbsp, 16g	95	8	76%
Sesame Butter/Tahini, 1 tsp	30	3	90%
1 Tbsp	90	8	80%
Sunflower Butter, 1 Tbsp	97	7	65%

"I've worked on vitamins for years and I've discovered that the three most important elements necessary to life are breakfast, lunch and dinner!"

SUPPLEMENTS

	C	F	%fc
Aloe Vera Juice, undil., 2 fl.oz	4	0	0%
Cod Liver Oil, 1 Tbsp	120	13	98%
Fiber Supplements:			
Tablets, average, each	1	0	0%
Metamucil, 1 packet	5	0	0%
Regular, 1 rounded Tbsp	34	0	0%
1 heaping tsp	14	0	0%
Sugar-Free, 1 med. Tbsp	6	0	0%
Fish Oil Capsules, aver., each	10	1	90%
Garlic Tablets/Capsules, each	3	0	0%
Lecithin Granules, 1 Tbsp, 10g	50	5	90%
Capsules, each	11	1	82%
Oyster Tablets/Pearls, each	3	0	0%
Pollen Granules/Meal, 1 Tbsp	35	<1	15%
Protein; Powders, aver., 1 oz	100	<1	45%
Tablets, 20 tabs., 1/2 oz	70	0	0%
Seaweed: Dried, 1 oz	85	<1	5%
Soaked, drained, 1 oz	15	<1	30%
Spirulina, 1 tablet	2	0	0%
Vitamins/Minerals:			
Tablets/Capsules, aver. each	<3	0	0%
Vitamin E Capsules, each	5	<1	90%
Yeast: Tablets, 2 tabs.	4	0	0%
Flakes, 1 heaping Tbsp, 1/3 oz	30	<1	15%
Powder, 1 heaping Tbsp, 1/2 oz	50	<1	9%

COUGH & PHARMACEUTICAL

	C	F	%fc
Cough/Cold Syrups: 1 tsp	36	0	0%
Regular, average, 1 Tbsp	120	0	0%
Sugar-free, 1 Tbsp	<1	0	0%
Cough Drops/Lozenges - See Page 104			
Antacids: Average, 1 tablet	4	0	0%
Liquid, 1 Tbsp	6	0	0%
Sudafed Syrup, 1 tsp	14	0	0%
Tylenol **Liquid:** Child, 1 tsp	17	0	0%
Extra Strength, 1 tsp	11	0	0%

Nut eaters are healthier and live longer say medical researchers. Nuts are a nutritious source of protein, vitamins, minerals and fiber.

Their fat content can help to lower blood cholesterol, but watch the quantity if overweight.

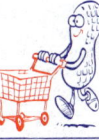

FRESH FRUIT

WEIGHTS AS PURCHASED	C	F	%fc
Acerola, 1 cup, 20 pcs, 3 1/2 oz	30	0	0%
Atemoya, 1/3 cup	95	0	0%
Apples: whole, average all varieties:			
1 small (4 per lb), 4 oz	70	0	0%
1 medium (3 per lb), 5 1/2 oz	90	0	0%
1 large (2 per lb), 8 oz	135	0	0%
1 extra large, 11 oz	170	0	0%
without skin, 1/2 medium	35	0	0%
Caramel Apple, 1 medium	170	0	0%
Nut Coated, 1 medium	230	5	20%
Apricots: 1 small (12 per lb)	17	0	0%
1 medium (8 per lb), 2 oz	25	0	0%
1 large (5-6 per lb), 3 oz	35	0	0%
Avocado (wt. w/out seed):			
Average, 1/2 medium	160	15	84%
California, 1/2 medium, 3 oz	150	15	90%
Mashed/Puree, 1/2 c., 4 oz	200	20	90%
Florida, 1/2 medium, 5 1/2 oz	170	13	70%
Mashed/Puree, 1/2 c., 4 oz	125	10	70%
1/2 cup cubed, 3 oz	95	8	70%

Note: Avocados are nutritious with no cholesterol. Fat is mainly monounsaturated and benefits blood cholesterol. Excellent substitute for butter or margarine on bread.

WEIGHTS AS PURCHASED	C	F	%fc
Banana: 1 small (4 lb), 4 oz	55	0	0%
1 medium (3 per lb), 5 oz	80	0	0%
1 large (2 1/2 per lb), 7 oz	105	0	0%
W/out skin, 1 medium., 3 1/4 oz	80	0	0%
1/2 cup, mashed, 4 oz	105	0	0%
Berries: Average all types (Black/Boysenberries/Blueberries)			
1/2 cup, 2 1/2 oz	40	0	0%
1 pint, 14 oz	220	1	0%
Breadfruit, 1/2 cup, 4 oz	115	0	0%
Cantaloupe, 1/2 med. (5" diam.)	100	0	0%
1 slice, 2 1/2 oz (w/out skin)	20	0	0%
1 cup pieces/balls, 5 1/2 oz	55	0	0%
Carambola (Star Fruit), 1 med	50	0	0%
Cassava, 1/3 cup	120	0	0%
Cherimoya (Custard Apple),			
1/4 only, 5 oz	130	0	0%
Cherries: Sweet, 8 fruit, 2 oz	40	0	0%
1/2 lb (30 cherries)	145	0	0%
Sour, 8 fruit, 2 oz	25	0	0%
1/2 lb (30 cherries)	100	0	0%
Coconut: Fresh, 1 piece, 1 oz	100	10	90%
Shredded, fresh, 1/2 cup	140	14	90%
Sweetened, dried, 1/2 cup	235	16	61%

WEIGHTS AS PURCHASED	C	F	%fc
Crab Apples, 1/2 cup slices, 2 oz	40	0	0%
Cranberries, 1/2 cup, 2 oz	20	0	0%
Currants (per 1/2 cup):			
European Black, raw, 2 oz	35	0	0%
Red & White, raw, 2 oz	30	0	0%
Dates — See Dried Fruits			
Durian, flesh, 4 oz	140	2	12%
Elderberries, 1/2 cup, 2 1/2 oz	55	0	0%
Feijoas, 1 medium, 2 1/2 oz	35	0	0%
Figs, green/black: 1 med., 2 oz	40	0	0%
1 large, 3 oz	60	0	0%
Fruit Salad, fresh, average,			
1/2 cup, 3 1/2 oz	60	0	0%
1 cup, 7 oz	120	0	0%
Gooseberries, raw, 1/2 c., 2 1/2 oz	30	0	0%
Grapefruit: average all types,			
1/2 fruit, 8 1/2 oz (4 1/2 oz flesh)	40	0	0%
1 cup sections w. juice, 8 oz	75	0	0%
Grapes: Average, 1 cup, 5 1/2 oz	100	0	0%
1 small bunch, 4 oz	70	0	0%
1 medium bunch, 7 oz	125	0	0%
1 large bunch, 1 lb	285	0	0%
Granadilla, flesh, 3 1/2 oz	95	0	0%
Groundcherries, 1/2 cup, 2 1/2 oz	35	0	0%
Guava: 1 fruit, 4 oz	80	0	0%
1/2 cup, 3 oz	40	0	0%
Honeydew, 1 wedge (7"x2" wide),			
8 oz (with skin)	45	0	0%
1 cup cubes/balls, 6 oz	60	0	0%
Honey Murcots, 1 only, 5 oz	45	0	0%
Jabotica, flesh, 4 oz	75	2	24%
Jackfruit, flesh, 1/8 average, 4 oz	105	0	0%
Jambos, flesh, 4 oz	35	0	0%
Java-Plum, 4 plums, 1/2 cup	25	0	0%
Jujube, 3 oz	65	0	0%
Kiwifruit, 1 medium, 3 oz	45	0	0%
1 large, 4 oz	60	0	0%
Kumquats, 5 medium, 3 1/2 oz	60	0	0%
Kiwano, 1/2 medium, 5 oz	35	0	0%
Langsat, Duku, 1 medium, 2 oz	25	0	0%
Lemon, 1 medium, 4 oz	20	0	0%
1 wedge, 1 oz	5	0	0%
Peel, 1 Tbsp	4	0	0%
Limes, 1 only, 2 oz	20	0	0%
Loganberries, froz., 1/2 c., 2 1/2 oz	40	0	0%
Logans, 5 fruit, 1/2 oz	10	0	0%
Loquats, 4 fruit, 2 1/4 oz	20	0	0%
Lychees, 4 fruit, 2 1/4 oz	25	0	0%

FRESH FRUIT CONT

WEIGHTS AS PURCHASED	C	F	%fc
Mamey Apple, 1 whole, 3 lb	430	4	8%
1/4 fruit (1 cup flesh), 7 oz	100	1	8%
Mandarin: 1 small, 3 oz	25	0	0%
1 medium, 4 oz	35	0	0%
1 large, 6 oz	55	0	0%
Mango, flesh, 1/2 cup sl., 3 oz	25	0	0%
1 whole, medium, 11 oz	140	0	0%
Melons: Average all types			
1 cup, cubes/balls, 6 oz	60	0	0%
Monstera Deliciosa (Taxonia),			
Edible part, 4 oz	50	0	0%
Mulberries, 20 fruit, 1 oz	15	0	0%
Nashi Fruit (Asian Pear),			
1 medium, 4 1/2 oz	50	0	0%
Nectarines, 1 medium, 4 oz	50	0	0%
1 large, 5 1/2 oz	70	0	0%
Oheloberries, 1/2 cup, 2 1/2 oz	20	0	0%
Olives: Pickled:			
Green, 10 large, 1 1/2 oz	45	5	90%
Ripe, Grk. Style, 10 med., 1 oz	70	7	90%
Ripe (Black), Californian:			
1 small/medium	4	<1	90%
1 large/extra large	6	<1	90%
1 jumbo	7	<1	90%
1 colossal	9	1	90%
1 super colossal	13	1	90%

WEIGHTS AS PURCHASED	C	F	%fc
Oranges, average all varieties:			
1 small, 5 oz	50	0	0%
1 medium, 8 oz	80	0	0%
1 large, 10 oz	95	0	0%
Californian: Valencias, 8 oz	85	0	0%
Navels (thick skin), 8 oz	70	0	0%
Flesh only, 1 cup, 6 oz	80	0	0%
Florida, 1 medium, 7 oz	70	0	0%
Peel, 1 Tbsp	4	0	0%
Papaya, 1/2 cup, cubed, 2 1/2 oz	30	0	0%
1 medium, 16 oz	120	0	0%
Passionfruit, 1 medium, 1 1/4 oz	20	0	0%
Peaches: 1 med. (4 per lb), 4 oz	35	0	0%
1 large, 6 oz	55	0	0%
Pears: Bartlett, 1 small, 4 oz	60	0	0%
1 medium, 6 oz	90	0	0%
1 large, 8 oz	120	0	0%
Bosc, 6 oz	90	0	0%
D'Anjou, 1 medium, 8 oz	120	0	0%
Red Pear, 5 oz	80	0	0%
Seckel (Wash'ton), 2 1/4 oz	35	0	0%
Asian (Nashi), 1 large, 7 oz	80	0	0%
Pepino, 1/2 medium, 4 oz	20	0	0%
Persimmons: Native, 1 oz	30	0	0%
Japan. (2 1/2"d. x 2 1/2"h), 7 oz	120	0	0%
Seedless (Maui), 1 md., 5 oz	100	0	0%
Pineapple (flesh only), 1 slice			
(3/4" thick, 3 1/2" diam.), 3 oz	40	0	0%
1 cup, diced, 5 1/2 oz	80	0	0%
1 medium, 4/2 lb	525	0	0%
Pitanga, 3 fruit, 1 oz	6	0	0%
Plaintains, 1/2 cup slices, 2 1/2 oz	90	0	0%
Plums, average all types:			
Mini/Damson, (1" diam.), 1/2 oz	8	0	0%
Small (1 3/4" diam.), 2 oz	30	0	0%
Medium (2 1/4" diam.), 3 oz	45	0	0%
Large (2 1/2" diam.), 4 oz	65	0	0%
Pomegranates, 1/2 fruit, 5 oz	55	0	0%
Pummelo, flesh, 1/2 cup, 4 oz	35	0	0%
Prickly Pears, 1 fruit, 5 oz	50	0	0%
Quinces, 1 fruit, 5 oz	50	0	0%
Rambutan (Rambotang),			
Red/Yellow, 1 med., 2 oz	15	0	0%
Raspberries, 1/2 cup, 2 oz	30	0	0%
Rhubarb, raw, 1/2 cup, 2 oz	15	0	0%

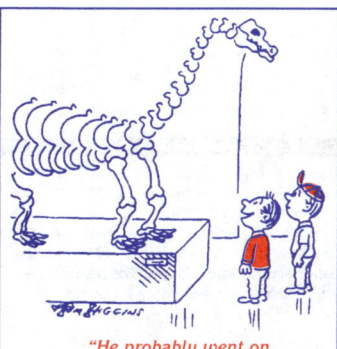

"He probably went on one of those crash diets and starved himself to death!"

FRESH FRUIT (CONT)

	C	F	%fc
WEIGHTS AS PURCHASED			
Sapodilla (Chico), 1 md., 7½ oz	140	2	12%
Sapotes, 1 medium, 11 oz	300	1	3%
Soursop, 1 cup pulp, 8 oz	150	0	0%
Strawberries: 1 cup, 5½ oz	45	0	0%
6 medium/3 large, 2 oz	15	0	0%
1 pint, 12 oz	95	0	0%
Sugar Apples, ½ cup pulp, 4 oz	120	0	0%
Tamarillo, 1 medium, 3 oz	20	0	0%
Tamarind: 1 fruit, ¼ oz	5	0	0%
Tangelo: 1 small, 4 oz	30	0	0%
1 medium, 5 oz	40	0	0%
1 large, 7 oz	55	0	0%
Tangerine, 1 fruit, 4 oz	35	0	0%
Tangor, 1 medium, 4 oz	35	0	0%
Tomato: Cherry, 1 med., ¾ oz	5	0	0%
1 small, 3 oz	25	0	0%
1 medium, 5 oz	35	0	0%
1 large, 7 oz	45	0	0%
1 medium slice	5	0	0%
Canned Tomatoes/Products ~ Page 68-71.			
Tree Tomato (Tamarillo)			
1 medium, 3 oz	20	0	0%
Ugli Fruit, Tangelo type, 5 oz	40	0	0%
Watermelon (flesh only): 1 sl, 8 oz	70	0	0%
1 cup cubed, 5½ oz	50	0	0%
Wax Jambu (Rose Apple),			
1 medium, 2 oz	10	0	0%

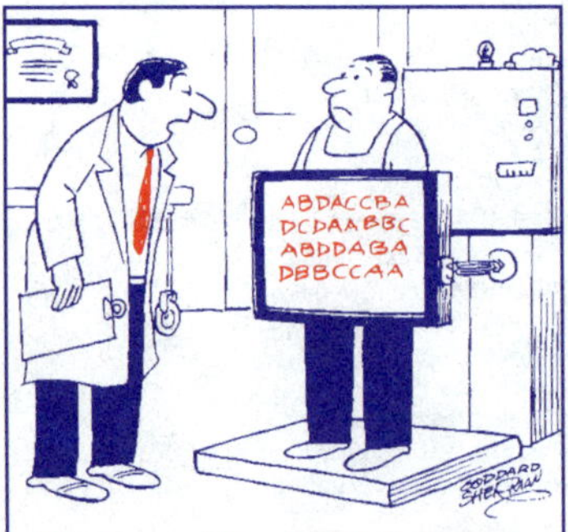

DRIED FRUIT

	C	F	%fc
Apples, 5 rings, 1 oz	75	0	0%
Apricots, 8 halves, 1 oz	65	0	0%
Banana Chips, ½ cup, 1½ oz	160	5	28%
Banana Flakes, 4 Tbsp, 1 oz	80	0	0%
Currants, ¼ cup, 1¼ oz	100	0	0%
Dates: 5 medium dates, 1½ oz	120	0	0%
Large Calif., 3 dates, 2 oz	160	0	0%
½ cup, chopped, 3 oz	240	0	0%
Figs, 3 medium figs, 2 oz	145	0	0%
Longans; Lychees, 1 oz	80	0	0%
Mango Slices, 4 strips, 1 oz	70	0	0%
Mixed Fruit, 1 oz	70	0	0%
Papaya Spears, 1 oz	75	0	0%
Peaches, 2 halves, 1 oz	60	0	0%
Pears, 3 halves, 2 oz	75	0	0%
Pineapple, 1 oz	80	0	0%
Prunes: with pits, 1 oz	60	0	0%
1 Medium (60/lb)	16	0	0%
1 Large (50/lb)	22	0	0%
1 Extra Large (40/lb)	27	0	0%
Without pits, 4 med., 1 oz	70	0	0%
Cooked: w. sugar, ½ c, 5 oz	200	0	0%
w/out sugar, ½ c, 4½ oz	125	0	0%
Raisins, 2 Tbsp, 1 oz package	85	0	0%
½ cup, 2½ oz	215	0	0%

CANDIED GLACE FRUIT

	C	F	%fc
Apricot, 1 medium, 1 oz	100	0	0%
Cherry, 3 large, ½ oz	50	0	0%
Citron/Fruit Peel, 1 oz	90	0	0%
Fig, 1 piece, 1 oz	90	0	0%
Ginger, 1 oz	95	0	0%
Pineapple, 1 slice, 1¼ oz	120	0	0%

FRUIT LEATHER/ROLLS

	C	F	%fc
Average all brands, 1 oz	100	0	0%
Fruit By The Foot, 1 leather	80	0	0%
Fruit Roll-Ups, 1 roll, ½ oz	50	0	0%
Stretch Island Leathers, 2 pces, 1 oz	90	0	0%
Sunkist Fruit Roll, 1 roll	75	0	0%
Other Fruit Confectionery/Snacks/Bars			
~ See Snacks/Granola Bars Page 106.			

"You have a Vitamin E deficiency"

CANNED FRUIT & SNACKS

CANNED FRUIT

	C	F	%fc
SOLIDS & LIQUIDS:			
Per 1/2 Cup (Approx. 4 1/2 oz)			
Apples: sweetened	70	0	0%
Apricots: In water/diet	35	0	0%
In juice/light	60	0	0%
In syrup	105	0	0%
Blackberries/Blueberries			
In heavy syrup	115	0	0%
Cherries, pitted, in water	55	0	0%
In light syrup	85	0	0%
In heavy syrup	110	0	0%
In extra heavy syrup	130	0	0%
Fruit Cocktail: In water/diet	40	0	0%
In juice/light	55	0	0%
In light syrup	80	0	0%
In heavy syrup	95	0	0%
Fruit Salad: In water/diet	35	0	0%
In juice/Light	60	0	0%
In heavy syrup	95	0	0%
Gooseberries: Light syrup	90	0	0%
Grapefruit: Juice pack	45	0	0%
In light syrup	75	0	0%
Mixed Fruit: In water/diet	40	0	0%
In fruit juices	60	0	0%
In light syrup	60	0	0%
In heavy syrup	100	0	0%
Mandarin Oranges: In water	40	0	0%
In light syrup	80	0	0%
Peaches (halves or slices):			
In water/diet	30	0	0%
In juice/light	50	0	0%
In light syrup	70	0	0%
drained, 1/2 peach	40	0	0%
In heavy syrup	100	0	0%
Pears: In water/diet	35	0	0%
In juice/light	60	0	0%
In heavy syrup	100	0	0%
Pineapple:			
(Chunks/Crushed/Spears/Wedges/Slices)			
In own juice	70	0	0%
In heavy syrup	90	0	0%
Slices, drained, 2 slices			
In own juice	30	0	0%
In heavy syrup	45	0	0%

	C	F	%fc
Per 1/2 Cup			
Plums: In water	50	0	0%
In juice	75	0	0%
In light syrup, 3 plums	85	0	0%
In heavy syrup, 1/2 cup, 3 plums	160	0	0%
	120	0	0%
Prunes: In heavy syrup	120	0	0%
4 prunes	70	0	0%
Raspberries, in heavy syrup	120	0	0%
Strawberries: In water	25	0	0%
In heavy syrup	120	0	0%
Tropical Fruit Salad:			
In light syrup	80	0	0%
In heavy syrup	95	0	0%

FRUIT SNACK CUPS

Del Monte Snack Cups

	C	F	%fc
EZ Open Lid (4 1/2 oz cup):			
Diced Peaches/Pears/Mixed,			
In heavy syrup	90	0	0%
In extra light syrup	60	0	0%
In fruit juices	60	0	0%
Plastic Cup (3 1/2 oz):			
Diced Peaches/Pears/Mixed			
In light syrup	70	0	0%

"And how long has celery been your basic diet?"

FRUIT & VEGETABLE JUICES

QUICK GUIDE
ORANGE JUICE

Per 8 fl.oz Unless Indicated

	C	F	%fc
Average ~ Fresh or Sweetened:			
1/2 Cup, 4 fl.oz	55	0	0%
Small Glass, 6 fl.oz	82	0	0%
Regular Glass, 8 fl.oz	110	0	0%
8 3/4 fl.oz Box	120	0	0%
10 fl.oz Bottle	140	0	0%
11 1/2 fl.oz Can	160	0	0%
16 fl.oz Bottle	220	0	0%
64 fl.oz Bottle	880	0	0%

OTHER JUICES

Per 8 fl.oz Unless Indicated

Average All Brands	C	F	%fc
Aloe Vera Juice, unsweet., 2 oz	5	0	0%
Apple Juice, 1/2 cup	58	0	0%
6 fl.oz	85	0	0%
8 fl.oz	115	0	0%
10 fl.oz Bottle	145	0	0%
64 fl.oz	920	0	0%
Blueberry Juice, 8 fl.oz	90	0	0%
Carrot Juice: Fresh, 6 fl.oz	60	0	0%
Sweetened, 6 fl.oz	75	0	0%
Cranberry Juice, Cocktail/Blend			
8 fl.oz	120	0	0%
Grape Juice, 8 fl.oz	130	0	0%
Grapefruit Juice, 8 fl.oz	100	0	0%
Lemon Juice: 1 Tbsp	4	0	0%
1 cup, 8 fl.oz	60	0	0%
Lime Juice, 1 Tbsp	4	0	0%
Orange Juice, 8 fl.oz	110	0	0%
Passion Fruit Juice (Fresh):			
Purple, 1 cup, 8 fl.oz	125	0	0%
Yellow, 1 cup, 8 fl.oz	150	0	0%
Papaya/Peach Nectar, 8 fl.oz	140	0	0%
Pear Nectar, 8 fl.oz	150	0	0%
Pineapple Juice, 8 fl.oz	110	0	0%
Prune Juice, 8 fl.oz	170	0	0%
Strawb./Raspberry Juice, 8 fl.oz	100	0	0%
Tangerine Juice, 8 fl.oz	100	0	0%
Tomato Juice, 8 fl.oz	50	0	0%
Vegetable Juice, 8 fl.oz	50	0	0%
Fruit Blends, average, 8 fl.oz	120	0	0%
Fruit Nectars, average, 8 fl.oz	140	0	0%

BRANDS

Per 8 fl.oz Unless Indicated

	C	F	%fc
AFTER THE FALL			
Amaretto Almond, 12 oz can	170	0	0%
American Pie Cherry, 12 oz can	190	0	0%
Apple Juice, 10 oz bottle	110	0	0%
Apple Apricot, 1 cup, 8 oz	100	0	0%
Apple Rasp./Strawberry, 10 oz bottle	120	0	0%
Banana Casablanca, 10 oz bottle	120	0	0%
Berrymeister, 12 oz can	160	0	0%
Capeland Cranberry, 10 oz bottle	130	0	0%
Grapefruit Juice (Pink), 10 oz can	100	0	0%
Spicy Lemon: 12 oz can	150	0	0%
BOKU			
Coolers, Fruit Drinks, aver., 8 oz	120	0	0%
BRIGHT & EARLY			
Orange Juice (Chilled/Frozen)	120	0	0%
Grape Juice (Frozen)	140	0	0%
CAMPBELL'S			
Tomato Juice, 8 fl.oz	50	0	0%
10.5 fl.oz	70	0	0%
V-8 Vegetable Juice	50	0	0%
CAPRI SUN			
Foil Pouch, 6.57 oz, all types	100	0	0%
CHIQUITA			
Frozen Concentrates, prep.			
Average all varieties, 8 fl.oz	130	0	0%
DEL MONTE			
Pineapple Juice: Fresh, 8 fl.oz	110	0	0%
From Concentrate, 8 fl.oz	130	0	0%
Prune Juice, 8 fl.oz	170	0	0%
Tomato Juice: Fresh, 8 fl.oz	40	0	0%
From Concentrate, 8 fl.oz	50	0	0%
DOLE			
Pineapple Juice, 8 fl.oz	110	0	0%
Frozen concentrates, prepared			
Average all varieties, 8 fl.oz	130	0	0%
FARMERS MARKET			
All varieties, average	120	0	0%

FRUIT & VEGETABLE JUICES CONT

Per 8 fl.oz Unless Indicated | C | F | %fc

FIVE ALIVE
Citrus beverage, 8 fl.oz — **120** / 0 / 0%

FRUITOPIA
Apple Raspb.; Trop. Consideration — **75** / 0 / 0%
Lemonade Love; Cranberry Lemon — **115** / 0 / 0%
Pink L'nade; Tangerine Wavelength — **118** / 0 / 0%
Other flavors, average — **125** / 0 / 0%
Iced Teas: See Page 123.

HAWAIIAN PUNCH
Fruit Juicy, Red, 8 fl. oz — **120** / 0 / 0%
  Box, 8.45fl. oz — **130** / 0 / 0%

HEINKE'S: Black Cherry — **180** / 0 / 0%
100% Cranberry — **60** / 0 / 0%
Other varieties, average — **120** / 0 / 0%

HI-C: Orange Juice
Chilled/Premium Choice, 8 fl. oz — **110** / 0 / 0%
  10 fl. oz bottle — **140** / 0 / 0%
Calcium Rich, 8 fl. oz — **120** / 0 / 0%
Other Juices Drinks
Average, 8 fl. oz — **130** / 0 / 0%
  8.45 fl. oz box, average — **135** / 0 / 0%
  11.5 fl. oz can — **180** / 0 / 0%

HOOD
Grapefruit Juice (Select) — **100** / 0 / 0%
Natural Blenders, average — **130** / 0 / 0%
Orange Juice: Select — **120** / 0 / 0%
  Calcium Rich — **120** / 0 / 0%

HOLLYWOOD
Carrot Juice, 12 oz Bottle — **120** / 0 / 0%

JUICY JUICE
Apple Grape, 8.45 fl. oz box — **120** / 0 / 0%
Berry, 8.45 fl. oz box — **130** / 0 / 0%
Cherry, 8.45 fl. oz box — **130** / 0 / 0%
Punch, 8.45 fl. oz box — **140** / 0 / 0%
Tropical, 8.45 fl. oz box — **150** / 0 / 0%

KERNS NECTARS
Pineapple Coconut Nectar, 8 fl. oz — **200** / 0 / 0%
  11.5 fl. oz box — **290** / 0 / 0%
Other nectars, average, 8 fl.oz — **150** / 0 / 0%

KOOL AID
Koolers, average, 8.45 fl. oz — **140** / 0 / 0%
Fruit Drinks, average, 8 fl. oz — **100** / 0 / 0%
  Sugar Free, 8 fl. oz — **3** / 0 / 0%

KNUDSEN
Fruit Juices: Apple — **110** / 0 / 0%
  Apple Blends, all varieties — **120** / 0 / 0%
  Black Cherry; Prunes — **180** / 0 / 0%
  Grape; Pomegranate — **150** / 0 / 0%
  Grapefruit — **100** / 0 / 0%
  Just Cranberry; Tomato — **60** / 0 / 0%
  Orange — **100** / 0 / 0%
  Pear — **120** / 0 / 0%
Nectars: Coconut — **140** / 5 / 30%
  Other Nectars, average — **130** / 0 / 0%
Blends: Coolers — **120** / 0 / 0%
  Cranberry flavors — **120** / 0 / 0%
  Lemon Ginger Echinecea — **100** / 0 / 0%
  Mango Peach; Or. Mango — **120** / 0 / 0%
  P'apple Coconut; Rain Forest — **125** / 0 / 0%
  Raspberry Hibiscus — **90** / 0 / 0%
  Raspberry/Strawberry flavors — **120** / 0 / 0%
  Strawb. Guava — **110** / 0 / 0%
  Strawb. Kiwi; Tropical Punch — **120** / 0 / 0%
Citrus Juices: Rio Rea Grapefruit — **140** / 0 / 0%
  Lemonade (Natural) — **120** / 0 / 0%
  Natural Breakfast Juice — **110** / 0 / 0%
Morning Blend: Vita Juice — **120** / 0 / 0%
Frozen Juice Concentrates:
  Black Cherry — **130** / 0 / 0%
  Cranberry — **70** / 0 / 0%
  Cranberry Nectar; Org. Grape — **150** / 0 / 0%
  Other flavors, average — **120** / 0 / 0%
Floats: Orange — **140** / 0 / 0%
Spritzers: Aver. all flavors, 12 oz — **170** / 0 / 0%
  Lights, all flavors, 12 oz — **110** / 0 / 0%
TeaZers: All flavors, 12 oz — **110** / 0 / 0%
Very Veggie, 8 fl. oz — **50** / 0 / 0%

L & A
Papaya Delight Juice, 8 fl.oz — **130** / 0 / 0%
Papaya Nectar, 8 fl.oz — **130** / 0 / 0%

LIBBY
Orange Juice, 8 fl.oz — **105** / 0 / 0%
Juicy Juice, 8 fl.oz — **130** / 0 / 0%
Nectar, 1 can, $11^{1}/_{2}$ fl.oz — **220** / 0 / 0%

FRUIT & VEGETABLE JUICES CONT

Per 8 fl.oz Unless Indicated — **C** **F** **%fc**   *Per 8 fl.oz Unless Indicated* — **C** **F** **%fc**

MAUNA LA'I
	C	F	%fc
All flavors, 8 fl.oz	130	0	0%
Grapefruit Juice, 10 fl. oz bottle	120	0	0%
Pink Cocktail, 8 fl. oz	160	0	0%

MINUTE MAID
100% Juices - Per 8 fl. oz
	C	F	%fc
Apple	112	0	0%
Lemon (Frozen)	50	0	0%
Orange Juice	114	0	0%
Pink Grapefruit	124	0	0%

Fruit Drinks/Punch - Per 8 fl. oz
	C	F	%fc
Cranberry Apple Raspb. Blend	123	0	0%
Concord Punch	127	0	0%
Fruit Punch	112	0	0%

Chilled Singles - 16 oz Bottle
	C	F	%fc
Berry Punch	240	0	0%
Lemonade	220	0	0%
Orange Juice	220	0	0%
Tropical Punch	240	0	0%

Multipak - Per 8 oz Bottle
	C	F	%fc
Fruit Punch	120	0	0%
Lemonade	110	0	0%
Orange Juice	110	0	0%
Tropical Punch	120	0	0%

Boxed Juices - Per 8.45 fl.oz
	C	F	%fc
Cherry Grape	130	0	0%
Orange Juice; Apple Juice	120	0	0%
Berry/Fruit/Tropical Punch	120	0	0%

MOTT'S
	C	F	%fc
Apple Raspberry, 10 fl. oz	140	0	0%
Apple Cranberry, P/apple Orange, 10 fl. oz	170	0	0%
Boxes, all flavors, 8.45 fl. oz	120	0	0%
Mini Motts, 4.23 oz	60	0	0%
Clamato Juice, 8 fl.oz	110	0	0%
Fruit Basket Cocktails, prep.	130	0	0%
Grapefruit (from conc.), prep.	120	0	0%
Orange Juice (from conc.)	105	0	0%
Vegetable Juice, prep, 8 fl. oz	60	0	0%

OCEAN SPRAY
Per 8 fl. oz
	C	F	%fc
Cranberry Grape	170	0	0%
Cranberry Juice Cocktail	140	0	0%
Reduced Calorie	50	0	0%
Light Style Low Calorie	40	0	0%

OCEAN SPRAY (Cont)
	C	F	%fc
Cranicot; Crantastic; Cranapple	160	0	0%
Cranberry- Raspb./Strawberry	140	0	0%
Other Cranberry flavors	160	0	0%
Reduced Calorie	50	0	0%
Fruit Punch	130	0	0%
Light Style Low Calorie	40	0	0%
Grapefruit: 100% Juice	100	0	0%
Pink Juice Cocktail	120	0	0%
Ruby Red Drink	130	0	0%
Refreshers flavors, average	130	0	0%
Ruby Red Tangerine Grapefruit	130	0	0%
Summer Cooler	120	0	0%
Vegetable Cocktail	70	0	0%

ODWALLA:
	C	F	%fc
Boyzenberry Mango	140	0	0%
C Monster	300	0	0%
Fruitshake Blackberry	160	0	0%
Grapefruit Juice	90	0	0%
Guanaba Dabba Doo!	130	0	0%
Lotta Colada	160	0	0%
Mango Tango	150	0	0%
Mo Beta	280	0	0%
Orange Juice	120	0	0%
Raspberry Smoothie	140	0	0%
Strawberry Smoothie	100	0	0%
Strawberry Banana Smoothie	100	0	0%
Strawberry Go Man Go	100	0	0%
Super Protein	400	0	0%
Vegetable Cocktail	70	0	0%

ORANGE JULIUS
Per 16 fl. oz
	C	F	%fc
Orange	265	0	0%
Pina Colada	300	0	0%
Strawberry	340	0	0%
Raspberry Cream Supreme	510	20	35%
Tropical Cream Supreme	510	25	44%

REALEMON - REALIME (Borden)
Lemon/Lime Juice (from concentrate)
	C	F	%fc
1 teaspoon	0	0	0%
2 Tbsp, 1 fl. oz	6	0	0%
1/2 cup, 4 fl.oz	24	0	0%

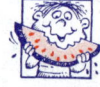

116

FRUIT & VEGETABLE JUICES CONT

Per 8 fl.oz Unless Indicated — **C** | **F** | **%fc**

Item	C	F	%fc
SANTA CRUZ Natural 100%			
Average all varieties, 8 fl. oz	120	0	0%
Sparkling varieties, 8 fl. oz	150	0	0%
SNAPPLE			
Cranberry Royal, 10 fl. oz	150	0	0%
Grapefruit Juice, 10 fl. oz	110	0	0%
Fruit Drink Blends, 8 fl. oz	120	0	0%
Orange Juice, 8 fl. oz	105	0	0%
Orangeade, 8 fl. oz	120	0	0%
SQUEEZIT			
Per 6.75 fl. oz Pkg			
Acrobat Apple, Cherry	90	0	0%
100 Berry, Lifesaver Watermelon	90	0	0%
Other flavors	90	0	0%
SUNNY DELIGHT			
Florida Citrus, 8 fl. oz	120	0	0%
Calcium Rich, 8 fl. oz	150	0	0%
Florida Citrus Punch, 8 fl. oz	120	0	0%
Tropical Fruit Punch, 8 fl. oz	120	0	0%
Sunny Delight Lite, 8 oz	20	0	0%
SUNSWEET			
Prune Juice, 8 fl. oz	180	0	0%
Prune Juice with Pulp	180	0	0%
S&W			
Apple Juice, 8 fl. oz	115	0	0%
Orange Juice, 8 fl. oz	110	0	0%
Grapefruit Juice, unswt'd, 8 fl. oz	105	0	0%
Tomato Juice, 5.5 fl. oz	30	0	0%
TANG			
Fruit Box (8 .45 fl. oz):			
Average all flavors	140	0	0%
Mix: Made up, 8 fl. oz			
Regular (2 Tbsp dry)	100	0	0%
Sugar Free	7	0	0%
TROPICANA			
Grapefruit Juice	90	0	0%
Orange Juice, 8 fl. oz	110	0	0%
10 fl. oz bottle	130	0	0%
Premium Plus:			
Orange Juice w. Calcium	110	0	0%
Punch: Berry; P'apple, 8 fl. oz	120	0	0%
Citrus; Cranberry, 8 fl. oz	140	0	0%
Fruit Punch, 8 fl. oz	130	0	0%
Seasons Best: Grape Juice	160	0	0%
Grapefruit Juice, 8 fl. oz	90	0	0%
10 fl. oz bottle	110	0	0%
11.5 fl. oz can	120	0	0%
Tropics: Aver. all flavors, 8 fl. oz	110	0	0%
Twister: Average, 8 fl. oz	120	0	0%
10 fl. oz bottle	150	0	0%
11.5 fl. oz can	160	0	0%
Light, average, 8 fl. oz	35	0	0%
10 fl. oz bottle	50	0	0%
TREE TOP: *Per 8 fl. oz*			
Apple Juice	120	0	0%
Apple Citrus/Pear	120	0	0%
Apple Cranberry/Grape	130	0	0%
Grape Juice or Sparkling	150	0	0%
Grapefruit Juice	105	0	0%
Orange Juice	120	0	0%
8.45 fl. oz Boxes, all varieties	120	0	0%
V-8 VEGETABLE JUICE			
V-8 Vegetable Juice, aver., all varieties			
1 cup, 8 fl oz	50	0	0%
11.5 oz Can	70	0	0%
VERYFINE: Apple Cranberry	130	0	0%
Cranberry Juice Drink	160	0	0%
Fruit Punch	130	0	0%
Grape Juice (100%)	150	0	0%
Grape Drink	130	0	0%
Grapefruit Juice (100%)	100	0	0%
Pink	120	0	0%
Guava Straw.; Lemon Lime	120	0	0%
Per 8 fl.oz Unless Indicated			
Orange Juice (100%)	120	0	0%
Orange Drink	140	0	0%
Papaya Punch	120	0	0%
Pineapple Orange	130	0	0%
WELCH'S: Regular Juices:			
Average all blends, 8 fl. oz	130	0	0%
8.45 fl. oz Box, average	150	0	0%
Frozen Juice Concentrates:			
(Reconstituted, Per 8 fl. oz)	130	0	0%
Grape	160	0	0%
White Grape Classic Raspberry	150	0	0%
Other flavors, average	130	0	0%
Lite Cranberry/Raspberry	50	0	0%

VEGETABLES - FRESH OR FROZEN

Edible Portion (Raw Weight Unless Indicated)	C	F	%fc
Alfalfa Sprouts, 1/2 cup, 1/2 oz	5	0	0%
Artichokes, Globe/French:			
1 medium, 4 1/2 oz	65	0	0%
Artichoke Heart, 1/2 cup, 3 oz	40	0	0%
Asparagus, raw/frozen:			
4 medium spears, 2 oz	15	0	0%
Cuts & tips, 1/2 cup, 3 oz	25	0	0%
Bamboo Shoots, ckd, 1/2 c, 4 oz	15	0	0%
Beans: Green/Snap, 1/2 c, 2 oz	20	0	0%
Broadbeans, ckd, 1/2 cup, 3 oz	90	0	0%
Butterbeans, 1/2 cup, 3 oz	90	0	0%
Lima, baby, 1/2 cup, 3 oz	90	0	0%
Dry Beans, average all types: (Kidney, Brown, Haricot, Lima, Mung, Navy, Pinto, Red, White)			
Raw, 2 Tbsp, 1 oz	95	<1	4%
1 cup, 7 oz	665	3	4%
Cooked, 1 oz	35	0	4%
1/2 cup, 3 oz	105	<1	4%
Soybeans: Mature, dry, 1 oz	110	5	40%
Dry, 1/2 cup, 3 1/2 oz	385	18	40%
Cooked, 1/2 cup, 3 oz	105	5	40%
Bean Sprouts, aver., 1/2 c., 3 oz	25	0	0%
Beets, cooked, 1/2 c, slices, 3 oz	25	0	0%
1 beet, 2" diam., 2 oz	17	0	0%
Beet Greens, ckd, 1/2 c., 2 1/2 oz	20	0	0%
Black Eyed Peas, ckd, 1/2 c., 2 oz	160	<1	5%
Bok Choy (Chinese Chard), 3 oz	12	0	0%
Broccoli: Raw, 1/2 cup, 1 1/2 oz	12	0	0%
1 spear (5 oz edible)	40	0	0%
Cooked, 1/2 cup, 3 oz	25	0	0%
Brussel Sprouts, ckd, 1/2 c, 3 oz	35	0	0%
Cabbage, average all varieties:			
Raw, shred., 1/2 cup, 1 1/4 oz	8	0	0%
Cooked, 1/2 cup, 2 1/2 oz	15	0	0%
Carrots: Ckd, 1/2 c. sl., 2 1/4 oz	35	0	0%
Raw, 1 medium (7 1/2"), 3 oz	33	0	0%
Raw, 1 lb, (5-6 med)	175	0	0%
4 sticks (4"), 1 1/2 oz	15	0	0%
Shredded, 1/2 cup, 2 oz	25	0	0%
Cauliflower, cooked:			
3 floret, 1/2 c. 1" pcs, 3 oz	15	0	0%
1/2 medium (15 oz raw)	100	0	0%
Celeriac, 1/2 cup, raw, 2 3/4 oz	30	0	0%
Celery, 1 stalk, 7 1/2", 1 1/2 oz	5	0	0%
Diced, 1/2 cup, 2 1/4 oz	10	0	0%
Chard (Swiss), 1/2 cup, ckd, 3 oz	20	0	0%

Edible Portion (Raw Weight Unless Indicated)	C	F	%fc
Chick Peas (Garbanzo Beans):			
Dry, 1 cup, 6 oz	550	10	15%
Cooked, 1 cup, 6 oz	270	4	15%
Chicory/Witlof — See Endive			
Chicory, Greens, 1/2 cup, 3 oz	20	0	0%
Chives, chopped, 1 Tbsp	1	0	0%
Collards, 1/2 cup, 3 oz	15	0	0%
Corn, yellow/white:			
Raw, kernels, 1/2 c., 2 3/4 oz	65	1	11%
Ear (5"x 1 3/4"), 5 1/2 oz	80	1	11%
Trimmed to 3 1/2" long	60	1	11%
Cooked, kernels, 1/4 c., 1 1/2 oz	35	<1	11%
(Also see Frozen & Canned Corn Page 121)			
Cress, Garden, 1/2 cup, 1 oz	10	0	0%
Cucumber, 1 whole, 11 oz	40	0	0%
1/2 cup slices, 2 oz	5	0	0%
Dandelion Greens, 1/2 cup, 1 oz	15	0	0%
Eggplant: 1 whole, 4 1/2 oz	40	0	0%
1/2 cup, 1" pieces, 1 1/2 oz	10	0	0%
1 slice, fried, 1 oz	40	4	90%
Endive, Belgian/French:			
1 med. head (6"), 2 1/2 oz	12	0	0%
Fennel, 2 oz	10	0	0%
Garlic, 1 clove	4	0	0%
Ginger: 1/4 cup slices, 1 oz	20	0	0%
Crystallized (sugared), 1 oz	95	0	0%
Horseradish, 1 pod, 3/4 oz	4	0	0%
Jerusalem Artichoke, 1/2 cup	60	0	0%
Jicama, raw, 1/2 cup	25	0	0%
Kale, 1/2 cup, 2 oz	20	0	0%
Kohlrabi, 1/2 cup, cooked, 3 oz	25	0	0%
Leeks, cooked, 1 whole, 4 oz	40	0	0%
Lentils, green/brown: Dry, 1 oz	95	0	0%
Dry, 1 cup, 6 1/2 oz	620	0	0%
Cooked, 1/2 cup, 3 1/2 oz	115	0	0%
Lettuce: 1 c., chop./shred., 2 1/2 oz	10	0	0%
Butterhead, 2 leaves, 1/2 oz	2	0	0%
Cos/Romaine, 1/2., shred., 2 1/2 oz	4	0	0%
Iceberg: 1 leaf, 3/4 oz	3	0	0%
1 medium head, 15-16 oz	60	0	0%
Lotus Root, 10 slices, ckd, 3 oz	60	0	0%
Mung Bean Sprouts, 1/2 cup	15	0	0%
Mushrooms: Raw, 1/2 cup, 1 oz	10	0	0%
Cooked, 1/2 cup, 2 1/2 oz	20	0	0%
Mustard Greens, 1/2 cup, 1 oz	7	0	0%
Okra, ckd., 1/2 cup, slices, 2 3/4 oz	25	0	0%

VEGETABLES - FRESH OR FROZEN CONT

Edible Portion (Raw Weight Unless Indicated)	C	F	%fc
Onions: Raw, 1 medium, 4 oz	45	0	0%
1/2 cup, chopped, 3 oz	30	0	0%
Dehydrated flakes, 1/4 c, 1/2 oz	45	0	0%
Rings, breaded/fried, 2 rings	80	5	56%
Scallions, 1/2 cup, 2 oz	15	0	0%
Spring, 1/4 cup, chopped, 1 oz	6	0	0%
Parsley, chopped, 1/2 cup, 1 oz	10	0	0%
Parsnips, 1 medium, 4 oz	80	0	0%
Cooked, 1/2 cup slices, 2 3/4 oz	65	0	0%
Peas: Green, 1/4 cup, 1 1/2 oz	35	0	0%
raw, with pods, 1/2 lb	70	0	0%
Snow Peas (8-9 pods), 1 oz	10	0	0%
Split, dry, hulled, 1 oz	50	0	0%
cooked, 1 cup, 7 oz	230	1	4%
Peppers: Bell, 1 med, 5 oz	25	0	0%
1/2 cup, chopped, raw, 1 3/4 oz	12	0	0%
1 ring (3" diam. x 1/4" thick)	2	0	0%
Sweet, 1 medium, 5 oz	35	0	0%
Chili: Green/Red, 1 1/2 oz	18	0	0%
Habanero, 1 only, 8g	11	0	0%
Pigeon Peas, cooked, 1/2 cup	85	1	9%
Pimientos, 3 medium, 3 1/2 oz	25	0	0%
Potatoes: Raw (with skin)			
1 Baby, Gourmet, 2 oz	45	0	0%
1 small, 3 oz	65	0	0%
1 medium, 5 oz	110	0	0%
1 peeled, 4 oz	90	0	0%
1 large, 8 oz	180	0	0%
1 Extra lge. (Russet), 12 oz	270	0	0%
Mashed with milk and fat			
1/2 cup, 3 1/2 oz	110	4	33%
Baked (no fat); large, 10 oz raw:			
Plain, with skin, 7 oz	220	0	0%
without skin, 5 1/2 oz	145	0	0%
With Toppings:			
+ 2 tsp fat	290	8	25%
+ Sour Cr./Chives, 2 Tbsp	270	6	13%
+ Plain Yoghurt, 2 Tbsp	240	1	4%
+ Grated Cheese, 1 oz	330	9	11%
+ Cottage Cheese, 2 oz	280	2	6%
Roasted (with fat), 3 oz	155	8	23%
French Fries:			
small serving, 2 1/2 oz	220	12	50%
medium serving, 4 oz	350	20	50%
Frozen, uncooked, 18 fries, 4 oz	185	7	34%
Oven-heated, 18 fries, 4 oz	185	7	34%
Fried, 18 fries, 3 oz	275	15	50%

Edible Portion (Raw Weight Unless Indicated)	C	F	%fc
Potatoes (Cont):			
Hash Browns:			
Homemade, 1/2 cup, 2 1/2 oz	165	10	55%
with Butter Sauce, 2 1/2 oz	125	6	43%
Au Gratin, 1/2 cup, 4.3 oz	160	9	43%
Pancakes, 1 only, 2 1/2 oz	495	13	24%
Puffs, fried, 4 puffs, 1 oz	65	3	42%
Scalloped, 1/2 cup, 4 1/4 oz	105	4	35%
Frozen Potatoes (As Purchased):			
Ore-Ida: Steak Fries, 3 oz	110	3.5	29%
Potato Wedges, 4 oz	120	4.5	34%
Frozen Crispers, 3 oz	220	13	53%
Crispy Crunchies, 3 oz	160	8	45%
Fast Fries, 3 oz	150	6	36%
Golden Crinkles, 3 oz	140	3.5	23%
Golden Patties, 1 patty, 3 oz	70	0	0%
Golden Twirls, 3 oz	150	6	36%
Hash Browns, 1 patty, 3 oz	70	0	0%
Country Style, 1 cup	60	0	0%
Mashed Potato w. Butter,			
3/4 cup	90	2.5	25%
Potatoes O'Brien, 3/4 cup	150	6	36%
Shoestrings, 3 oz	150	5	30%
Sweet Potatoes			
5 slices, 5 1/2 oz	190	0	0%
Tater Tots, 9 pces, 3 oz	160	8	45%
Taters 3 oz	150	7	42%
Texas Crispers, 3 oz	150	7	42%
Zesties, 3 oz	160	9	50%
Simp: Microwave French Fries,			
3 oz	220	10	40%
Potato Salad, 1/2 cup, 4 1/2 oz	180	10	50%
Poi, 1/2 cup, 4 1/4 oz	135	0	0%
Pumpkin, mashed, 1/2 c., 4 oz	25	0	0%
Purslane, cooked, 1/2 c., 2 oz	10	0	0%
Radish: aver., 10 only, 1 1/2 oz	10	0	0%
Oriental, 1/2 c. slices, 1 1/2 oz	10	0	0%
Rutabagas, ckd., 1/2 c. cubes, 3 oz	30	0	0%
Salsify, ckd, 1/2 c. slices, 2 1/2 oz	45	0	0%
Sauerkraut, 1/2 cup, 4 oz	25	0	0%
Seaweed, average all types:			
Dried, 1 oz	50	0	0%
Soaked, drained, 1 oz	15	0	0%
Nori/Laver, dried, 6 sheets, 1/2 oz	35	0	0%

VEGETABLES - FRESH OR FROZEN cont

Edible Portion
(Raw Weight Unless Indicated)

Item	C	F	%fc
Shallots, chopped, 1 Tbsp	7	0	0%
Soybeans ~ See Beans Page 57-62,118			
(Soy Products/Tofu/Tempeh ~See Pages 60)			
Sorrel, raw, 1/2 cup, 4 oz	20	0	0%
Spinach, cooked, 1/2 cup, 3 oz	20	0	0%
Squash: Summer, average			
raw, 1/2 cup slices, 2 1/4 oz	13	0	0%
cooked, 1/2 cup slices, 3 oz	18	0	0%
Winter, cooked:			
Acorn, 1/2 cup cubes, 3 1/2 oz	55	0	0%
1/2 medium (10 oz raw wt.)	85	0	0%
Butternut, 1/2 c. cubes, 3 1/2 oz	40	0	0%
1/4 medium (9 oz raw wt.)	95	0	0%
Hubbard, 1/2 c. cubes, 3 1/2 oz	50	0	0%
Spaghetti, 1/2 cup, 2 3/4 oz	23	0	0%
Succotash, ckd, 1/2 cup, 3 1/3 oz	110	1	8%
Sweetcorn — See Corn.			
Sweet Potatoes: Cooked with Skin			
No fat, 1 only, 4 oz	120	0	0%
No skin, mash, 1/2 c., 5 1/2 oz	170	0	0%
Swedes, 1/2 cup, 3 oz	45	0	0%
Taro, cooked, 1/2 cup, 2 oz	95	0	0%
Tomatoes: See Fruit ~ Page 112			
1 medium, 5 oz	35	0	0%
1 large, 7 oz	45	0	0%
Cooked, 1/2 cup, 4 1/4 oz	30	0	0%
Fried, 1 small, 3 oz	60	4	60%
Tomatillo, 1 oz	7	0	0%
Turnips: White, ckd, 1/2 cup, 3 oz	15	0	0%
Greens, ckd, 1/2 cup, 2 1/2 oz	15	0	0%
Water Chestnuts, 4 nuts	40	0	0%
1/2 cup slices, 2 1/4 oz	65	0	0%
Watercress, 10 sprigs, 1 oz	4	0	0%
Yam, cooked, 1/2 cup, 2 1/2 oz	80	0	0%
Mountain (Hawaii), ckd, 1/2 cup	60	0	0%
Yardlong Bean, 1 pod, 1/2 oz	7	0	0%
Zucchini, 1 medium, 10 oz	45	0	0%
1/2 cup slices, cooked, 3 oz	13	0	0%

FROZEN VEGETABLES - MIXED

Item	C	F	%fc
BIG VALLEY			
Stew Vegetables, 2/3 cup, 3 oz	40	0	0%
Other varieties, 3/4 cup, 3 oz	25	0	0%
BIRDS EYE			
Combination Vegetables: *Per Serve*			
French Beans s/Almonds, 3 oz	50	2	36%
Peas with Pearl Onions, 3 1/2 oz	70	0	0%
Peas & Potatoes w. Cr. Sce, 5 oz	190	12	56%
Cheese Sauce Combination Veges:			
Average all types, 5 oz	130	6	40%
Internationals: *Per 3 1/2 oz*			
Bavarian; Californian	90	5	50%
Austrian; French	70	4	51%
New England	100	5	45%
Japanese	60	3	45%
Stir Fry: Average 3.3 oz	35	0	0%
International Rice: Country	90	0	0%
French; Spanish, 3.3 oz	35	0	0%
Farm Fresh Mixtures: *Per 4 oz (3/4 cup)*			
Broccoli/Carrots/W. Chestnuts	40	0	0%
Broccoli/Corn/Red Peppers	60	1	15%
Broccoli, Other mixes, average	35	0	0%
Brussels Sprouts/Cauli./Carrots	40	0	0%
Cauliflower/Carrots/Snow Peas	40	0	0%
FRESHLIKE			
Chuckwagon, Mixed Veges, 3 1/2 oz	70	0	0%
Peas & Carrots, 3 1/2 oz	65	0	0%
Other varieties, average, 3 1/2 oz	30	0	0%
GREEN GIANT			
American Mixtures: *Per 3/4 Cup*			
Corn, Broccoli, Red Pepper	60	0	0%
Gr. Beans, Pots, Onion, Red Pepper	45	1	20%
Sweet Peas, Potatoes, Carrots, 2/3 c.	70	1.5	19%
Other mixtures, aver., 3/4 cup	30	0	0%
Butter Sauce Vegetables: *Per Serving*			
Baby Brussel Sprouts, 2/3 cup	60	1.5	23%
Lima Beans, 2/3 cup	120	2.5	19%
Broc, Caulif, Carrots, Corn, Peas, 3/4 cup	60	2	30%
Broc, Pasta, Peas, Corn, Red Peppers, 3/4 cup	70	2	25%
Broccoli Spears, 4 oz	50	1.5	28%
Cut Leaf Spinach, cup	40	1.5	35%

Continued Next Page.

VEGETABLES - CANNED/BOTTLED

	C	F	%fc
FROZEN VEGES (Cont)			
GREEN GIANT (Cont)			
Butter Sauce Vegetables (Cont):			
Peas, all varieties, 3/4 cup	100	2	18%
Mixed Vegetables, 3/4 cup	70	2	25%
Corn: Niblets, 2/3 cup	130	3	20%
Shoepeg White, 3/4 cup	120	2.5	18%
Cheese & Cream Sauce Veg: *Per Serving*			
In Cheese Sauce: Cauliflower, 1/2 c.	60	2.5	38%
Broccoli varieties, 2/3 cup	80	2.5	28%
Cream Style Corn, 1/2 cup	110	1	6%
Creamed Spinach, 1/2 cup	80	3	33%
Create A Meal! Vegetables			
Aver. all varieties, prep., 1/3 pkg	330	11	30%
Sw. & Sr. Stir Fry, prep., 1/3 pkg	270	7	20%
Teriyaki Stir Fry, prep., 1/3 pkg	240	6	20%
Harvest Fresh:			
Gr. Beans & Almonds, 2/3 cup	60	3	45%
Sweetcorn & Pearl Onions, 1/2 c.	50	0	0%
LA CHOY			
Mixed Fancy Vegetables, 1/2 cup	12	0	0%

CANNED/BOTTLED

	C	F	%fc
Solids & Liquid			
Artichoke Hearts, plain, 1 oz (1)	30	0	0%
Marinated, 1 oz	60	5	75%
Asparagus (Tips/Cuts/Spears), 1/2 cup, 4 1/2 oz	20	0	0%
Bamboo Shoots, 1 cup, 4 1/2 oz	25	0	0%
Bean Salad, 1/2 cup, 3 oz	90	0	0%
Bean Sprouts, 2/3 cup	10	0	0%
Beans: Green, 1/2 cup, 4 1/4 oz	20	0	0%
Baked Beans, 1/2 cup, 4 1/2 oz	120	<1	3%
Butter Beans, 1/2 cup, 4 1/2 oz	90	0	0%
Italian, cut, 1/2 cup, 4 1/2 oz	30	0	0%
Kidney Beans, 1/2 cup, 4 1/2 oz	105	<1	3%
Lima Beans, 1/2 cup, 4 1/2 oz	80	0	0%
Pinto Beans, 1/2 cup, 4 1/2 oz	100	<1	3%
Wax Beans, cut, 1/2 cup, 4 1/2 oz	20	0	0%
(Also see Canned Products ~ Pages 57-58)			
Beets: Sliced/Whole, 1/2 c., 4 1/2 oz	35	0	0%
Crinkle/Pickled (*Del Monte*) 1/2 c.	80	0	0%
Carrots, sliced, 1/2 cup	35	0	0%
Corn: Whole kernel, sweet: 1/2 cup, 4 1/2 oz	80	0.5	5%
Drained Solids, 1/2 cup, 3 oz	65	0.5	6%
Creamed style, 1/2 cup, 4 1/2 oz	100	0.5	5%
Dill Pickles - See Page 71.			

	C	F	%fc
CANNED (Cont)			
Eggplant, 2 Tbsp, 1 oz	25	2	72%
Garbanzo/Chick Peas, 3 oz	100	2	15%
Green Chilies, diced, 2 Tbsp, 1 oz	5	0	0%
Hearts of Palm, (1), 1.2 oz	9	0	0%
1 cup, 5 oz	40	<1	12%
Mushrooms: 1/2 cup, 2 1/2 oz	20	0	0%
in Butter Sauce, 2 oz	30	1	30%
Olive Salad (*Progresso*), drain, 2 T.	25	2.5	90%
Onions: Pickled, 1 med., 3/4 oz	10	0	0%
Cocktail, 1 onion	2	0	0%
Peas, 1/2 cup, 3 oz	60	0	0%
Peppers: Hot Chilli, 1 only, 1 oz	8	0	0%
Sweet, undrained, 2 1/2 oz	15	0	0%
Jalapeno, w. liq., 1/2 c. chopped	17	0	0%
Cherry (*Progresso*), dr., 2 T., 1 oz	25	2	72%
Fried, drain, 2 Tbsp, 1 oz	60	5	75%
Hot Cherry; Rst; Tuscan, dr., 1 oz	10	0	0%
Pepper Salad (*Progresso*), dr., 2 T.	15	1	60%
Potatoes, 1/2 cup, 3 oz	55	0	0%
Salsa: Average all types, 2 Tbsp	15	0	0%
Sauerkraut, undrained, 1/2 c., 4 oz	25	0	0%
Spinach, 1/2 cup, 3 1/2 oz	25	0	0%
Succotash: Per 1/2 cup, 4 1/2 oz			
w. Cream Style Corn	100	<1	3%
w. whole kernels, undrained	80	<1	3%
Sweetcorn: See Corn.			
Sweet Potato, 1/2 cup, 3 1/2 oz	105	0	0%
Tomatoes: Sundried			
Natural, 5-6 pces, 0.4 oz	22	0	0%
In Oil, drained, 6 pces, 1/2 oz	60	4	60%
Tomato Products ~ See Page 68 - 71.			
Vegetables, mixed, 1/2 cup, 4 oz	45	0	0%
Yams in Light Syrup, 1/2 cup, 4 oz	105	0	0%
Zucchini in Tom. Sce., 1/2 cup, 4 oz	30	0	0%

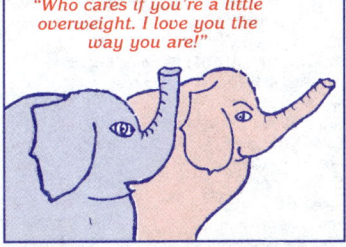

"Who cares if you're a little overweight. I love you the way you are!"

SALADS - FRESH, DELI, RESTAURANT

Average All Outlets
Per Serving

	C	F	%fc
Ambrosia Salad, 1/2 cup	230	15	58%
Antipasto Salad, 1 cup	140	10	64%
Bean Salad, 1/2 cup	110	5	42%
Bulgur Salad, 1/2 cup	70	2	22%
Caesar Salad, Classic, 1 cup	200	14	63%
Side Salad, no dressing	25	0	0%
Carrot Raisin: No dress., 1/2 cup	20	0	0%
with dressing, 1/2 cup	65	5	69%
Chef Salad: Regular, no dressing	620	37	54%
w. 2 oz 1000 Island	860	61	64%
Chicken Salad Platter, 6 oz	200	8	26%
Coleslaw: Traditional, 1/2 cup	150	8	48%
w. low cal dressing	60	1	15%
Corn, Mexican, 1/2 cup	240	12	45%
Cucumber, non-oil dress, 1/2 cup	60	0	0%
w. Oil dressing, 1/2 cup	140	12	77%
Eggplant Salad, 1/2 cup	75	2	24%
Fettucini w. veges, 1/2 cup	110	5	42%
Garden Salad: No dressing	35	0	0%
Greek Salad, 1 cup	120	9	67%
Greek Vegetables, 1/2 cup	125	12	85%
Lettuce, hearts, 1/4 head	20	0	0%
Lobster Salad Platter, 6 oz	200	8	36%
Macaroni Salad, 1/2 cup	140	8	50%
Pasta Salad, 1/2 cup	160	8	45%
Pineapple Coconut Slaw, 1/2 cup	150	10	60%
Potato Salad: Dijon	140	7	45%
w. Mayonnaise, 1/2 cup	170	10	52%
w. Yogurt dressing, 1/2 cup	140	3	19%
Rice Salad, 1/2 cup	150	9	53%
Saffrono Rice, 1/2 cup	130	3	21%
Spinach Salad	180	13	65%
Tomato & Mozzarella, 1/2 cup	180	14	70%
Tabouli, 1/2 cup	150	6	34%
Three Bean Salad, 1/2 cup	80	5	53%
Tortelini w. Basil, 1/2 cup	170	10	52%
Waldorf w. mayo, 1/2 cup	160	12	67%

SIGNATURE SALADS: Per 6 oz Serving
(Supplied to Deli's and Institutions)

	C	F	%fc
Antipasto Salad, 6 oz	510	50	88%
Artichoke Salad, marinated	400	41	92%
California Medley	120	7	52%
Cheese Agnolotti	250	8	28%
Chicken Salad	420	33	70%
Crabmeat Flavored	450	38	76%
Egg Salad	300	23	69%
Fresh Button Mushroom	190	16	75%

SIGNATURE SALADS (Cont)

	C	F	%fc
Garden Olive, 6 oz	630	67	95%
Ham Salad	400	32	72%
Prima Pasta Salad	360	29	72%
Seafood Pasta Del Mar	170	10	53%
Seafood with Crab & Shrimp	420	34	72%
Shrimp Salad	360	32	80%
Tuna Salad	450	36	72%

FAST-FOOD/RESTAURANT CHAINS
(See *Arby's, Boston Market, Denny's, Kenny Rogers, Olive Garden, McDonald's, Cousins Subs, Sizzler, Souplantation, Sweet Tomatoes, Subway, Taco John's, Wendy's*)

FRESH SALAD PACKS

Pre-Packaged (Supermarkets)
DOLE: *Lunch For One*

	C	F	%fc
Caesar, Fat Free, 6 oz	300	24	72%
Classic; Ranch, 7 oz	340	29	76%
Italian, Fat Free, 7 oz	110	0	0%
Regular Salad Packs:			
Classic Coleslaw, no dress., 3 oz	25	0	0%
Herb Ranch, 3 1/2 oz	50	10	1%
Oriental, 3 1/2 oz	120	6	45%
Raspberry & Romaine, 3 1/2 oz	50	0.5	1%
Sunflower Ranch, 3 1/2 oz	170	16	84%
Zesty Italian, 7 oz	110	0	0%

FRESH EXPRESS

	C	F	%fc
Caesar Salad Kit, 2 cups	160	12	67%
Creamy Mexican, 1 1/2 cups	110	8	87%
Fiesta Salad Kit, 1 1/2 cups	100	8	72%
Ranch; F.F.Hidden Valley, 1 1/2 c.	80	0	0%

READY PAC: Aver. all types, 3 c. | **15** | **0** | 0%

SALAD TIME: *Salad In-A-Bowl*

	C	F	%fc
Caesar w. Aged Parmesan, 5.6 oz	220	15	61%
Italian Dry Salami, 5.9 oz	240	15	56%
Sante Fe Salad, 5.8oz	230	14	55%

WEIGHT WATCHERS

	C	F	%fc
Caesar Salad, 1 cup + 2 T. Dress.	160	3	16%
European Salad, 1 cup + 2 T. Dress.	160	3	16%

SALAD TOPPINGS

	C	F	%fc
Bacon Bits, aver., 1 Tbsp	30	1.5	45%
Croutons, 2 Tbsp, 10g	35	1	25%
Chow Mein Noodles, dry, 1/2 c.	120	3	22%
Olives, 5 medium	25	2	70%
Sunflower Seeds, 1 Tbsp, 8 g	45	4	80%
Potato Chips, 1 oz	150	10	60%
Tortilla Chips, 1 oz	150	8	48%

COFFEE

INSTANT COFFEE

	C	F	%fc
(Powder/Granules):			
Regular or Decaffeinated,			
1 level tsp	2	0	0%
1 rounded tsp	4	0	0%
Ground, 1 Tbsp	5	0	
Brewed/Percolated,			
1 cup, 8 fl. oz	5	0	0%
Coffee With Milk/Cream/Creamers:			
w. Whole Milk: Dash, 1 Tbsp	15	0.5	32%
2 Tbsp, 1 fl. oz	25	1	35%
w. 2% Milk, 2 Tbsp	20	0.5	25%
w. 1% Milk, 2 Tbsp	15	0.3	18%
w. Nonfat milk, 2 Tbsp	14	0	0%
w. Half & Half: 1 Tbsp	25	2	70%
2 Tbsp	45	4	70%
w. Cream (light coffee): 1 Tbsp	35	3	75%
2 Tbsp	65	6	75%
w. *Coffee Mate:* Liquid, reg., 1Tbsp	25	1	35%
Liquid Fat Free, 1 Tbsp	15	0	0%
Powder, 1 heaping tsp	20	1	45%
Sugar ~ add extra: 1 heap. tsp	25	0	0%
Single portion, 1 pkt	25	0	0%
Flavored Coffee Mixes - *Per Serving*			
General Foods, Cafe International:			
Regular	60	3	45%
Sugar-free	35	2	50%
Hills Bros Cafe Coffees: Reg., aver.	60	2	30%
Sugar-free, 1 cup	40	2	45%
Maxwell House: Hot Cappuccino,	60	1	15%
Cappio Coffee Iced, 8 oz	120	3	22%
Cappio Mocha Iced, 8 oz	130	2	14%
Chicory: Instant Coffee, 1 tsp	6	0	0%
Coffee Essence, 1 tsp	16	0	0%

COFFEE SHOPS/RESTAURANTS

Per 8 fl. oz Cup Unless Indicated

	C	F	%fc
Coffee (Regular/Percolated/Filtered)	5	0	0%
Drip Coffee; Americano, 1 cup	5	0	0%
Caffe Latte: w. Whole Milk	100	5	45%
w. 2% Milk	80	2.5	28%
w. Nonfat Milk	60	0	0%
Tall Glass, 12 oz: w/Whole Milk	180	10	50%
w. Nonfat Milk	110	0.5	4%
Grande Size, 16 fl. oz, whole	220	11	45%
w. Nonfat Milk	130	0.5	4%
Cafe Mocha (Mochaccino):			
1 cup, 8 fl. oz	120	3	23%
Tall Glass, 12 fl. oz	180	4.5	23%
Grande Size, 16 fl. oz	240	6	23%
Mocha, with Cream, 8 fl. oz:			
w. Whole Milk	180	12	60%
w. Nonfat Milk	150	8	48%
Tall, 12 fl. oz: Whole Milk	290	18	56%
w. Nonfat Milk	230	11	43%
Iced Mocha (no cream)			
Tall, 12 fl. oz: w/Whole Milk	190	9	43%
w. Nonfat Milk	140	2	13%
Cappuccino, 1 cup, 8 fl. oz:			
w. Whole Milk	70	3.5	45%
w. 2% Milk	60	2	30%
w. Nonfat Milk	40	0	0%
Large/Tall, 12 fl. oz:			
w. Whole Milk	110	6	49%
w. 2% Milk	80	3	34%
w. Nonfat Milk	60	0	0%
Espresso: Regular	4	0	0%
Doppio (Double)	8	0	0%
Espresso Con Panna			
(w. dollop whipped cream)	40	4	90%
Espresso Macchiato	15	0.5	30%
Frappucino: Tall, 12 fl. oz	180	2	10%
Grande, 16 fl. oz	250	3	11%
Frappucino Mocha:			
Large/Tall, 12 fl. oz	210	2	8%
Grande, 16 fl. oz	280	3	9%
Iced Latte: Similar to Caffe Latte			

IRISH & LIQUEUR COFFEES

	C	F	%fc
Irish Coffee (no sugar)	175	10	51%
Liqueur Coffee, aver. all types	200	10	45%

COCOA/CHOCOLATE

	C	F	%fc
Cocoa (w. Whipping Cream -*Starbucks*):			
1 cup, 8 fl. oz, Whole Milk	210	14	60%
w. Nonfat Milk	80	8	90%
Tall (16 fl. oz) Whole Milk	300	19	57%
w. Nonfat Milk	100	11	99%
Hot Chocolate: Whole Milk, 8oz	200	10	45%
w. Nonfat Milk, 8 fl. oz	140	2	13%
Tall, 12 fl. oz, Whole Milk	300	15	45%
w. Nonfat Milk	210	3	13%

COFFEE SUBSTITUTES

	C	F	%fc
Cafix Instant Beverage, 1 tsp	6	0	0%
Kaffree Roma (Natural Touch) , 1 tsp	6	0	0%
Postum, Instant Hot Beverage:			
Regular/Coffee Flavor, 1 tsp	12	0	0%
Teeccino Caffe, 1 tsp	10	0	0%

Caffeine Guide & Counter ~ Page 224-225

TEA & ICED TEAS

TEAS

	C	F	%fc
Regular: Bag, Loose or Instant			
Brewed, 1 cup, 8 fl. oz	1	0	0%
(Add extra for sugar/milk)			
Herbal: Average all varieties, 1 cup	1	0	0%
Bigelow: Apple Orchard, 1 cup	5	0	0%
Other Varieties	2	0	0%
Celestial Seasonings:			
Bengal Spice	5	0	0%
Lemon Zinger	4	0	0%
Roastaroma	10	0	0%
Spearmint	5	0	0%
Other varieties	2	0	0%

ICED TEA - QUICK CHECK

	C	F	%fc
Average All Brands			
Pre-Sweetened: 8 fl. oz	100	0	0%
12 fl. oz	150	0	0%
16 fl. oz	200	0	0%
Unsweetened: 8 fl. oz	2	0	0%

ICED TEA MIXES

	C	F	%fc
Per Serving			
4C Instant	90	0	0%
Bigelow, Nice Over Ice	1	0	0%
Celestial Seasonings, Iced Delight	4	0	0%
Crystal Light, Sugar Free	3	0	0%
Lipton: Instant	0	0	0%
Instant Lemon/Raspberry	3	0	0%
Lemon	55	0	0%
Peach/Raspb, SugarFree	5	0	0%
Nestea: 100% Instant	2	0	0%
Ice Teasers, all flavors	6	0	0%
Lemon	6	0	0%
Peach, Raspberry	90	0	0%

A woman is like a teabag.

You never know her strength until she's in hot water.

— Nancy Reagan

BOTTLED ICED TEA

	C	F	%fc
Per 8 fl. oz unless indicated			
Apple & Eve	100	0	0%
Arizona: Average all varieties	95	0	0%
Ginseng	60	0	0%
Low Calorie	40	0	0%
Fruitopia: Born Strawb.Passion	120	0	0%
Peaceable Peach	110	0	0%
Knudsen: Coolers, all flavors	90	0	0%
Lipton: average, all flavors	80	0	0%
Diet, Lemon	3	0	0%
Nestea Iced Tea:			
Cool from Nestea, 1 cup	80	0	0%
12 fl. oz	120	0	0%
Diet Cool from Nestea	2	0	0%
Diet Lemon	3	0	0%
Earl Grey	70	0	0%
Lemon Sweetened	80	0	0%
Pitcher Style: Extra Swet	100	0	0%
Lightly Sweetened	55	0	0%
Unsweetened	1	0	0%
Sweetened Ice Tea	65	0	0%
Royal Mistic:			
Regular, 12 fl. oz	145	0	0%
Diet, 12 fl. oz	8	0	0%
Schweppes, 8 fl. oz	90	0	0%
Shasta, 8 fl. oz	80	0	0%
Snapple: Regular, sweetened	70	0	0%
Diet/Unsweetened	0	0	0%
Lemon, Peach, Raspberry	100	0	0%
Diet	0	0	0%
Kiwi Strawberry, regular	120	0	0%
Diet	20	0	0%
Ssips (Johanna Farms), 8.45 fl. oz	100	0	0%
Tropicana: Lemonfruit	100	0	0%
Diet Lemon Fruit	15	0	0%
Peach/Rasp./Tangerine, 8 fl. oz	120	0	0%
10 fl. oz Bottle	140	0	0%
11.5 fl. oz can	160	0	0%
Twister, Apple Berry, 8 fl. oz	100	0	0%
Lemon Citrus	110	0	0%
Turkey Hill: Regular	90	0	0%
Raspberry Cooler	110	0	0%
Diet Decaffeinated	0	0	0%
Veryfine: Regular	80	0	0%
Lemon	90	0	0%
Raspberry	100	0	0%

SPORTS DRINKS & SHAKES

SPORTS DRINKS

(Fluid Replacement, Carbohydrate Rich)
Per 8 fl. oz Unless Indicated

	C	F	%fc
All Sport, all flavors, 8 fl. oz	70	0	0%
Amino Force, 22 oz	390	0	0%
Blue Thunder, 22 oz	400	0	0%
Body Fuel (w. NutraSweet), 8 fl.oz	4	0	0%
Body Works (Shasta), 12 fl.oz	90	0	0%
Exceed, Powder, 2 Tbsp	70	0	0%
Liquid, 12 fl. oz box	105	0	0%
Gatorade: Regular, 8 fl. oz	50	0	0%
8.45 fl.oz Box, all flavors	60	0	0%
Light, Lemon-Lime	25	0	0%
GatorLode, 11.6 fl. oz can	280	0	0%
GatorPro, 11 fl. oz can	360	6	15%
Knudsen, Isotonic Sports	60	0	0%
Max, made-up, 8 fl. oz	96	0	0%
Pavilion Select Winners	50	0	0%
Powerade, all flavors, 8 fl. oz	70	0	0%
Pro-formance, all flavors	100	0	0%
Recharge (Knudsen), all flavors	70	0	0%
Relode, 0.75 oz pkt.	80	0	0%
Ripped Force, 16 oz	90	0	0%
Snapple Sport, all flavors	80	0	0%
Super Shake, 12 oz	265	0	0%
The Juice, 11 fl. oz	260	0	0%
Thermo Force, 16 oz	260	0	0%
Tiger's Milk (mix):			
Energy Booster, 3 heap Tbsp.	120	0	0%
Protein Booster, 3 heap Tbsp	90	0	0%
Twin Lab Ultra Fuel, 16 oz	400	0	0%
Upper Deck: All flavors	80	0	0%

NUTRITIONAL SHAKES, DRINKS

	C	F	%fc
Appeal Lite (IDN), 1 pkt, 43g	140	1	6%
Bariatrix Shakes, 1 serving	100	2	18%
Proti-Max Meal, 67g	250	3	11%
Fruit Drinks (High Protein), 20g	70	1	11%
Boost: Ready-To-Drink, 8 oz	240	4	15%
Carnation: Inst. Brkfast, 10 oz	220	2.5	10%
Dynatrim, w. 1% milk, 8 fl. oz	220	4	16%
Ensure: Eggnog, 8 oz	250	6	22%
High Protein, 8 oz	225	6	24%
Ensure Plus, all varieties, 8 oz	355	13	33%
Powder, 8 oz	250	9	28%
w. Fiber: Pecan; Vanilla, 8 oz	250	6	22%
Chocolate	260	9	31%
Herbalife, (Thermogetics F.1), 1oz	100	1	9%

NUTRITIONAL SHAKES, DRINKS (Cont)

	C	F	%fc
HMR 500 Shakes, 1 pkt	100	0	2%
HMR 120, 1 serving	120	2	15%
Met-Pro (Universal), 80g	270	0	0%
Met-Rx: Nutrition Drink Mix, 72g	260	2	7%
Nestle Sweet Success:			
Aver. all flavors, 10 fl. oz box	200	3	13%
Powder, all flavors, 1 scoop	90	1	10%
Nutra/Shake: All flavors, 4 fl. oz	200	6	20%
High Fiber Nutra/Shakes 6 fl. oz	300	6	18%
Free (no Added Sugar), 4 fl.oz	200	8	36%
Citrus Nutra/Shakes, 4 oz	200	0	0%
Juice Plus Fibre,, 10 fl. oz	150	0.5	2%
Phosphagain, 58g	170	1.5	7%
Pro-Cal 100 (R-Kane),			
Shake/Pudding, 1 pkt	103	2	17%
Pro-Performance:			
Weight Gainer 2200	2200	1	1%
Resource: Fructose Swtnd., 1 ctn.	250	11	40%
Fruit Beverage, 1 ctn.	180	0	0%
Health Shake (Aspartame swtnd.)			
w. *Benefiber*, 4 fl.oz ctn.	190	6	28%
Shake, 1 ctn., 6 oz	250	9	30%
Shake Plus, French Vanilla, 8 oz	360	11	28%
Sego: Lite, all flavors, 10 fl. oz	150	4	24%
Very Chocolate/Malt, 10 fl. oz	225	1	4%
Very Strawb./Vanilla, 10 fl. oz	225	5	20%
Slim-Fast, all flavors, 1 scoop	100	1	9%
Prepared w.Skim milk, 8 fl. oz	190	1	4%
Sustacal: Liquid, 8 fl.oz can	240	5.5	20%
Basic, 8 fl.oz can	250	9	32%
Plus, 8 fl.oz	360	13.5	34%
Powder, 2 oz + water	200	1	3%
Vanilla, 8 oz	240	6	23%
Twin Lab RxFuel, 1 pkt	250	0	0%
Ultra Slim-Fast: Powder, 1 scp.	120	0.5	4%
Ready-To-Drink, 11 oz can	220	3	12%
Universal Designer Protein, 22g	85	1	10%
Weider: Dry Mixes			
Dynamic: Body Shaper, 1/3 cup	140	0.5	2%
Muscle Builder, 1/3 cup	190	0	0%
Weight Gainer, 1/2 cup	330	0.5	1%
Carbo Energizer, 4 scoops	230	0	0%
N2itro-Fire Protein, 2 Tbsp	110	1	8%
Victory: Creative EFX, 58g	142	0	0%
Giant Mega Mass 4000	1640	4	2%
Pure Egg Protein, 1 serving	80	0	0%

Nutrition Bars: Page 107

SOFT DRINKS & SODA

COCA COLA & PEPSI

BOTH CONTAIN ZERO FAT **C**

Coca Cola Classic or *Pepsi:*
8 fl. oz Bottle	100
12 fl. oz Can	150
16 fl. oz Bottle	200
20 fl. oz Contour Bottle	250
1 Litre Bottle	400
2 Litre Bottle	800

Diet Coke, Diet Pepsi:
12 fl. oz Can	10

QUICK CHECK

ALL CONTAIN ZERO FAT

	C PER 8 fl.oz	C PER 12 fl.oz
Average All Brands		
Cola: Regular	105	160
Diet (no Added Sugar)	<1	1
Club Soda	0	0
Club Soda Cream	115	170
Diet Soft Drinks: Average	<2	<4
Ginger Ale	80	120
Lemon Lime	145	220
Orange	120	180
Root Beer	110	165
Tonic Water	90	135
Mineral Water: Plain	0	0
Sweetened/flavored	100	150
w. Fruit Juice	80	120
Seltzers: Plain/Diet	0	0
Sweetened/flavored	100	150
w. Fruit Juice	80	120

SODA BRANDS

ALL CONTAIN ZERO FAT

	C PER 8 fl.oz	C PER 12 fl.oz
A&W: Cream Soda	110	165
Cream Soda/Root Beer, 'Diet'	<1	1
Root Beer	110	165
Barq's Root Beer	110	165
Barrelhead: Rootbeer	110	165
Bodyworks (Shasta), all flav.	60	90
Canada Dry: Birch Beer	110	165
Cactus Cooler	110	165
Club Soda	0	0
Collins Mixer	80	120
Ginger Ale, all flavors	100	150
Diet, all flavors	0	0

ALL CONTAIN ZERO FAT

	C PER 8 fl.oz	C PER 12 fl.oz
Canada Dry (Cont)		
Half & Half	110	165
Hi-Spot	110	165
Lemon Sour	100	150
Seltzer, all flavors	0	0
Sour Mixer	90	135
Tahitian Treat	150	225
Tonic Water/Twist Lime	100	150
Diet	0	0
Wild Cherry	110	165
Clearly Canadian, average	95	140
Coca Cola: Classic	100	150
Coke II	105	160
Diet Coke	<1	1
Cherry Coca Cola	105	160
Diet Cherry	<1	1
Cragmont: Cola	110	165
Cherry	120	180
Diet, all flavors	0	0
Crush, all flavors	140	210
Crystal Light, all flavors	5	8
Diet Rite, all flavors	<1	1
Doc Shasta	105	160
Dr Diablo, Cola	95	140
Dr Nehi	100	150
Dr Pepper: Regular	110	165
Diet	2	3
Fanta: Orange	120	180
Ginger Ale	86	130
Grape	120	180
Root Beer	110	165
Fresca	3	4
Health Valley: Ginger Ale	100	150
Sarsaparilla Rootbeer	100	150
Rootbeer Old Fashioned	80	120
Wild Berry	95	142
Hires: Cream	120	180
Root Beer	120	180
Jolt Cola	100	150
Kick (Royal Crown)	120	180
Knudsen: Spritzers, average	110	170
Lights, all flavors	75	110
Lucozade, 7 fl. oz	136	-
Manishewitz Seltzer	0	0
Mello Yello: Regular	120	180
Diet	4	5

126

SOFT DRINKS & SODA cont

ALL CONTAIN ZERO FAT	C 8 fl.oz	C 12 fl.oz
Minute Maid: Orange	120	180
Diet Orange	2	3
Berry; Black Cherry	110	165
Fruit Punch; Grape	120	180
Grapefruit	110	165
Lemonade	106	160
Peach; Pineapple; Raspberry	110	165
Strawberry	122	185
Mountain Dew	110	165
Mr Pibb: Regular	100	150
Diet	1	2
Mug: Root Beer	110	165
Natural Brew: Apple, Cream	112	170
Cafe Mocha, Cherry Amaretto	105	160
Ginseng Cola, Ginger Ale	112	170
Nehi (Royal Crown): Cream	120	180
Ginger Ale, Quinine Water	90	135
Other flavors, average	130	195
Orangina, 10 fl. oz Bottle	-	120
Pepsi: Regular; Caffeine Free	100	150
Diet Pepsi	0	0
Pepsi Kona	105	160
Wild Cherry Cola	105	160
Perrier: Regular or flavors	0	0
Ramblin' Root Beer	120	180
RC Cola	100	150
Diet Cola	<1	1
Cherry	110	165
Royal Mistic:		
Caribbean Fruit Punch, 16 fl. oz	-	230
'N Juice, average	102	155
Sparkling, average, 11.1 fl. oz	-	115
Schweppes: Bitter Lemon	110	165
Ginger Ale, regular	80	120
Raspberry	80	120
Ginger Beer	100	150
Grapefruit	110	165
Lemon Lime	100	150
Lemon Sour	110	165
Seltzer	0	0
Tonic: Regular	80	120
Diet	0	0
7UP: Regular	95	145
Cherry, Gold	102	155
Santa Cruz: Sparkling, all types	100	150
Orange	130	195
Sensa (Guarana flavored)	90	135

ALL CONTAIN ZERO FAT	C 8 fl.oz	C 12 fl.oz
Shasta: Black Cherry	110	165
Cherry Cola	105	160
Club Soda; Diet, all flavors	0	0
Cola, regular	110	170
Caffeine Free	105	160
Doc Shasta	105	160
Fruit Punch, Pineapple	133	200
Ginger Ale	90	130
Shasta Plus: all flavors	110	170
Slice: Lemon Lime	100	150
Diet Lemon Lime	0	0
Dr. Slice	95	140
Mandarin Orange, Fruit Punch	130	195
Grape; Pineapple; Red	125	190
CherryLime; Slice Cola	105	160
Snapple: Average all flavors	120	180
Spree (Shasta): all flavors	112	170
Sprite: Regular	100	150
Diet	3	4
Squirt: Regular Soda	100	150
Ruby Red Soda	120	180
Sunkist: Average all flavors	140	210
Diet Citrus	0	0
Diet Orange	5	7
Surge Citrus	100	150
TAB	<1	1
Upper 10 (RC): Regular	100	150
Diet	3	4
Vernor's: Ginger Ale	100	150
Wink	130	195
Welch's: Sparkling, average	120	180

FRUITOPIA

(Contain 10% Fruit Juice)	8 fl.oz	12 fl.oz
Apple Raspb.; Trop. Consideration	75	115
Lemonade Love; Cranberry Lemon	115	170
Pink Lemonade; Tangerine Wave.	118	175
Other flavors, average	125	190

KOOL-AID, TANG

Per 6 fl.oz Serving	C	F	%fc
Bright & Early, 6 fl.oz	90	0	0%
Kool-Aid, all flav., unsweetened	2	0	0%
Sugar, sweetened	80	0	0%
Sugar Free (NutraSweet)	4	0	0%
Tang, all flavors, 6 fl.oz	90	0	0%
Sugar-Free, 6 fl.oz	6	0	0%

ALCOHOL GUIDE

▸ **Health Hazards: Excess alcohol** contributes to obesity, high blood pressure, stroke, heart and liver disease, some cancers, and even impotence. **Concentration and short-term memory** are reduced as well as sporting performance.

Other alcohol hazards include stomach upsets, menstrual problems, anxiety, headaches, insomnia, work absenteeism and family arguments.

▸ **Alcohol contributes to obesity** through its high calories and by lessening the body's ability to burn fat. Fat storage is promoted, particularly in the belly - a danger zone.

▸ **Alcohol is potentially more harmful while dieting.** Blood sugar levels may drop with resultant tiredness and further impairment of concentration, reflexes and driving skills - and maybe the dieter's resolve!

SAFE ALCOHOL LIMITS
(Dietary Guidelines for Americans, 1990)
Women: No more than **1 drink** per day.
Men: No more than **2 drinks** per day.
1 Drink = 12 fl.oz regular beer, **or** 5 fl.oz wine,
or 1 1/2 fl.oz spirits (80 proof).
Each drink contains approx. **14g alcohol.**

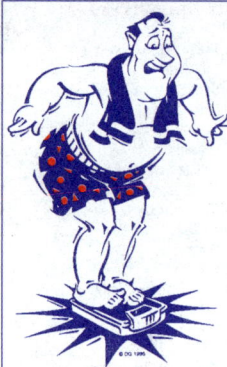

Excess alcohol contributes to obesity and high blood pressure.

For some people, safe drinking will mean no alcohol drinks at all. (Even one drink may impair driving skills; and 3-4 drinks daily has been linked to brain shrinkage in some social drinkers).

▸ **It is advisable not to drink at all if you are:**
- pregnant or trying to conceive
- taking drug medication (unless approved by your doctor or pharmacist)
- have a condition such as liver or heart disease
- planning to drive or use machinery
- studying or needing to concentrate
- a child or adolescent

▸ **Women and adolescents are more prone** to alcohol's ill-effects due to their lower body weight, smaller livers and lesser capacity to metabolise alcohol.

Note: You cannot save daily drinks for one occasion.
Binge drinking is particularly harmful ~
4 drinks 'in a row' for males or 3 drinks for females.

HOW TO CALCULATE ALCOHOL CONTENT

Percent alcohol on label refers to alcohol volume (ml alcohol/100ml).

To convert to grams (weight) of alcohol, multiply the percent volume by 0.8 - since 1 ml of alcohol weighs only 0.8 grams (actually 0.789g).

EXAMPLE
12 fl.oz Can Beer (5% alcohol)
5% alc.volume = 5% of 12 fl.oz
= 0.6 fl.oz
= 18ml alcohol
(1 fl.oz=30ml)
Weight (18x0.8)
= 14.4g alcohol

BEERS • ALES • MALT LIQUORS

QUICK GUIDE

BEER CONTAINS ZERO FAT

Alc ~ Alcohol (Grams)

Average All Brands

	C	Alc
MALT LIQUOR/ALE (5.6% Alc. Vol.)		
12 fl. oz Can/Bottle/Glass	180	16
22 fl. oz Can/Bottle/Glass	330	29
REGULAR BEER (5% Alc. Vol.)		
7 fl. oz Glass	80	8.5
12 fl. oz Bottle/Can/Glass	140	14
16 fl. oz Bottle/Can	185	19
22 fl. oz Bottle	260	26
32 fl. oz Bottle	370	37
40 fl. oz Bottle	470	47
LIGHT BEER (4.2% Alc. Vol.)		
7 fl. oz Glass	65	7
12 fl. oz Bottle/Can/Glass	110	12
16 fl. oz Bottle/Can	145	16
22 fl. oz Bottle	200	22
LOW ALCOHOL BEER (2.3% Alc. Vol)		
(Example: *Blatz LA*), 12 fl. oz	75	7
NON-ALCOHOL/NEAR BEER		
(Less than 0.5% alcohol by volume)		
Average All Brands, 12 fl. oz	70	1

BRANDS

Per 12 fl. oz Serving
Percentage alcohol listed below is by volume - not by weight.

	C	Alc
Amber Ice (5.3% alcohol)	130	15
Anchor Steam (4.6%)	155	13
Anheuser Light (3.2% alcohol)	75	9
Artic Ice (5.3%)	150	15
Artic Ice Light 3.2 (3.9%)	100	11
Augsburger Bock (4.9%)	170	14
Augsburger Golden/Dark (4.9%)	170	14
Augsburger Red (4.9%)	160	14
Ballard Bitter (4.7%)	180	14
Beck's (5%)	150	14
Big Sky (4.8%)	150	14
Big Sky Light (4.5%)	105	13
Black & Tan (4.5%)	185	13
Black Label (5.6%)	155	16
Black Label Light (3.7%)	100	11
Blackhook Porter (4.9%)	160	14
Blatz (4.3%)	135	12
Blatz LA (2.3%)	75	7

BRANDS (CONT)

BEER CONTAINS ZERO FAT

	C	Alc
Blatz Light (3.7%), 12 fl.oz	100	11
Blue Moon Ale: Belgian (4.8%)	160	14
Honey Blond Ale (5.5%)	200	16
Nut Brown Ale (5.1%)	180	15
Raspberry Cream Ale (4.9%)	190	14
Bud Dry (4.9%)	130	14
Bud Light (4.2%)	110	12
Bud Ice (5.5%)	150	16
Bud Ice Light (4.1%)	95	12
Budweiser (4.9%)	150	14
Busch (4.9%)	145	14
Busch Light (4.2%)	110	12
Carling (4.4%)	140	13
Carlsberg (5%)	135	13
Castlemaine XXXX (4.7%)	140	13
Colt 45 MM (5.6%)	155	16
Coors (4.9%)	150	14
Coors Dry (4.9%)	120	14
Coors Light 3.2 (4%)	100	11
Corona Extra (4.6%)	130	13
Dos Equis Lager (5%)	130	14
Elk Mountain Amber Ale (5.5%)	190	16
Elk Mountain Red (4.9%)	160	14
Extra Gold (4.9%)	150	14
Extra Gold 3.2 (4%)	120	11
Faust (5%)	170	14
First Reserve (4.9%)	170	14
Fosters Lager (4.9%)	135	14
Goebel (4.1%)	130	12
Goebel Light (3.9%)	110	11
Grolsch Premium (5%)	140	14
Guinness Draught (4.3%)	155	12
Heileman's: Old Style (4.9%)	147	14
Old Style Light (4.1%)	110	12
Heineken (5.4%)	170	15
Heineken Dark (5.2%)	175	15
Herman Joseph's		
Special Premium (4.9%)	150	14
Highland Ale: Black (5.6%)	180	16
Amber (5.2%)	160	15
Hurricane (5.5%)	150	16
Icehouse, Miller (5.0%)	135	14
Icehouse, Miller (5.5%)	150	16
Keystone Regular/Dry (4.9%)	125	14
Ice (5.3%)	145	15
Light, 3.2 (4%)	100	10
Amber Light (3.8%)	110	11

BEERS • ALES • MALT LIQUORS

BRANDS (CONT)

BEER CONTAINS ZERO FAT
Per 12 fl. oz Serving

Brand	C	Alc
Killian's: Irish Brown Ale (5.2%)	185	15
Irish Red (5%)	160	14
Wilde Honey Ale (5.3%)	170	15
King Cobra (5.9%)	180	17
Kirin Lager (Japan) (4.8%)	135	13
Labatt's Blue (5%)	145	14
Lowenbrau Dark/Special (4.9%)	160	14
Magnum Malt Liquor (5.9%)	155	17
Meister Brau (4.5%)	130	13
Meister Brau Light (4.5%)	105	13
Memphis Brown (4.6%)	120	13
Michelob: Regular (5%)	160	14
Light (4.3%)	135	12
Dry (4.9%)	130	14
Amber Bock (5%)	150	14
Centennial (5.5%)	175	16
Classic Dark (5%)	160	14
Golden Draft (4.8%)	150	14
Golden Draft Light (4.2%)	110	12
Hefeweizen (5%)	165	14
Malt (5.8%)	160	17
Miller, Regular (5%)	150	14
Miller Genuine Draft (5%)	145	14
Light (4.5%)	100	13
Miller High Life (5%)	145	14
Miller High Life Ice (5.5%)	142	16
Miller High Life Light (4.5%)	100	13
Miller Lite (4.5%)	95	13
Miller Lite Ice (5.5%)	125	16
Miller Lite Ice (5%)	115	14
Milwaukee's Best (4.5%)	130	13
Milwaukee's Best Ice (5.5%)	135	16
Milwaukee's Best Light (4.5%)	100	13
Minnesota's Best (4.9%)	140	14
Moosehead (5%)	125	14
Natural Ice, Budweiser (5.9%)	180	17
Natural Light, Budweiser (4.2%)	110	12
Natural Pilsner, Buswieser (4.9%)	150	14
Newcastle Brown Ale (4.5%)	140	12
Northstone Amber Ale (4.9%)	150	14
Old Milwaukee (4.5%)	145	13
Light (4.3%)	122	12
Ice (5.5%)	155	16
Red (4.5%)	135	13
Pabst (5%)	155	14
Pete's Wicked Ale (5%)	180	14
Piels (4.7%)	135	13
Piels Light (4.5%)	127	13

BEER CONTAINS ZERO FAT

Brand	C	Alc
Primo (4.3%), 12 fl.oz	140	12
Ranier (4.6%)	142	13
Red Bull Malt (7%)	192	20
Red Dog (5%)	150	14
Red Hook ESB (5.4%)	175	16
Red Hook Rye (5%)	155	14
Red Light (4.1%)	105	12
Red River Valley (4.9%)	165	14
Red Wolf (5.5%)	155	16
Samuel Adams (4.6%)	170	13
Samuel Adams Lager (4.7%)	180	13
Sapporo Draft (Japan) (4.5%)	140	12
Schaefer (4.3%)	140	12
Schaefer Light (3.9%)	110	11
Schlitz Ice (4.6%)	145	13
Schlitz Ice Light (4.3%)	120	12
Schlitz Malt (5.9%)	180	17
Schmidt (4.6%)	142	13
Sheaf Stout, 5.7%	180	16
Sierra Nevada: Pale Ale (5.6%)	175	16
Big Foot Ale (10.1%)	210	29
Pale Bock (6.6%)	190	19
Porter (6%)	185	17
Silver Thunder (5.9%)	165	17
Stella Artois, 5%, 330ml	135	14
Southpaw Light (5%)	125	14
Stroh's (4.4%)	145	13
Stroh's Light (4.3%)	115	13
Stroh's Signature (4.9%)	160	14
Wheat Hook (4.8%)	150	14
Winterfest (5.7%)	185	16
Zeigenbock (5%)	155	14
Zima Clear Malt (4.7%)	150	14

Homebrewed Beer: Similar to regular beers, according to alcohol content.

NON-ALCOHOLIC BREWS

Per 12 fl. oz Serving

Brand	C	Alc
Busch, Kingsbury, Sharp's	60	1
Coors Cutter (0.5%)	80	1.5
Kaliber, Haakebeck, O'Douls	70	1
Hamm's, Pabst	55	1
Old Milwaukee NA, Stroh's NA	70	1
Texas Select	70	1

CIDER

Alcoholic Cider, average, 5.5% alc.

	C	Alc
Dry, 12 fl oz	130	16
Sweet, 12 fl. oz	160	16

WINE • LIQUOR • COOLERS

TABLE WINE QUICK GUIDE

WINE CONTAINS ZERO FAT

Average All Varieties (11.5% Alcohol)	C	Alc
4 fl. oz (½ filled wine glass)	85	11
6 fl. oz (fuller wine glass)	125	16
½ Carafe/Bottle, 375ml	265	34
1 Bottle, 750ml	530	68

TABLE WINES

Alc ~ Alcohol (Grams)

Per 4 fl. oz Serving	C	Alc
Red: Claret/Burgundy/Chianti	80	11
Sparkling Reds	90	11
Rose: Medium, 4 fl. oz	80	11
White: Dry (Chablis/Hock/Riesling)	75	11
Sweet (Moselle/Sauterne)	85	11
Sparkling	95	11
Champagne: *Per 4 fl. oz Serving*		
Average 1 glass, 4 fl. oz	85	11
w. Orange Jce (3:1 orange)	75	8
w. Orange Jce (1:1 orange)	65	5
Cold Duck, 4 fl. oz	108	11
Sake: Rice Wine (16% Alc.), 4 oz	125	15
Mulled Wine: (Gluhwein), 4 oz	180	14
Non-Alcoholic Wine, average, 4 oz	50	0

DESSERT WINES

	C	Alc
Madeira (18% alc), 2 oz	85	9
Marsala (18%), 2 oz	110	9
Port, Muscatel, (18%), 2 oz	85	9
Sherry (18%), 2 oz		
Dry, 1 Sherry glass	65	9
Sweet/Cream, average	85	9
Vermouth: Dry (18%), 2 oz	65	9
Sweet (15%), 2 oz	85	7

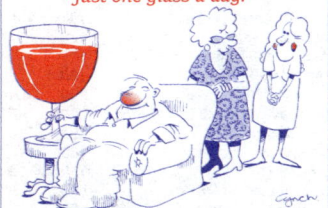

"The doctor told him to cut down to just one glass a day."

SPIRITS • LIQUORS

ALL CONTAIN ZERO FAT
Includes Bourbon, Brandy, Gin, Rum, Scotch, Tequila, Vodka, Whiskey.
Note: All spirits with same proof (alcohol) have similar calories and zero fat.

Average All Brands:	C	Alc
80 Proof (40% Alcohol by Volume):		
1 fl. oz	65	9.5
1½ fl. oz Jigger	100	14.5
½ Bottle, 375 ml	810	120
1 Bottle, 750 ml	1620	240
86 Proof (43% Alcohol):		
1 fl. oz	70	10
1½ fl. oz Jigger	105	15
½ Bottle, 375 ml	870	125
1 Bottle, 750 ml	1750	250
100 Proof (50% Alcohol):		
1 fl. oz	82	12
1½ fl. oz Jigger	125	18
½ Bottle, 375 ml	1025	150
1 Bottle	2050	300

COOLERS & PREMIX COCKTAILS

ZERO FAT UNLESS INDICATED

Bacardi Fruit Mixers (Frozen Conc.)	C	Alc
Made up (2oz mix + 1oz Rum + Ice)		
Margarita	160	10
Pina Colada	230	10
Other varieties, average	200	10
(If 2 oz Rum used, add extra 70 cals/10g alcohol)		
Bartles & Jaymes:		
Wine Cooler/Cocktails (5%), *Per 12 fl. oz:*		
Berry; Peach; Strawberry	220	14
Original; Black Cherry	200	14
Fuzzy Navel; Mai Tai	250	14
Long Island Tea	250	14
Margarita; Pina Colada	270	14
Strawberry Daiquiri; Tropical	230	14
Malt Based Coolers (3.9% alc.), 12 fl. oz:		
Berry; Peach; Strawberry	210	11
Original; Bl. Cherry; Red Sangria	200	11
Cranb. Raspb; Kiwi Strawberry	220	11
Fuzzy Navel; Strawb. Daiquiri	230	11
Long Island Tea	250	11
Mai Tai; Cranberry Lemonade	250	11
Margarita; Pina Colada	260	11

Continued Next Page

COOLERS • COCKTAILS

COOLERS/PREMIX COCKTAILS (Cont)
ZERO FAT UNLESS INDICATED — C | Alc

Boone's Farm Wine Coolers:
	C	Alc
Snow Creek Berry; Sun Peach (5%)	150	10
Wild Island (5%)	160	10
Sangria; Strawberry Hill (7.5%)	190	14

Breezer By Bacardi (3.2% alc):
	C	Alc
Passionfruit; Calypso Berry, 12 fl.oz	220	9
Pina Colada; Strawb. Daiquiri	250	9
Tahitian Tangerine, 12 fl. oz	200	9

Hueblein Premium Classics:
	C	Alc
Long Is. Ice Tea (15% alc), 2 oz	n/a	7
Manhattan (22.5%), 2 oz + ice	n/a	11
Mai Tai (22%), 2 oz + ice	n/a	11
Pina Colada, 4 oz (10g fat) + ice	280	4

Jack Daniels Country Cocktails (5.9%):
	C	Alc
All flavors, 200ml	n/a	9.5

Jose Cueruo Cocktails (5.9%):
	C	Alc
Margarita, Margarita Lime, 200ml	n/a	9.5
Strawberry, 200ml bottle	n/a	9.5

TGI Friday's Frozen Cocktails (12.5%):
Per Serving (3 fl.oz Premix & Ice):
	C	Alc
Margarita; Strawberry Daiquiri	145	9

Note: All drinks below contain 6g fat/serving.
	C	Alc
B52; Strawberry Shortcake	230	9
Mint Choc. Chip; P.Colada; Almond	250	9
Mudslide; Orange Dream	240	9

The Club (Premix Cocktails): *Per 4 oz*
	C	Alc
Censored On The Beach	n/a	7
Long Island Ice Tea; Manhattan	n/a	16
Margarita;Screwdriver; Vod. Martini	n/a	7
Mudslide (9g fat)	270	12
Pina Colada; Or. Craze; Whiskey Sour	n/a	10

Tropical Freezes (5.9%):
	C	Alc
All flavors, 8 oz/230ml pouch	230	11

FLAVORINGS/SYRUPS

Non-Alcoholic, Fat Free
	C	Alc
Angostura Bitters, 1/4 tsp	3	0
Grenadine/Cassis, 2 Tbsp, 1 oz	70	0
Lime Juice, 2 Tbsp, 1 oz	10	0
Sugar Syrup, 2 Tbsp, 1 oz	70	0
Soda Water	0	0
Tonic Water, 8 fl. oz	90	0

COCKTAILS
ZERO FAT UNLESS INDICATED
(Made to Standard Recipes)

	C	Alc
Bloody Mary	120	14
Bourbon & Soda	110	15
Brandy Alexander (contains 16g fat)	300	16
Cerebral Hemorrhage	290	17
Collins (w. 2 oz gin)	180	19
Daiquiri	110	14
Gin & Tonic	170	16
Harvey Wallbanger (2 oz Vodka)	250	29
Highball (1½ oz Whiskey)	110	14
Irish Coffee (contains 9g fat)	210	14
Leprechaun's Libation	285	31
Mai Tai (2 oz Rum)	260	27
Manhattan	130	17
Martini	160	22
Mind Eraser	160	17
Mint Julep	165	19
Pina Colada (contains 12g fat)	260	14
Screwdriver	180	14
Spritzer (3 oz Wine)	70	8
Tequila Sunrise	190	19
Tom Collins	120	16
Whiskey Sour	125	15

SHOOTERS
	C	Alc
Kamakazi	150	20
Mud Slide	160	13
Fuzzy Navel	120	13
Pineapple Bomber	130	11
Turbo	110	14

LIQUEURS/CORDIALS

Per 1 fl. oz Unless Indicated
	C	Alc
Bailey Irish Cream (34 Proof) (5g fat)	95	4
Lite (30 Proof), (2g fat)	75	4
Coffee Liqueur (53 Proof)	90	6.5
Amaretto (56 Proof)	110	6
Benedictine (80 Proof)	90	10
Cointreau (80 Proof)	100	10
Creme de Cacao (54 Proof)	100	6
Creme de Menthe (60 Proof)	120	7
Drambuie (80 Proof)	105	10
Grand Marnier (80 Proof)	100	10
Kahlua (53 Proof)	90	6.5
Midori, average all types, (42 Proof)	80	5
Ouzo (80 Proof)	90	10
Sambuca (84 Proof)	100	10
Schnapps (80 Proof)	100	10
Southern Comfort (78 Proof)	76	9
Triple Sec (60 Proof)	80	7

SANDWICHES & WRAPS

SANDWICHES

	C	F	%fc
No Butter/Mayo/Dressings			
(Includes 2 slices Bread):			
BLT (3 strips Bacon, 1 Tbsp Mayo)	350	22	57%
Bologna (3 oz)	410	26	57%
Cheese (3 slices, 3 oz)	470	29	56%
Cheese (2 oz) & Bacon (2 slices)	440	26	47%
Cheese (2 oz) & Ham (2 oz)	470	26	50%
Chicken Salad (8 oz)	540	30	50%
Chopped Liver (3 oz) & Egg	460	17	33%
Corned Beef (4 oz)	420	22	47%
Cream Cheese (2 Tbsp, 1 oz)	240	12	45%
with Olives (5 large)	270	13	43%
Egg, boiled (1 Jumbo, 2 1/4 oz)	240	9	34%
w. Bacon (2 slices)	320	15	42%
w. Salami (6 slices, 2 oz)	380	21	50%
Ham (4 oz)	350	14	36%
Ham (4 oz) & Cheese (4 sl., 4 oz)	800	56	54%
Liverwurst (3 oz)	430	26	54%
Lobster Salad (1/2 cup, 4 oz)	360	15	38%
Meatball w/Tomato Sce (4 oz)	490	27	50%
Pastrami, overstuffed (5 oz)	640	42	59%
Peanut Butter (2 Tbsp)	310	16	46%
with Jelly (1 Tbsp)	370	16	39%
Polish (Kielbasa) Sausage (4 oz)	480	30	56%
Roast Pork (4 oz)	420	19	41%
Roast Beef (4 oz)	410	17	37%
Reuben (6 oz Corned Beef, 2 oz Chse, 2 Tbsp Sauerkraut, 2 T. Dress)	920	60	59%
Sloppy Joe w. Sce (7 oz)	520	29	50%
Steak Sandwich (5 oz ckd)	610	31	46%
Tongue (4 oz)	460	25	49%
Tuna Salad (1/2 cup, 4 oz)	440	26	53%
with Egg (1 Jumbo, 2 1/4 oz)	540	33	55%
Turkey (4 oz) & Cranb. (2 Tbsp)	370	7	17%
Club Sandwich (Includes 3 slices Bread):			
Ham (3 oz) & Cheese (3 sl.)	700	40	51%
Chicken Salad (6 oz)	630	36	51%
& Bacon (3 pce)	740	45	55%
Egg Salad (6 oz)	510	26	46%
& Bacon (3 pce)	620	25	36%
Lobster Salad (1/2 cup)	430	16	33%
& Bacon (3 pce)	540	25	42%
Shrimp Salad (4 oz)	450	23	46%
& Bacon (3 pce)	560	32	51%
Turkey (4 oz) & Bacon (3 pce)	520	18	31%
Tuna Salad (4 oz) & Egg (1)	610	34	50%
Bagel: w. 2 Tbsp Cream Cheese	260	12	42%
w. 2 oz Lox (Smoked Salmon)	230	3.5	14%

	C	F	%fc
Croissants:			
Unfilled, med, 1 1/2 oz	180	10	50%
w. Ham (2 oz), Cheese (2 oz)	470	30	57%
w. Chick (2 oz) Chse (2 oz)	470	30	57%
w. Turkey/Ham/Chse (2 oz ea.)	580	36	56%
Hot Dogs: See Page 41.			
Extras: Butter/Margarine, 2 tsp	70	8	100%
Oil, 2 tsp	90	10	100%
Mayonnaise, 1 Tbsp, 1/2 oz	100	11	99%
1000 Island, 1 Tbsp, 1/2 oz	50	5	90%
Ranch Dressing, 1 Tbsp, 1/2 oz	70	8	100%
Cheese, 1 slice, 1 oz	110	9	74%
Cream Cheese, 2 Tbsp, 1 oz	100	10	90%
Avocado, 1/4 medium	80	7.5	84%
Coleslaw, 1/2 cup, 4 oz	150	8	48%
Potato Salad, 1/2 cup, 4 oz	170	10	53%
Potato Chips, 1 oz	150	10	60%
Dill Pickle, 1 pickle	10	0	0%
Mustard, 1 tsp 5	0	0	0%
Tartar Sauce, 1 Tbsp	75	7	84%
Salad (Lettuce; Tomato; Carrot)	15	0	0%

WRAPS & ROLL-UPS

	C	F	%fc
Average all Types			
(Meat/Chicken/Fish/Vegetables)			
Regular size, approx 9 oz	500	25	45%
Large, approx 15 oz	830	40	45%
Jumbo, approx 22 oz	1400	70	45%
Au Bon Pain Wraps:			
Chicken Caesar, 10 oz	630	31	44%
Southwestern Tuna, 15 oz	950	64	60%
Summer Turkey, 12 oz	550	12	20%
Ground Round Wraps:			
Mediterranean Chicken, 11 oz	600	23	35%
Southwestern Chicken, 14 oz	800	42	47%
Thai Vegetable Roll, 10 oz	450	9	18%
Long John Silver's Wraps:			
Aver. all wraps: Regular, 11 oz	720	35	45%
Large wrap, 22 oz	1400	70	45%
Taco Bell Fajita Wraps:			
Chicken/Steak (Regular), 8 oz	460	21	41%
Chicken/Steak (Supreme), 9 oz	500	25	45%
Veggio Supreme, 9 oz	460	23	45%
TGI Friday's Wrappers:			
Grilled Chicken, 9 oz	460	22	43%
Veggie Wrapper, 13 oz	850	55	58%
Wendy's Pitas:			
Chicken Caesar Pita, 8 1/2 oz	500	17	31%
Classic Greek Pita, 8 1/2 oz	430	19	40%
Garden Ranch Chicken, 10 oz	480	17	32%
Garden Veggie Pita, 9 oz	400	16	36%

RESTAURANT & ETHNIC FOODS

Note: Calories of these dishes are only a guide. Large variations occur with serving size, recipe ingredients and cooking methods.

CHINESE & ASIAN DISHES

APPETIZERS

	C	F	%fc
Curried Meat Triangles, 1 pce	150	5	30%
Dim Sum (Dumplings), 1 ball	65	2	28%
Egg Rolls, mini, 3 rolls	100	3	30%
Spring Roll, Small, 1½ oz	100	7	63%
Medium, 3 oz	200	12	54%
Large, 5 oz	350	15	39%
Wonton, 1 only	55	3	49%
Soup: Clear, 1 bowl	30	1	30%
with Noodles	100	3	27%
Chicken & Corn	150	8	48%
Fortune Cookie: each	25	<1	18%

ENTREES & MAIN DISHES
Per Whole Dish (2-3 Serves)

	C	F	%fc
Beef with Broccoli, 16 oz	650	30	42%
Beef in Black Bean Sce, 17 oz	530	33	56%
Chicken & Almonds, 18 oz	685	49	64%
Chop Suey: Chicken, 20 oz	560	37	59%
Pork, 20 oz	680	49	65%
Chow Mein: Beef/Chick., 24 oz	940	59	56%
Crispy Fried Chicken, 8 oz	485	33	61%
Lemon Chicken, 10 oz	580	32	50%
Omelet: Chick/Shrimp, 16 oz	990	82	75%
Sweet & Sour: Fish, 20 oz	1160	58	45%
Pork, 18 oz	950	49	46%
Duck, 18 oz	1120	71	57%
Vegetable Combination	250	17	61%
Extra Listings: See Frozen Entrees/Meals.			
RICE: Plain: 1 cup, 5 oz	170	0	0%
Fried: 1 cup, 5 oz	320	13	37%
Large dish, 16 oz	1010	40	36%
Noodles: Chinese Egg, boiled, 1 cup	200	3	14%

*C*onfucious say:
"Man who eat with one chopstick never have problem with obesity!"

CAJUN & CREOLE

Per Serving

	C	F	%fc
Alligator, 1 oz, ckd	40	0.5	11%
Baked Herb Chicken	850	53	56%
Bouillabaisse	350	11	28%
Cajun Fried Turkey	630	25	36%
Cocktail Sauce, 1 Tbsp	15	0	0%
Couche-couche, 2 cups	80	0	0%
Crawfish Bisque	500	10	18%
Crawfish, cooked, 2 oz	45	0.5	10%
Creole Jambalaya	550	29	47%
Dove, cooked, 1 oz	60	3.5	53%
Frog's Legs, steamed (2)	45	0	4%
Guinea Fowl, flesh, 1 oz, ckd	40	1	23%
Hogshead Cheese, ¼ cup	80	5.5	62%
Jambalaya, Shrimp & Crabmeat	520	14	24%
Red Beans & Rice	400	17	38%
Roasted Quail, w/Bacon on Toast	550	25	41%
Remoulade Sauce, 1 Tbsp	55	5.5	90%
Shrimp Creole	450	20	40%
Stuffed Smothered Steak, w. 1 cup, rice	890	49	50%
Squab, flesh, 1 oz, cooked	60	3.5	53%
Turtle, cooked, 1½ oz	60	1.5	23%

FRENCH

	C	F	%fc
Blanquetted d'Agneau (Lamb Stew w. Veg)	800	30	34%
Brioche, 1 cake	280	14	45%
Bouillabaise (Fish Stew)	400	15	34%
Coq au Vin (Chicken in Wine)	800	30	34%
Coquilles St. Jacques, fried, 6 lge	300	14	42%
Creme Caramel (Caram. Custard)	260	10	35%
Crepe Suzette, 1x 6"crepe/sauce	220	10	41%
Duck a l'Orange	780	35	40%
Escargots (Snails), in garlic but., (6)	200	18	81%
Frogs Legs, fried, 4 med. pairs	400	20	45%
Lamb Noisettes, fried, 2 chops	500	40	72%
Mousse au Chocolat	380	15	36%
Potage Creme Crecy (Carrot Soup)	360	18	45%
Salade Nicoise (Tuna/Oliv./Veg.)	450	13	26%
Veal Cordon Bleu (Veal/Ham/Ch)	650	25	35%
Vichyssoise (Pot./Leek Soup), 1 c.	200	9	41%

RESTAURANT & ETHNIC FOODS CONT

GERMAN

	C	F	%fc
Bavarian Brd. Dumpling, 3 small	330	9	25%
Beef: Goulash with Veges	520	20	35%
Black Forest Cake, 1 slice	380	16	38%
Chicken: Fried, Viennese-style	530	20	34%
Livers w. Apple/On., 6 oz	460	28	55%
Herring, Pickled: Rollmops, 4 oz	260	16	55%
with Sour Cream, 4 oz	310	20	58%
Hot Sausage Curry	300	7	21%
Kugelhupf (Yeast Cake), 1 lge sl.	400	12	27%
Pastry-Wrap. Bratwurst, 1 med.	250	10	36%
Sauerbraten Pork (Pot Roast)	650	35	48%
Torte: Linzer (Alm./Raspb. Jam)	430	18	38%
Sacher (Choc./Apricot Jam)	260	12	42%
Weiner Schnitzel, 1 med.	750	35	42%

GREEK FOODS

	C	F	%fc
Baklava Pastry, 1 only, 3 3/4 oz	400	21	47%
Calamari, deep fried, 1 cup	300	13	39%
Galactobureko, 1 only (Filo, Custard, Pastry in Syrup)	360	15	38%
Kataifi, (Filo, Nut, Pastry in Syrup)	350	11	28%
Moussaka, 1 serve, 8 oz	350	22	57%
Souvlakia (Lamb), each, 2 oz	120	6	45%
Stuffed Tomatoes, 2 only	250	12	43%
Taramosalata, 1 Tbsp, 1/2 oz	40	3	68%
Tyropita (Filo/Egg/Cheese Pastry)	350	26	67%
Tzatziki (Cucumber/Yog Dip), 1 T.	20	1	45%
Vine Leaves, stuffd., 3 rolls, 6 oz	200	5	23%

INDIAN & PAKISTAN

Per Serving
(Meat dishes allow 4 oz meat/serving)

	C	F	%fc
Aloo Samosa, each (Savory Pastries w. Potato fill.)	150	12	72%
Alu Gosht Kari (Meat/Pot. Curry)	600	40	60%
Aviyal, 1/2 cup	80	2	23%
Bhona Gosht (Mint Brld. Lamb)	560	28	45%
Chicken Pilaf (Murgh Biriyani)	700	53	68%
Chapati/Roti, 7" diam. piece (Baked Whole Wheat Bread)	60	<1	7%
Dal (Lentil Puree), 1 cup, no oil	230	1	4%
1 Tbsp Tadka (oil topping)	120	13	98%
Dhakla, 1 oz	105	5	43%
Dhansak, 1/2 cup	105	3.5	30%
Fish Jhol (Fish in Gravy)	230	10	39%

INDIAN & PAKISTAN (Cont)

	C	F	%fc
Gosht Kari (Meat Curry/Tom./Pot.)	460	25	49%
Idli, 3 1/2 oz	70	0	0%
Lamb Pilaf	520	35	61%
Masala Gosht (Beef/Tom./Gravy)	400	25	56%
Matki Usual, 1/2 cup	105	6	51%
Mulligatawney Soup, average	300	15	45%
Naan, 1/2 cup	75	2	24%
Pappadom, 1 large/2 small	50	3	54%
Pesrattu, 9" crepe	130	5	35%
Pork Vendaloo Curry	620	47	68%
Rajmah (Kidney Bean Curry)	400	17	38%
Rogan Josh (Lamb/Yoghurt Sce.)	500	30	54%
Saag Gosht (Beef/Spinach Sce.)	430	26	54%
Sambar, 1/2 cup	90	1	10%
Shahi Korma (Braised Lamb)	430	28	59%
Tandoori Chicken: Breast	260	13	45%
Leg/Thigh portion	300	17	51%

ITALIAN DISHES

	C	F	%fc
Cannelloni, 1 tube, 6 oz	280	15	48%
Chicken Cacciatore	370	22	54%
Gnocchi, Spinach	300	18	54%
Lasagne with meat, 10 oz	400	17	38%
Manicotti, cheese/tomato	230	14	55%
Minestrone Soup, 1 cup	260	6	21%
Osso Buco (Veal/Tom./Mushr.)	550	28	46%
Ravioli, 8 oz	300	12	36%
Risotto (Chicken)	420	14	30%
Spaghetti:			
Plain, 1 cup, 5 oz	185	1	5%
Restaurant: 2 cups	370	2	5%
w. Bolognese (Meat Sce)	650	16	22%
w. Marinara (Seafoods)	700	20	26%
w. Napoletana (Tom. Sce)	540	13	22%
Saltimbocca (Veal/Ham/Cheese)	430	28	59%
Tortellini, 20 pieces	530	20	34%
Veal Marsala	400	20	45%
Veal Parmigiana	350	20	51%
Pizza: Per 1/2Pizza (12")			
Vegetarian/Cheese:			
Thin Crust	650	26	36%
Thick Crust	850	24	25%
Sausage/Pepperoni:			
Thin Crust	700	42	54%
Thick Crust	900	40	40%

(Also see *Pizza Hut, Domino's, Shakey's, Godfather's Pizza* ~ **Fast Foods Section.**)

Restaurant & Ethnic Foods cont

JAPANESE

SUSHI	C	F	%fc
Lunch Menu (Assorted Sushi)			
Regular, 1 serving	330	3	8%
Deluxe, 1 serving	430	4	8%
Sushi Rice, ckd, 1 Tbsp	25	<1	4%
1 cup, 5¼ oz	380	3	7%
Nigiri-Zushi: (Fish wrapped Sushi)			
Per 1 oz piece:			
Ebi-zushi (Jumbo Shrimp)	20	<1	13%
Kani-zushi (Surimi Crab)	30	<1	15%
Maguro-zushi (Tuna)	25	<1	18%
Sake-zushi (Salmon)	35	1	26%
Suzume-zushi (Baby Snapper)	30	<1	15%
Tai-zushi (Red Snapper)	30	<1	15%
Nori-Maki-Zushi: *Per Piece*			
(Seaweed-wrapped Sushi Rolls)			
Anago-maki (Conger Eel)	20	1	45%
California-maki (Crab/Caviar/Avocado)			
½ roll	70	1	13%
Futo-maki (Egg Omelet, Shellfish, Veg.),			
1 piece.	70	1	13%
Kobana-maki (Egg Omelet, Cucum.)	35	<1	13%
Kappa-maki (Cucumber)	15	0	0%
Tekka-maki (Tuna)	20	<1	22%
Uni-maki (Sea Urchin)	20	<1	22%
Inari-Zushi (Bean Curd Pouches w. Sushi)			
1 pouch, 3 oz	130	2	14%
Tamago-Yaki (Omelet-wrapped Sushi)			
1 piece	45	1	20%
Sashimi (Slice Raw Seafood/Beef)			
Ika (Squid), 4 oz	105	2	17%
Hamachi (Yellowtail), 4 oz	165	6	33%
Naguro (Yellowfin Tuna), 4 oz	120	1	8%
Niku (Beef), 4 oz	200	10	45%
Saba (Mackerel), 4 oz	160	7	39%
Suzuki (Sea Bass), 4 oz	110	<1	4%
Tako (Octopus), 4 oz	95	1	9%
Dipping Sauces: Aver., 2 Tbsp	30	0	0%
Ginger Vinegar Dress., 2 Tbsp	20	0	0%
Miso Soup w. tofu pces, 1 cup	85	3	32%
Sukiyaki (Beef/Tofu/Veg.), 8 oz	400	24	77%
Tempura (Batter-fried Shrimp & Veges.)			
3 large shrimp & veges	320	18	51%
1 shrimp only	60	4	60%
Teppan Yaki (Steak, Seafood & Veges.)			
10 oz serving	470	30	57%
Teriyaki Beef, 4 oz serving	350	25	64%
Sake Wine (16% alc.), 3 fl. oz	115	0	0%

JEWISH/DELI FOODS

	C	F	%fc
Bagel/Bialy,			
½ small, 1 oz	80	1	11%
Beiglach (Cheese Knish)	350	17	44%
Blintzes, average, 1 only	120	4	30%
w. Sour Crm. & Preserves	370	10	24%
Borscht, (no cream), 1 cup	85	6	64%
Diet/Reduced Cal., 1 cup	30	1	30%
Cabbage Roll (meat/rice), 5 oz	170	6	32%
Chicken Broth, 1 cup	80	8	90%
with vegetables	100	8	72%
with noodles	150	9	54%
Lowfat, plain, 1 cup	25	1	36%
Cholent, 1 med serve, 1 cup	350	26	67%
Chopped Liver: 1 serve, 3 oz	110	6	49%
with Egg Salad, ¼ cup	100	7	63%
Farfel, dry, 1 cup	90	<1	5%
Hallah (Yeast Bread), 1 sl., 1 oz	85	2	21%
Gefilte Fish Balls:			
Regular, medium, 2oz	55	2	33%
with jelled broth	80	2	23%
Cocktail size, 1 oz	30	1	30%
Sweet, medium, 2 oz	65	2	28%
with jelled broth	95	2	19%
Herring: Smoked, 2 oz	120	8	60%
in Sour Cream, 2oz	150	10	60%
Kasha, cooked, ½ cup	100	<1	5%
Kipfel (Vanilla/Almd. Cookie), 1 pce.	60	4	60%
Knaidlach, 1 ball	40	2	45%
Knish: Kasha/Potato, 1 only	130	8	55%
Cheese, 1 only	350	17	44%
Kreplach, beef, 1 piece	40	1	23%
Kugel, potato/noodle, 1 serve	150	7	33%
Latkes (Potato Pancake), 2 oz	200	11	22%
3 Latkes w. Sour Cr./Apple Sce	750	20	24%
Lochshen: Plain, 1 cup	130	5	35%
Pudding, 1 cup	380	13	31%
Lox (Smoked Salmon), 2 oz	65	2	28%
Mandelbrot (Almond Bread), 1 slice,			
¼" thick	45	2	40%
Matzo: 1 board, 1 oz	110	<1	4%
(Also see Matzoh ~ Page 84)			
Matzo Balls, 2 small, 1 large	90	3	30%
Soup, with 1 large ball	180	7	35%
New York Cheesecake, 4 oz	350	24	62%
Pierogi, potato/cheese, 1 pce	90	4	40%
Reuben Sandwich	920	60	59%
Schmaltz (Rend'd chick. fat), 1 Tbsp	90	10	1%

RESTAURANT & ETHNIC FOODS CONT

LEBANESE - MIDDLE EAST

	C	F	%fc
Baba Ghannouj, 2 Tbsp, 1 oz			
(Eggplant/Seasame Dip)	70	6	77%
Baklava, 1 pastry, 1 3/4 oz			
(Pastry, Nuts, Syrup)	245	18	66%
Cabbage Rolls, 1 roll, 3 oz			
(Cabbage Leaf, Meat, Rice)	100	3	27%
Cous Cous, 1 serve			
(Semolina, Milk, Fruit, Nuts)	400	21	47%
Felafel (Chick Pea Fritter):			
Fried, 1 medium, 1 oz	60	4	60%
Hummus, 1/4 cup, 2.2 oz	105	3	26%
Fried Kibbi, 1 piece, 3 oz			
(Wheat, Meat, Pinenuts)	180	8	40%
Kafta, 1 skewer, 1 1/2 oz			
(Ground Lamb Saus. on Skewer)	85	5	53%
Kibbeh Naye, 1 cup, 9 oz			
(Raw Lamb, Bulgur & Spices)	450	18	36%
Lebanese Omelet, 1 serving, 4 oz			
(Egg, Spinach, Pinenuts, Onion)	200	12	54%
Pilaf, 1 cup			
(Rice, Onion, Rais., Apr. Spice)	680	11	15%
Shawourma, 1 serve, 4 oz			
(Spit Roast Beef)	280	15	48%
Shish Kabob, 1 stick, 2 1/2 oz	130	7	48%
Spinach Pie, 1 piece	290	21	65%
Sweet Almond Sanbusak, 1 pce			
(Pastry, Almonds, Spices)	200	15	68%
Tabouli, 1 serve, 4 oz	170	14	74%
Tahini Sauce, aver., 1 Tbsp	90	8	80%

MEXICAN

	C	F	%fc
Black Bean Soup, 1 bowl	200	7	32%
Bueso Fresco, 1/4 cup	80	4.5	51%
Burritos (*Taco Bell*): Bean	370	11	27%
Big Beef Supreme	510	22	39%
Chili, plain, 1/4 cup	90	6	60%
Chili con Carne, w. Beans, 1 cup	310	17	49%
w/out Beans, 1 cup	370	28	68%
Corn Chips, 1/2 cup, 1 oz	160	10	56%
Empanadas, average, 1 small	230	10	39%
Enchilada, average	330	10	27%
Enchirito (*Taco Bell*)	380	20	47%
Fajitas: Chicken/Steak	200	7	32%
Guacamole, 2 Tbsp, 1 oz	110	12	98%
Margarita (w. 1 1/2 oz Tequila)	160	0	0%
Menudo, 1/2 cup	55	1.5	25%

MEXICAN (Cont)

	C	F	%fc
Nachos: *Taco Bell*, Big Beef	430	24	50%
Bellgrande (Taco Bell)	740	39	47%
Del Taco: Regular	450	29	53%
Macho Nachos	1090	61	50%
Pan Dulce, 1 only, 3 1/2 oz	385	12	28%
Refried Beans, 3/4 cup, 6 oz	210	5	21%
Sopaipillas (flky. pstry.puffs), 1 pc	100	7	63%
w. honey & cream	200	14	63%
Taco (*Taco Bell*): Regular	170	10	53%
Chicken	250	11	40%
Taco Supreme	260	13	45%
Big Border Taco	285	16	51%
Taco Salad w. Salsa	850	52	55%
Taco Sauce, average, 1/4 cup	15	0	0%
Taco Shell, regular	50	2	36%
Tamales, Van Camp's (can), 1/2 c	150	8	48%
Tostada (Taco Bell)	240	11	41%
Tortilla, corn, 6" diam.	70	1	13%
Tortilla Chips, 1 oz	150	8	48%

Extra Listings of Mexican Dishes:
• Frozen Entrees/Meals (Banquet/Patio etc)
• Fast Foods Section (Taco Bell, Del Taco,
• Canned Bean/Chili Products ~ See Page 57.

POLISH

	C	F	%fc
Cabbage Rolls w. Sour Cr., 2 sm.	220	10	41%
Chicken Casserole w. Mush., 1 c.	520	17	29%
Kielbasa (Sausages, Onions,			
fried, 2 lge.)	350	28	72%
Meatballs in Sour Cream,			
3 x 1 1/2" balls	300	16	48%
Pierogi, Fruit/Veg, 3" ball	80	2	23%
Pork Goulash (Pork/Veg. Stew)	550	21	34%
Pot Roast with Vegetables	630	21	30%

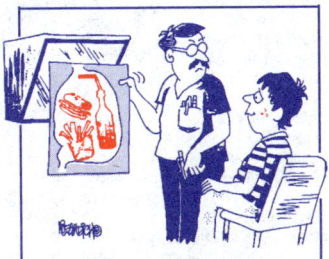

Restaurant & Ethnic Foods cont

SOUL FOODS

	C	F	%fc
Breakfast Sausage, fried, 2 patties	250	17	60%
Cornbread, homemade, 3 oz	200	7.5	34%
Fatback, raw, 1/4 oz	60	6.5	98%
Ham Hock, 1 oz	90	6.5	65%
Hog Maw, 1 oz	45	2.5	50%
Hominy, 3/4 cup	85	1	11%
Hush Puppies, 5 pces, 3 oz	260	12	42%
Kale, ckd, 1/2 cup	20	0.5	23%
Neck Bones, Pork, 1 oz	65	4	55%
Opossum, 1 oz	65	3	42%
Oxtail, 1 oz	70	3.5	45%
Pig Ear, 1/4 ear	50	3	54%
Pig Foot, 1/2 foot	70	4.5	58%
Pig Tail, 1/3 tail	115	10	78%
Poke Salad, ckd, 1/2 cup	15	0.5	30%
Pork Brains, 1 oz	40	2.5	56%
Pork Cracklings, 1 Tbsp	60	5	75%
Pork Chitterlings, simmered, 3 oz	260	25	85%
Pork Skin, 1 cup	70	4.5	58%
Sousemeat, 1 oz	60	4.5	68%
Succotash, 1/2 cup	80	1	11%
Sweet Potato Pie, 1/8 of 9" pie	250	12	43%
Tongue Pork, 1/3 tongue	75	5.5	66%
Tripe, 2 oz	55	2	33%
Vienna Sausage, 2 small	90	8	80%

THAI FOODS

	C	F	%fc
Appetizers: Satay Pork, 30g	100	7	70%
Spring Roll, 35g	110	6	55%
Soups: Tom Yam (Hot & Sour):			
with Seafood, 1 cup	100	3	27%
Vegetarian, 1 cup	50	0	0%
Mud Crab w. Coconut, 1 cup	400	37	83%
Curries: Per 1 Cup			
Chicken w. Ginger	390	34	78%
Thick Red Curry w. Beef	600	50	75%
Thai Chicken Curry	340	23	60%
Massaman Curry	680	57	75%
Green Curry w. Pork	480	44	83%
Stir Fry: Per 1 Cup			
(Combinations include Meat & Seafood)			
Comb. w. Fried Rice Noodles	470	33	63%
Comb. w. Steamed Rice Noodles	360	20	50%
Comb. Stir Fry & Veges (no rice)	410	30	66%
Stir Fry Vegetables	100	9	81%
Salads: Thai Chicken, 1 serving	330	9	25%
Thai Beef Salad, 1 serving	260	9	31%

SPANISH FOODS

	C	F	%fc
Per Serving			
Arroz Abanda (Fish with Rice)	340	8	21%
Arroz Con Pollo (Rice/Chick. Sal)	500	23	41%
Clams Marinera, 8 clams	330	16	44%
Cochifrito (Lamb w. Lemon/Garlic)	650	25	35%
Cochinillo Asado, 2 sl. (Rst Suckling Pig)	300	15	45%
Cocido Madrileno (Madrid-Style Boiled Dinner)	450	27	54%
Flan de Leche (Caramel Custard)	325	9	25%
Fritadera de Ternera (Sauteed Veal)	450	27	54%
Gazpacho, 1 bowl	60	0	0%
Paella a la Valenciana (Chicken & Shellfish Rice)	900	42	42%
Pollo a la Espanola (Chicken)	475	30	57%
Ternera al Jerez (Veal w. Sherry)	660	29	40%
Zarzuela (Fish & Shellfish Medley)	530	27	46%

VIETNAMESE

	C	F	%fc
Bo Xao Dau Phong (Per Whole Dish) (Ginger Beef w.Onion, Fish Sce.)	750	30	36%
Bo Nuong (Beef Satay), 2 sticks	265	9	31%
Ca Chien Gung (Whole Snapper w. Ginger)	600	16	24%
Canh Chay (Veg./Tofu Soup)	80	3	34%
Cuu Xao Lan (Curried Lamb, Veges in Coconut)	900	35	35%
Ga Chien (Crsp. Chick + Plum Sce)	900	40	40%
Ga Nuong (Chicken Satay + Sce.)	240	11	41%
Ga Xao Rau (Marinated Chicken Braised w.Veg.)	800	26	29%
Rau Cai Xao Chay (Stir Fried Vege., Soy Sauce.)	400	25	56%
Thit Heo Goi Baup Cai, each (Spicy Cabbage Rolls w.Pork)	200	7	32%

GOURMET & MISCELLANEOUS

	C	F	%fc
Ants Eggs/Larvae, 1 Tbsp	20	0	0%
Ants, Choc. coated, 3 Tbsp	140	7	45%
Bee Maggots, canned, 3 Tbsp	65	2	28%
Caviar, black/red, 1 Tbsp	40	3	68%
Caterpillars, canned, 60g	60	2	30%
Frogs Legs, fried, 1 pair (large)	125	7	50%
Haggis, boiled, 4 oz	350	24	62%
Locusts, raw, 1 oz	35	1	26%
Silkworms, raw, 1 oz	60	2	30%
Snails (Escargots) — See French			
Snake, roasted, 4 oz	160	6	34%

FAST-FOOD CHAINS & RESTAURANTS
FULL ANALYSIS

- **Cal** Calories
- **Fat** Fat/grams
- **%fc** Percent Fat Calories
- **S.Fat** Saturated Fat
- **Chol** Cholesterol (mg)
- **Sod** Sodium (mg)
- **Pro** Protein (grams)
- **Carb** Carbohydrates (g)

Arby's	140-141	Hardees	174-175	Red Lobster	196
Au Bon Pain	142-144	Harveys	176	Round Table Pizza	197
Baskin Robbins	144-147	IHOP	176	Roy Rogers	198-199
Big Boy	148	I Can't Believe It's Yogurt	177	Shakey's	199
Blimpie	148	Jack In The Box	178-179	7-Eleven	200
Bojangles	149	Kenny Rogers Roasters	180	Shoney's	201
Boston Market	150	KFC	181	Skipper's	202
Burger King	151-152	Krystal	182	Sizzler	203-204
Captain D's Seafood	153	Little Caesars	185	Souplantation	205-207
Carl's Jr	154-155	Long John Silver	183	Sonic Drive-In	208
Carvel Icecream	152	McDonald's	186-187	Sub Station II	208
Chick-Fil-A	155	Mrs Fields Cookies	184	Steak 'N Shake	209
Church's Fried Chicken	156	Mrs Winner's Chicken	184	Subway	210-211
Cousins Subs	156-157	Nathan's Famous	188	Sweet Tomatoes	211
Dairy Queen/Brazier	158	Olive Garden	188	Taco Bell	211-212
Del Taco	160	Papa John's Pizza	188	Taco John's	213
Denny's	161-165	Perkins	189	Taco Time	214
Domino's	165-166	Peter Piper Pizza	190	TCBY Treats	214
Dunkin Donuts	167-169	Pizza Hut	191-192	Wendy's	215-216
El Pollo Loco	170	Pizzeria Uno	192	Weinerschnitzel	217
Fazoli's	171	Popeye's	193	Whataburger	217
Godfather's Pizza	172	Quincy's Steakhouse	193-194	White Castle	218
Golden Corral	172	Rally's	195	Yoshinoya Beef Bowl	218
Haagen-Dazs	172-174	Rax	195	Zantiago	218

COPYRIGHT © 1997 ALLAN BORUSHEK

ARBY'S

	Cal	Fat (%Fc)	S.Fat	Chol	Sod	Pro	Carb
Breakfast Items							
Bacon, 2 strips	90	7 (70%)	3	15	220	5	0
Biscuit (Plain)	280	15 (48%)	3	0	730	6	34
Croissant (Plain)	220	12 (49%)	7	25	230	4	25
Egg	95	8 (76%)	2	180	55	0.5	0.5
French-Toastix, 6 pieces	430	21 (44%)	5	0	550	10	52
Ham	45	1 (20%)	<1	20	405	7	0
Sausage	165	15 (82%)	6	25	320	7	0
Swiss Cheese, 1 slice	45	3 (60%)	2	12	175	4	0.5
Table Syrup	100	0 (0%)	0	0	30	0	25
Roast Beef Sandwiches							
Arby's Melt w. Cheddar	370	18 (44%)	6	31	940	18	36
Arby-Q	430	18 (38%)	6	37	1320	22	48
Beef'n Cheddar	490	28 (52%)	9	50	1215	25	40
Giant Roast Beef	555	28 (45%)	11	71	1560	35	43
Junior Roast Beef	325	14 (39%)	5	30	780	17	35
Regular Roast Beef	390	19 (44%)	7	43	1010	23	33
Super Roast Beef	525	27 (46%)	9	43	1190	25	50
Chicken Sandwiches							
Breaded Chicken Fillet	535	28 (47%)	5	45	1015	28	46
Chicken Cordon Bleu	620	33 (48%)	8	77	1595	38	46
Chicken Fingers (2 Pieces)	290	16 (50%)	2	32	675	16	20
Grilled Chicken Deluxe	430	20 (42%)	4	61	850	23	41
Light Rst Chicken	275	7 (23%)	-	33	780	-	-
Sub Shop Sandwiches							
French Dip	475	22 (42%)	8	55	1410	30	40
Hot Ham 'n Cheese	500	23 (41%)	7	68	1665	30	43
Italian Sub	675	36 (48%)	13	83	2090	30	46
Philly Beef 'n Swiss	755	47 (56%)	15	91	2025	39	48
Roast Beef Sub	700	42 (54%)	14	84	2035	38	44
Turkey Sub	550	27 (44%)	7	65	2085	31	47
Light Menu: Garden Salad	60	0.5 (7%)	0	0	40	3	12
Roast Beef Deluxe	295	10 (31%)	3	42	825	18	33
Roast Chicken Deluxe	280	7 (23%)	2	33	775	20	33
Roast Turkey Deluxe	260	6 (21%)	2	33	1260	20	33
Roast Chicken Salad	150	2 (12%)	<1	29	420	20	12
Side Salad	25	0.3 (12%)	0	0	15	1	4
Crouton 1 pkt	60	2 (30%)	<1	1	155	2	9
Potatoes: Curly Fries	300	15 (45%)	3	0	850	4	38
Cheddar Curly Fries w. Sce	335	18 (48%)	4	3	1015	5	40
French Fries	245	13 (48%)	3	0	115	2	30
Potato Cakes	205	12 (53%)	2	0	400	2	20
Baked Potato (Plain)	355	0.3 (0%)	0	0	25	7	82
w. Marg/Sour Cream	580	24 (37%)	9	25	210	9	85
w. Broccoli 'n Cheddar	570	20 (32%)	5	12	565	14	89
Deluxe Baked Potato	735	36 (44%)	16	59	500	19	86

ARBY'S CONT

	Cal	Fat (%Fc)	S.Fat	Chol	Sod	Pro	Carb
Soups							
Cream of Broccoli	160	8 (45%)	4	25	1005	7	15
Boston Clam Chowder	190	9 (43%)	3	25	965	9	18
Lumberjack Mixed Vegetable	90	4 (40%)	2	5	1150	2	10
Old Fashioned Chicken Noodle	80	2 (22%)	0	20	850	6	11
Potato with Bacon	170	7 (37%)	3	20	905	6	23
Desserts							
Apple Turnover	330	14 (38%)	7	0	180	4	48
Cherry Turnover	320	13 (37%)	5	0	190	4	46
Cheesecake (Plain)	320	23 (65%)	14	95	240	5	23
Chocolate Chip Cookie	125	6 (43%)	2	10	85	2	16
Chocolate Shake	450	12 (24%)	3	35	240	15	76
Jamocha Shake	385	10 (23%)	3	36	260	15	62
Vanilla Shake	360	12 (30%)	4	36	280	15	50
Polar Swirl: Butterfinger	460	18 (35%)	8	28	320	15	62
Heath	545	22 (36%)	5	39	345	15	76
Oreo	480	22 (41%)	10	35	520	15	66
Peanut Butter Cup	515	24 (42%)	8	34	385	20	61
Snickers	510	19 (33%)	7	33	350	15	73
Dressings/Sauces							
Arby's Sauce	15	0.2 (12%)	0	0	115	0	4
Beef Stock Au Jus	10	0 (0%)	0	0	440	0	1
Barbeque Sauce	30	0 (0%)	0	0	185	0	7
Blue Cheese	290	31 (96%)	6	50	580	2	2
Cheddar Cheese Sauce	35	3 (77%)	1	4	140	1	1
Honey French	280	23 (74%)	3	0	400	0	18
Horsey Sauce	60	5 (75%)	1	5	150	0	2
Ketchup	16	0 (0%)	0	0	145	0	4
Mayonnaise	110	12 (98%)	7	5	80	0	0
Light Cholesterol Free	12	1 (75%)	0	0	65	0	0.5
Mustard, German Style	5	0 (0%)	0	0	70	0	1
Italian Sub Sauce	70	7 (90%)	1	0	240	0	1
Parmesan Cheese Sauce	70	7 (90%)	1	5	130	1	2
Red Ranch Dressing	75	6 (72%)	1	0	115	0	5
Tartar Sauce	140	15 (96%)	2	30	220	0	0
Thousand Island Dressing	260	26 (90%)	4	30	420	0	7
Reduced Calorie:							
Honey Mayonnaise	70	7 (90%)	1	20	135	0	1
Italian	20	1 (45%)	0	0	1,000	0	3
Buttermilk Ranch	50	0 (0%)	0	0	710	0	12

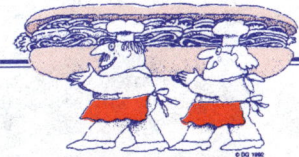

AU BON PAIN

	Cal	Fat (%Fc)	S.Fat	Chol	Sod	Pro	Carb
Bagels (each)							
Sesame	425	5 (11%)	1	0	665	17	81
Other types, average	390	2 (5%)	<1	0	665	16	81.0
Bread							
Baguette, 1 loaf	810	2 (2%)	<1	0	1830	27	166
Cheese, 1 loaf	1670	29 (16%)	9	75	4140	70	269
Four Grain, 1 loaf	1420	11 (7%)	<1	1	3050	57	262
Onion Herb, 1 loaf	1430	13 (8%)	<1	0	2390	52	263
Pita Pocket, 2 slices	80	<1 (3%)	na	na	na	3	18
Ponsienne, 1 loaf	1490	4 (2%)	<1	0	3380	49	166
Sandwich, Multigrain 2 slices	390	3 (7%)	1	1	2040	16	77
Sandwich, Rye 2 slices	375	4 (10%)	1	na	2170	14	73
Croissants: Almond	420	25 (54%)	12	95	250	8	41
Apple	250	10 (36%)	6	25	150	4	38
Blueberry Cheese	380	20 (47%)	12	60	280	7	44
Chocolate	400	24 (54%)	14	35	220	5	46
Cinnamon Raisin	390	13 (30%)	8	35	240	7	60
Coconut Pecan	440	23 (47%)	12	45	290	7	51
Hazelnut Chocolate	480	28 (53%)	14	35	220	6	56
Plain	220	10 (41%)	6	25	240	5	29
Raspberry/Strawberry Cheese	400	20 (45%)	12	60	280	7	49
Sweet Cheese	420	23 (49%)	14	70	310	8	45
w.Ham & Cheese	370	20 (49%)	12	55	280	10	38
w.Spinach & Cheese	290	16 (50%)	10	45	310	9	29
w.Turkey & Cheddar/Havarti	410	22 (48%)	13	70	680	16	38
Rolls: Alpine	220	3 (12%)	na	0	810	8	43
Country Seed	220	4 (16%)	na	8	460	9	37
Hearth	250	2 (7%)	na	0	510	10	42
Petit Pain	220	<1 (2%)	na	0	490	7	44
Pumpernickel	210	2 (9%)	na	0	1005	8	42
Rye	230	2 (8%)	na	0	na	8	44
Sandwich, braided	390	11 (26%)	3	34	1540	10	64
Sandwich, croissant	300	14 (42%)	8	35	240	7	38
Sandwich, French	320	<1 (1%)	na	0	710	10	65
Sandwich, hearth	370	3 (7%)	na	0	600	16	69
Sandwich, soft	310	8 (23%)	na	0	410	8	50
3 Seed Raisin	250	4 (14%)	na	0	480	8	46
Vegetable	230	5 (20%)	na	0	410	6	40
Soup: Per Serving							
Beef Barley, 1 bowl	110	3 (24%)	na	18	900	9	15
1 cup	75	2 (24%)	na	12	600	6	10
Broccoli, 1 bowl	300	26 (77%)	12	54	220	8	18
1 cup	200	17 (76%)	8	36	145	5	12
Chicken Noodle, 1 bowl	120	2 (15%)	<1	26	745	12	14
1 cup	80	1 (11%)	<1	17	495	8	9
Chili, 1 bowl	210	4 (17%)	<1	0	765	9	37
1 cup	140	3 (19%)	<1	0	510	6	24

AU BON PAIN CONT

	Cal	Fat	(%Fc)	S.Fat	Chol	Sod	Pro	Carb
Soup (Cont)								
Clam Chowder, 1 bowl	435	27	(56%)	15	90	1030	17	36
1 cup	290	18	(56%)	9	60	680	11	24
Minestrone, 1 cup	105	2	(17%)	na	1	265	5	20
Split Pea, 1 bowl	265	2	(7%)	na	1	455	18	45
1 cup	175	1	(5%)	na	1	305	12	3
Tomato, 1 bowl	90	2	(20%)	<1	0	220	4	15
1 cup	60	1	(15%)	<1	0	145	3	10
Vegetarian, 1 bowl	45	0.2	(4%)	<1	0	90	2	9
1 cup	30	0.1	(3%)	<1	0	60	1	6
Chicken Pot Pie, 1 serving	440	21	(43%)	7	45	1110	18	46
Chicken Sandwiches: *each*								
Cracked Pepper: on French Roll	440	3	(6%)	na	50	1390	33	66
on Hearth Roll	490	5	(9%)	na	50	1280	39	70
on Soft Roll	430	10	(21%)	na	50	1090	31	51
Grilled: on French Roll	450	5	(10%)	na	60	1320	33	66
on Hearth Roll	500	7	(13%)	na	60	1210	39	70
on Soft Roll	440	12	(25%)	na	60	1015	31	51
Tarragon: on French Roll	590	16	(24%)	na	70	1015	34	68
on Hearth Roll	640	18	(25%)	na	70	905	40	72
on Soft Roll	580	23	(36%)	na	70	715	32	53
Ham Sandwiches: *each*								
Country Ham on French Roll	470	8	(15%)	na	115	1680	27	68
on Hearth Roll	520	10	(17%)	na	115	1570	33	72
on Soft Roll	460	15	(29%)	na	115	1380	25	53
Roast Beef Sandwiches: *each*								
on French Roll	500	9	(16%)	na	60	1020	34	66
on Hearth Roll	550	11	(18%)	na	60	910	40	70
on Soft Roll	490	16	(29%)	na	60	720	32	51
Turkey Sandwiches: *each*								
Smoked: on French Roll	420	2	(4%)	na	35	1660	32	65
on Hearth Roll	470	4	(8%)	na	35	1550	38	69
on Soft Roll	410	9	(20%)	na	35	1360	30	50
Sandwich Fillings: Per Serving								
Boursin	290	29	(90%)	18		390	6	2
Brie	300	24	(72%)	15	85	510	18	3
Cheddar	110	9	(74%)	5	30	150	7	1
Provolone	155	13	(75%)	7	36	180	10	<1
Swiss	330	24	(65%)	15	80	230	25	3
Salads: Per Serving								
Garden: Small	20	<1	(0%)	na	0	10	5	5
Large	40	<1	(0%)	<1	0	20	3	8
Chicken Tarragon	310	15	(44%)	na	70	330	24	11
Cracked Pepper Chicken	100	2	(18%)	na	25	360	14	9
Grilled Chicken	110	2	(16%)	na	30	330	14	9
Shrimp	100	2	(18%)	na	105	195	11	8
Tuna	350	25	(64%)	4	40	480	21	11
Italian, low-calorie	70	6	(79%)	na	5	360	0	3

AU BON PAIN CONT

	Cal	Fat	(%Fc)	S.Fat	Chol	Sod	Pro	Carb
Muffins: Bran	390	11	(25%)	na	20	940	7	73
Blueberry	390	4	(9%)	na	40	410	8	66
Carrot	450	22	(44%)	5	15	610	7	58
Corn	460	17	(33%)	3	25	510	8	71
Cranberry Walnut	350	13	(33%)	na	15	730	7	53
Oat Bran Apple	400	2	(5%)	na	0	590	7	71
Pumpkin	410	16	(35%)	2	20	500	6	63
Whole Grain	440	16	(33%)	2	30	310	10	68
Danish Pastries: Cheese	390	22	(51%)	12	78	530	8	43
Cherry; Raspberry	335	16	(43%)	8	50	480	7	42
Cherry Dumpling	360	13	(33%)	2	0	255	5	59
Cookies, each:								
Chocolate Chip	280	15	(48%)	9	25	70	2	37
Chocolate Chunk Pecan	290	17	(53%)	6	10	200	3	37
Oatmeal Raisin	250	9	(32%)	na	10	230	4	41
Peanut Butter	290	15	(47%)	6	10	250	7	33
Shortbread	425	26	(55%)	16	68	385	5	46
White Choc. Chunk Pecan	300	17	(51%)	6	10	200	3	37

BASKIN ROBBINS

	Cal	Fat	(%Fc)	S.Fat	Chol	Sod	Pro	Carb
Deluxe: Per Regular Scoop								
Banana Nut	260	17	(58%)	8	50	70	4	26
Banana Strawberry	240	12	(45%)	8	50	75	3	30
Baseball Nut	280	16	(51%)	8	50	95	4	31
Black Walnut	280	19	(61%)	10	55	85	5	23
Blueberry Cheesecake	260	12	(42%)	7	45	140	3.5	35
Butterfinger	300	15	(45%)	7	31	120	4	39
Caramel Choc. Crunch	290	17	(53%)	11	50	150	4	33
Cherry Cheesecake	260	12	(42%)	7	25	45	4	35
Cherries Jubilee	240	13	(49%)	8	50	75	3	29
Chewy Babe Ruth	300	17	(51%)	11	55	115	4	32
Choc O The Irish	280	17	(55%)	11	55	105	4	30
Chocoholic's Resolution	300	16	(48%)	10	50	115	4	37
Chocolate	270	16	(53%)	10	55	110	4	31
Chocolate Almond	310	20	(58%)	10	50	100	6	30
Chocolate Chip	270	18	(60%)	11	60	85	4	26
Chocolate Chip Cookie Dough	300	17	(51%)	10	60	125	4	35
Chocolate Fudge	290	15	(47%)	8	41	180	4	34
Chocolate Mousse Royale	310	18	(52%)	9	50	105	4	35
Chocolate Raspberry Truffle	280	14	(45%)	9	50	95	4	36
Chocolate Ribbon	250	13	(47%)	9	50	80	3	30
Chunka Cherry Burn Love	250	13	(47%)	8	50	80	3	29
Chunky Heath Bar	300	18	(54%)	11	50	125	3	33
Cinnamon Tax Crunch	280	14	(45%)	7	45	125	4	35
Cookies 'n Cream	300	19	(57%)	12	55	140	4	29

BASKIN ROBBINS CONT

	Cal	Fat	(%Fc)	S.Fat	Chol	Sod	Pro	Carb
Deluxe: Per Regular Scoop								
Coconut	280	19	(61%)	13	60	85	4	24
Decorating Vanilla	250	16	(58%)	10	65	85	3	24
English Toffee	290	16	(50%)	10	55	125	3	34
French Vanilla	280	18	(58%)	10	90	90	4	25
Fudge Brownie	310	19	(55%)	11	50	130	5	35
German Choc Cake	310	15	(44%)	7	32	100	5	39
Gold Medal Ribbon	270	13	(43%)	8	50	170	3	35
Here Comes The Judge	270	13	(42%)	9	36	100	4	36
Jamoca	250	15	(54%)	10	60	85	3	25
Jamoca Almond Fudge	280	16	(51%)	8	45	70	4	30
Kahlua & Choc. Cream	270	14	48%	9	55	90	4	29
Lemon Custard	260	15	(52%)	9	80	100	4	29
Martian Mint	260	15	(52%)	9	40	140	3	30
Mint Choc Chip	270	18	(60%)	11	60	85	4	26
Naughty New Year's Resol,	310	20	(58%)	9	45	125	6	40
New York Cheesecake	270	16	(54%)	11	45	135	4	30
Nutty Coconut	310	21	(61%)	10	50	85	4	27
Nutty or Nice	290	16	(50%)	9	50	130	4	36
Old Fashion Butter Pecan	290	20	(62%)	10	60	90	4	23
Oregan Blackberry	230	12	(47%)	8	51	69	4	28
Peach	240	12	(45%)	8	50	70	3	28
Peanut Butter 'n Cookie	330	22	(60%)	10	50	170	6	29
Peppermint	270	14	(47%)	9	55	80	3	33
Pink Bubblegum	270	14	(47%)	9	55	75	3	34
Pistachio-Almond	300	21	(63%)	10	55	80	6	23
Pralines 'n Cream	290	16	(50%)	8	50	135	3	34
Pumpkin Patch	250	13	(47%)	8	45	90	3	31
Quarterback Crunch	290	17	(53%)	12	50	135	3	32
Red, White & Boo	260	12	(42%)	12	45	80	3	36
Reeses Peanut Butter	310	19	(55%)	11	55	125	5	30
Rocky Road	300	17	(51%)	9	50	105	5	34
Rudolph's Red Raspberry								
Cranberry Sorbet	140	0	(0%)	0	0	10	0	36
Rum Raisin	250	13	(47%)	8	50	70	3	32
S'Crunch Ous Crunch	310	16	(46%)	10	45	110	4	40
S'Mores	300	13	(39%)	8	29	100	4	41
Snickidy Doo Dah	300	16	(48%)	9	50	160	4	35
Strawberry Cheesecake	270	14	(47%)	9	45	130	3	34
Strawberry Shortcake	280	16	(51%)	10	50	125	3	32
Triple Chocolate Passion	290	18	(56%)	10	55	110	5	34
Vanilla	240	14	(52%)	9	52	115	4	24
Very Berry Strawberry	220	10	(41%)	5	30	95	3	30
Winter White Chocolate	270	16	(53%)	11	45	90	3	31
Winter Wondermint	270	14	(47%)	9	55	80	3	33
World Class Chocolate	280	16	(51%)	9	55	105	4	32

Continued Next Page

BASKIN ROBBINS CONT

	Cal	Fat	(%Fc)	S.Fat	Chol	Sod	Pro	Carb
Light Icecream: Regular Serving								
Almond Butterscotch	260	9	(30%)	4.5	22	120	9	39
Choc Caramel Nut	260	6	(21%)	4.5	11	165	9	44
Double Raspberry	200	5	(20%)	2	22	90	6	35
Espresso 'n Cream	220	6	(25%)	2	11	135	6	39
Pistachio Creme Chip	265	9	(30%)	5	22	120	9	37
Praline Dream	240	6	(23%)	4.5	11	160	9	39
Rocky Path	290	9	(28%)	3	22	120	9	42
Non Fat Icecream: Regular Serving								
Caramel Banana Surprise	240	0	(0%)	0	0	210	6	53
Chocolate Marshmallow	265	0	(0%)	0	11	165	2	57
Chocolate Wonder	200	0	(0%)	0	6	160	9	44
Jamoca Swirl	240	0	(0%)	0	11	230	6	51
Just Peachy	220	0	(0%)	0	0	200	6	48
Kookaberry Kiwi	200	0	(0%)	0	0	200	6	44
Peanut Butter Cream	220	0	(0%)	0	0	240	9	46
Pineapple Cheesecake	240	0	(0%)	0	4	220	6	53
Vanilla Bean	220	0	(0%)	0	0	240	9	44
Vanilla Marble	240	0	(0%)	0	4	240	9	51
No Sugar Added: Regular Serving								
Berries 'n Banana	175	2	(10%)	2	11	120	6	33
Call Me Nuts	220	5	(20%)	2	11	120	6	42
Cherry Cordial	220	5	(20%)	5	11	120	6	42
Chocolate Chip	220	6	(25%)	3	120	160	9	37
Chocolate Choc Chip	220	6	(25%)	3	11	160	9	37
Chunky Banana	200	5	(23%)	2	11	120	6	35
Coconut Fudge	240	5	(19%)	2	11	130	6	44
Jamoca Swiss Almond	220	6	(25%)	5	11	140	6	35
Pineapple Coconut	200	3	(14%)	2	11	130	6	35
Raspberry Revelation	220	2	(8%)	11	11	120	6	44
Thin Mint	220	6	(25%)	5	11	160	9	37
Vanilla Swiss Almond	240	5	(19%)	3	11	130	6	44
Soft Serving Icecream: Regular Serving								
Caramel Praline	260	0	(0%)	0	6	190	9	55
Vanilla	260	0	(0%)	0	6	190	11	55
Ices, Sherbets, Sorbets: Regular Serving								
Ices: Daquiri	240	0	(0%)	0	0	20	0	59
Grape	220	0	(0%)	0	0	20	0	59
Margarita	240	0	(0%)	0	0	20	0	61
Sherbets: Rainbow/Orange	260	5	(17%)	2	11	55	2	57
Sorbets:								
Pink Raspberry Lemonade	260	0	(0%)	0	0	20	0	64
Red Raspberry	260	0	(0%)	0	0	20	0	66

BASKIN ROBBINS CONT

	Cal	Fat	(%Fc)	S.Fat	Chol	Sod	Pro	Carb
Yogurt Gone Crazy								
For Heaven's Cake	260	5	(17%)	3	20	165	6	53
Have Your Cake	240	5	(19%)	2	11	220	9	48
Maui Brownie Madness	310	6	(17%)	2	11	220	9	48
Perils of Praline	310	6	(17%)	4	11	230	9	55
Raspberry Cheese Louse	290	6	(19%)	4	20	200	9	53
Frozen Yogurt: Reg. Scoop								
Low Fat: All flavors, aver.	260	4	(14%)	2	15	165	9	50
Non Fat: All flavors, aver.	240	0	(0%)	0	0	120	6	50
Truly Free; average	200	0	(0%)	0	11	180	9	40
Novelties: Per Serving								
Chillyburger, all types	220	11	(45%)	7	25	100	4	27
Sundae Bars: Per Serving								
Jamoca Almond Fudge	280	17	(55%)	9	20	60	5	28
Peanut Butter Choc	340	27	(71%)	11	20	115	7	22
Pralines 'n Cream	280	17	(55%)	10	10	105	4	28
Tiny Toon Bars								
All varieties, 1 serving	240	17	(64%)	11	25	40	3	20
Cappy Blast Bars								
All varieties, average	120	4	(30%)	3	15	35	2	20
Fountain Drinks								
Cappy Blast	290	10	(31%)	7	50	105	6	42
w.Whipped Cream, 2 tsp	320	13	(37%)	9	55	105	0	43
Mocha Cappy Blast	330	11	(30%)	7	50	130	6	55
w.Whipped Cream, 2 tsp	360	14	(35%)	9	55	130	0	56
Paradise Blast/Pina Colada	330	9	(25%)	5	40	55	3	55
Paradise Blast/Stawberry	300	6	(18%)	4	25	775	2	56
Malt Shake/Vanilla IC	660	31	(42%)	19	145	250	15	84
Malt Powder	110	1.5	(12%)	1	0	80	2	23
Toppings								
Butterscotch, 2 oz	200	2	(9%)	na	6	160	0	47
Hot Fudge, 1 oz	100	3	(27%)	na	4	45	1	17
No Sug.Add/Fat Free	90	0	(0%)	0	2	95	2	20
Praline Caramel, 1 oz	90	0	(0%)	0	0	105	0	19
Strawberry, 1 oz	60	0	(0%)	0	0	5	0	14
Whipped Cream, 2 tsp	30	3	(90%)	2	5	0	0	1
White & Colored Sprinkles	20	0.5	(22%)	0	0	0	0	3
Baby Gummy Bears, 75 pieces	130	0	(0%)	0	0	15	3	30
Cones: Sugar	60	3	(45%)	0	0	50	1	7
Cake	25	0.5	(18%)	0	0	55	1	4
Waffle Cone., large	120	1.5	(11%)	0	0	55	0	14
Fresh Baked	145	2	(12%)	0.5	13	5	2	30
Smoothies: Per 8 fl oz								
Blueberry Strawberry	150	0	(0%)	0	0	70	4	31
Orange Banana	120	0	(0%)	0	5	75	5	24
Strawberry Banana	170	0	(0%)	0	5	75	4	39

BIG BOY

	Cal	Fat	(%Fc)	S.Fat	Chol	Sod	Pro	Carb
Sandwiches								
Turkey	225	5	(20%)	na	75	835	22	24
Chicken w. Mozzarella	405	13	(29%)	na	76	420	42	26
Dinners (w.Bread; No Dressing):								
Chicken Breast: w.Salad	350	13	(34%)	na	65	340	38	20
w.Mozzarella & Salad	370	12	(29%)	na	76	355	42	24
Cajun & Salad	350	13	(34%)	na	65	610	38	20
Chckn. & Veg. stir-fry(no bread)	560	14	(22%)	na	68	750	43	68
Fish:Cod Baked; Dijon, Salad	430	18	(38%)	na	68	570	44	21
w.Salad	365	12	(30%)	na	68	370	43	20
Cod Broiled; Dijon, Salad	430	18	(38%)	na	68	570	44	21
w.Salad	365	12	(30%)	na	68	370	43	20
Cod, Cajun, Salad	365	12	(30%)	na	68	460	43	20
Spaghetti Marinara & Salad	450	6	(12%)	na	8	760	15	87
Soup: Cabbage, 1 bowl	45	1	(21%)	na	1	730	2	9
1 cup	40	0	(0%)	0	1	625	2	8
Vegetables: Vege. Stir-fry	410	10	(22%)	na	0	705	9	74
Beans, green	30	0	(0%)	0	0	0	2	6
Carrots	35	0	(0%)	0	0	40	1	8
Corn	90	1	(10%)	na	0	0	3	21
Mixed Vegetables	30	0	(0%)	0	0	40	2	5
Peas	80	0	(0%)	0	0	130	6	13
Potato, Baked	165	0	(0%)	0	0	10	5	37
Rice	115	0	(0%)	0	0	640	3	25
Roll	140	0	(0%)	0	2	185	3	30
Salad: Chicken Breast, Dijon	390	11	(25%)	na	65	415	42	31
Dinner, without Dressing	20	0	(0%)	na	0	10	1	4
Dressing: Buttermilk	35	2	(50%)	na	10	150	0	4
Desserts: 'No-no' frozen dessert	75	0	(0%)	0	0	35	2	17
Yogurt, frozen, regular	70	0	(0%)	0	0	30	2	16
Shake	185	0	(0%)	na	2	130	8	36

BLIMPIE

	Cal	Fat	(%Fc)	S.Fat	Chol	Sod	Pro	Carb
Subs: Per 6" sub								
Blimpie Best	410	13	(29%)	5	50	1480	26	47
Cheese Trio	510	23	(41%)	13	60	1060	26	51
Club	450	13	(26%)	6	40	1350	30	53
Grilled Chicken	400	9	(20%)	2	30	950	28	52
5 Meatball	500	22	(40%)	8	25	970	23	52
Ham & Swiss	400	13	(29%)	7	35	970	25	47
Ham, Salami. Provolone	590	28	(43%)	11	70	1880	32	52
Roast Beef	340	4.5	(13%)	1	20	870	27	47
Steak & Cheese	550	26	(42%)	4	70	1080	27	51
Tuna	570	32	(50%)	5	50	790	21	50
Turkey	320	4.5	(14%)	1	10	890	19	51
Salad: Grilled Chick., no dress.	350	12	(31%)	0	140	1190	47	13

BOJANGLES

	Cal	Fat	(%Fc)	S.Fat	Chol	Sod	Pro	Carb
Cajun Spiced Chicken								
Breast	280	17	(55%)	na	75	565	18	12
Leg	265	16	(55%)	na	96	530	19	11
Thigh	310	23	(67%)	na	67	465	15	11
Wing	355	25	(63%)	na	94	630	21	11
Cajun Roast Chicken								
Breast, without skin	145	5	(31%)	na	84	560	24	<1
Leg, without skin	160	8	(45%)	na	125	570	23	<1
Thigh, without skin	215	15	(63%)	na	95	430	20	<1
Wing, without skin	230	15	(59%)	na	117	620	22	3
Southern Style Chicken								
Breast	260	16	(55%)	na	76	700	16	12
Leg	260	15	(52%)	na	94	445	19	11
Thigh	310	21	(61%)	na	78	630	16	14
Wing	340	21	(56%)	na	86	685	17	19
Sandwiches/Nuggets								
Cajun Fillet	680	48	(63%)	9	43	735	22	41
Grilled Fillet	395	21	(48%)	3	54	810	20	33
Chicken Bites	180	5	(25%)	2	105	690	27	5
Biscuit Sandwiches								
Biscuit (plain)	295	16	(49%)	4	<1	740	6	33
Bacon	430	28	(59%)	8	25	1120	14	30
Bacon, Egg & Cheese	700	54	(69%)	17	173	1560	23	31
Cajun Filet	630	43	(61%)	10	31	990	21	41
Country Ham	330	18	(49%)	4	34	1465	14	30
Egg	425	31	(66%)	7	123	705	8	30
Sausage	510	36	(64%)	11	41	1150	15	30
Smoked Sausage	405	27	(60%)	9	20	1020	11	32
Steak	650	49	(68%)	13	34	1125	14	37
Fixins'								
Bo Rounds	390	31	(72%)	8	0	375	3	27
Cajun Pintos	100	0.2	(1%)	<1	0	735	5	19
Marinated Cole Slaw	135	3	(20%)	0	0	455	1	26
Corn on the Cob	140	2	(13%)	0	0	20	5	34
Dirty Rice	450	22	(44%)	6	24	1800	9	52
Green Beans	30	0	(0%)	0	0	555	1	6
Macaroni & Cheese	200	14	(63%)	5	26	420	7	12
Potatoes, no Gravy	110	3	(25%)	<1	0	435	2	18
Seasoned Fries	360	19	(47%)	6	0	1790	5	46
Sweet Biscuits: each								
Apple Cinnamon	395	19	(43%)	4	<1	785	6	50
Bo Berry	400	19	(43%)	5	<1	750	6	51
Cinnamon	370	19	(46%)	4	<1	775	6	45

BOSTON MARKET

	Cal	Fat	(%Fc)	S.Fat	Chol	Sod	Pro	Carb
Entrees								
Chicken: 1/4 white meat w. skin	330	7	(46%)	4.5	175	530	43	2
No skin or wing	160	3.5	(20%)	1	95	350	31	0
1/4 dark meat w. skin	330	22	(60%)	6	180	460	31	2
No skin	210	10	(43%)	2.5	150	320	28	1
1/2 chicken w. skin	630	37	(53%)	19	370	960	74	2
Original Pot Pie, 1 pie	750	34	(41%)	9	115	2380	34	78
Chunky Chicken Salad	390	30	(69%)	4.5	145	790	27	3
Ham w. Cinnamon Apples	350	13	(33%)	2.5	75	1750	25	35
Meat Loaf w. Tom Sauce	370	18	(44%)	8	120	1170	30	22
Meat Loaf w. Gravy	390	22	(51%)	8	120	1040	30	19
Turkey Breast, no skin	170	1	(5%)	0.5	100	850	36	1
Soup								
Chicken, 3/4 cup	80	3	(34%)	1	25	470	9	4
Chicken Tortilla, 1 cup	220	11	(45%)	4	35	1410	10	19
Salads								
Caesar, 10 oz	520	43	(74%)	12	40	1420	20	16
Caesar, no dressing, 8 oz	240	13	(49%)	7	25	780	19	14
Chicken Caesar, 13 oz	670	47	(63%)	13	120	1860	45	16
Sandwiches								
Chicken Salad	680	33	(44%)	4	145	1350	38	63
Chicken w. Cheese & Sauce	760	32	(38%)	11	160	1810	46	71
No Cheese or Sauce	430	3.5	(7%)	1	95	350	39	51
Ham w. Cheese & Sauce	760	35	(41%)	13	100	1880	38	71
No Cheese or Sauce	450	9	(18%)	3	45	1600	25	66
Meat Loaf w. Cheese	860	33	(35%)	18	165	2270	46	95
No Cheese	690	21	(27%)	7	120	1610	40	85
Ham & Trky Club w/Ch & Sce	890	43	(43%)	20	150	2310	47	79
No Cheese or Sauce	430	6	(13%)	2	55	1330	29	64
Turkey w. Cheese & Sauce	710	28	(35%)	10	110	1390	45	68
No Cheese or Sauce	400	3.5	(8%)	1	60	1070	32	51
Side Dishes								
Corn, 3/4 cup	190	4	(19%)	1	0	130	5	39
Coleslaw, 3/4 cup	280	16	(51%)	2.5	25	520	2	32
Hot Cinnamon Apples, 3/4 cup	250	4.5	(16%)	0.5	0	45	0	56
Macaroni Cheese, 3/4 cup	280	10	(32%)	6	20	760	12	36
Mash Potatoes & Gravy, 3/4 c.	200	9	(40%)	5	25	560	3	27
Rice Pilaf, 2/3 cup	180	5	(25%)	1	0	600	5	32
Stuffing, 3/4 cup	310	12	(35%)	2	0	1140	5	44
Mediterranean Pasta Salad, 3/4 cup	170	10	(53%)	2.5	10	490	4	16
Tortellini Salad, 3/4 cup	380	24	(57%)	4.5	90	530	14	29
Baked Goods: Brownie	450	27	(54%)	7	80	190	6	47
Corn Bread, 1 loaf	200	6	(27%)	1.5	25	390	3	33
Choc Chip Cookie	340	17	(45%)	6	25	240	4	48
Oatmeal Raisin Cookie	320	13	(37%)	2.5	25	260	4	48

BURGER KING

	Cal	Fat	(%Fc)	S.Fat	Chol	Sod	Pro	Carb
Breakfast: Biscuit w.Sausage	590	40	(61%)	13	45	1390	16	41
Biscuit w.Bacon,Egg,Cheese	510	31	(55%)	10	225	1530	19	39
Croissan'wich								
Sausage/Egg/Chse	600	46	(69%)	16	260	1140	22	25
French Toast Sticks	500	27	(49%)	7	0	490	4	60
Hash Browns	220	12	(49%)	3	0	320	2	25
A.M. Express Grape/Strawb.	30	0	(0%)	0	0	0	0	7
Burgers: Whopper Sandwich	640	39	(55%)	11	90	870	27	45
w. Cheese	730	46	(57%)	16	115	1350	33	46
Double Whopper Sandwich	870	56	(58%)	19	170	940	46	45
w. Cheese	960	63	(59%)	24	195	1420	52	46
Whopper JR Sandwich	420	24	(51%)	8	60	530	21	29
w.Cheese Sandwich	460	28	(54%)	10	75	770	23	29
Hamburger	330	15	(41%)	6	55	530	20	28
Cheeseburger	380	19	(45%)	9	65	770	23	28
Double Cheeseburger	600	36	(54%)	17	135	1060	41	28
w. Bacon	640	39	(55%)	18	145	1240	44	28
Sandwich/Side Orders								
BK Big Fish Sandwich	700	41	(53%)	6	90	980	26	56
BK Broiler Chicken Sandwich	550	29	(47%)	6	80	480	30	41
no Mayonnaise	340	6	(16%)	3	60	320	0	41
Chicken Sandwich	710	43	(55%)	9	60	1400	26	54
Chicken Tenders (8 piece)	310	17	(49%)	4	45	710	22	19
Broiled Chicken Salad	200	10	(45%)	4	60	110	21	7
Garden Salad, 9 oz	100	5	(45%)	3	15	110	6	8
Side Salad	60	3	(45%)	2	5	55	3	4
French Fries: Small, 2.6 oz	240	13	(49%)	3	0	155	3	28
Medium, salted: 4 oz	370	20	(49%)	5	0	240	5	43
Coated, $3^{1}/_{2}$ oz	340	17	(45%)	5	0	680	4	43
Large, 5 oz	460	25	(49%)	6	0	300	6	54
Onion Rings	310	14	(41%)	2	0	810	4	41
Dutch Apple Pie	300	15	(45%)	3	0	230	3	39
Condiments/Toppings								
American Cheese, 2 slices	90	8	(80%)	5	25	420	6	0
Lettuce	0	0	(0%)	0	0	0	0	0
Tomato, 2 slices	5	0	(0%)	0	0	0	0	1
Onion, $^{1}/_{2}$ oz	5	0	(0%)	0	0	0	0	1
Pickles, 4 slices	0	0	(0%)	0	0	140	0	0
Ketchup, $^{1}/_{2}$ oz	15	0	(0%)	0	0	180	0	4
Mustard, 3g	0	0	(0%)	0	0	40	0	0
Mayonnaise, 1 oz	210	23	(99%)	3	20	160	0	<1
Tartar Sauce, 1 oz	180	19	(95%)	3	15	220	0	0
Land O'Lakes Whipped	65	7	(97%)	1	0	75	0	0
Bull's Eye BBQ Sauce, $^{1}/_{2}$ oz	20	0	(0%)	0	0	140	0	5
Bacon Bits, 3 g	15	1	(60%)	<1	5	0	1	0
Croutons, $^{1}/_{4}$ oz	30	1	(30%)	0	0	75	<1	4

BURGER KING CONT

	Cal	Fat	(%Fc)	S.Fat	Chol	Sod	Pro	Carb
Salad Dressings, 1 oz: French	140	10	(64%)	2	0	190	0	11
Thousand Island	140	12	(77%)	3	15	190	0	7
Ranch	180	19	(95%)	4	10	170	<1	2
Bleu Cheese	160	16	(90%)	4	30	260	2	1
Reduced Calorie Light Italian	15	0.5	(30%)	0	0	50	0	3
Dipping Sauces, 1 oz: Ranch	170	17	(90%)	3	0	200	0	2
A.M.Exprs Dip; Honey, average	90	0	(0%)	0	0	20	0	21
Barbeque	35	0	(0%)	0	0	400	0	9
Sweet & Sour	45	0	(0%)	0	0	50	0	11
Shakes: Vanilla, Small, 16 fl oz	310	6.5	(19%)	3.5	15	240	10	53
Medium, 22 fl. oz	430	9	(19%)	5	20	330	14	73
Large, 32 fl. oz	625	13	(19%)	7	30	480	20	106
Choc/Strawb: Small, 16 fl. oz	410	7	(16%)	4	20	250	10	76
Medium, 22 fl. oz	560	10	(16%)	5.5	30	340	14	105
Large, 32 fl. oz	815	15	(16%)	8	45	495	20	153
Coca-Cola Classic, med, 22 oz	280	0	(0%)	0	0	5	0	70
Sprite, medium, 22 fl. oz	260	0	(0%)	0	0	5	0	66
Tropicana Orange Juice, 11 oz	140	0	(0%)	0	0	0	2	33
Milk - 2% Low Fat	120	5	(37%)	3	20	120	8	12

CARVEL ICECREAM

	Cal	Fat	(%Fc)	S.Fat	Chol	Sod	Pro	Carb
Soft Serving: Chocolate; Small	290	16	(50%)	10	65	90	7	33
Regular	395	22	(50%)	13	88	120	9	46
Large	510	28	(49%)	17	112	160	11	59
No Fat; Small	145	0	(0%)	0	0	110	5	30
Regular	200	0	(0%)	0	0	160	7	42
Large	250	0	(0%)	0	0	200	8	53
Vanilla; Small	305	16	(47%)	10	80	110	8	34
Regular	420	22	(47%)	13	110	160	11	46
Large	530	28	(47%)	17	140	200	14	59
No Fat; Small	190	0	(0%)	0	8	150	8	38
Regular	265	0	(0%)	0	11	210	11	53
Large	335	0	(0%)	0	14	270	14	67
Vanilla Yogurt; Small	160	3	(17%)	2	16	110	6.5	19
Regular	220	5	(17%)	2.5	22	150	9	26
Large	280	6	(17%)	3	28	190	11	34
Sherbet, all flavors; Small	240	1.5	(6%)	<1	8	50	1.5	53
Regular	330	2	(6%)	1	11	80	2	73
Large	420	3	(6%)	1.5	14	100	3	92
Novelties: Flying Saucers	240	10	(37%)	5	40	150	5	33
Chipsters	380	18	(43%)	9	30	240	6	50
Brown Bonnet Cone	380	21	(50%)	15	40	150	6	43
Ice Cream Cupcakes	210	10	(43%)	6	30	100	4	24
Ice Cream Cake, 4 oz	230	12	(47%)	8	35	95	4	27

CAPTAIN D's SEAFOOD

	Cal	Fat	(%Fc)	S.Fat	Chol	Sod	Pro	Carb
Platters								
Broiled Shrimp	720	8	(10%)	1	155	1760	32	131
Broiled Chicken	800	10	(11%)	2	82	1650	46	131
Broiled Fish	740	7	(8%)	1	49	1645	36	131
Fish & Chicken	780	10	(12%)	1	66	1650	41	131
Lunches								
Broiled Shrimp	420	7	(15%)	1	155	1725	25	64
Broiled Chicken	500	9	(16%)	2	82	1615	39	65
Broiled Fish	435	7	(14%)	1	49	1610	28	65
Broiled Fish & Chicken	480	8	(15%)	1	66	1610	34	68
Stuffed Crab:								
w. French Fries & Coleslaw	550	28	(46%)	na	16	650	14	77
Sandwiches								
Broiled Chicken	450	19	(38%)	na	105	860	40	29
Side Items								
Baked Potato	280	0	(0%)	0	0	20	6	64
Breadstick	110	4	(33%)	0	0	210	3	16
Cole Slaw	160	12	(68%)	na	16	250	3	12
Corn on the Cob	250	2	(7%)	na	0	15	9	60
Cracklins, 1 oz	220	17	(70%)	na	0	740	1	16
Dinner Salad	20	0	(0%)	0	0	15	1	4
French Fries,	300	10	(30%)	na	0	150	3	50
Fried Okra	300	16	(48%)	na	0	450	7	34
Green Beans	45	2	(39%)	na	4	750	2	5
Hushpuppy	125	4	(29%)	na	0	465	2	20
Rice	185	0	(0%)	0	0	1220	1	45
Vegetable Medley	35	1	(25%)	0	0	115	1	6
White Beans	125	0.2	(1%)	na	2	100	8	22
Salad Dressings: Per Serving								
Blue Cheese	110	12	(98%)	na	14	100	<1	<1
French	110	11	(89%)	na	7	190	<1	4
Light Italian	15	0.5	(28%)	0	0	470	0	3
Ranch	90	10	(98%)	na	15	230	<1	<1
Sour Cream, Imitation	30	3	(90%)	3	0	na	0	1
Sauces: Cocktail	35	0.3	(8%)	na	0	250	<1	8
Sweet & Sour	50	0	(0%)	0	0	5	0	13
Tartar	75	7	(84%)	na	10	160	<1	3
Desserts								
Carrot Cake	435	23	(48%)	na	32	415	8	49
Cheesecake	420	31	(66%)	na	141	480	7	30
Chocolate Cake	305	10	(30%)	na	20	260	4	49
Pecan Pie	460	20	(39%)	na	4	375	5	64

CARL'S JR

	Cal	Fat	(%Fc)	S.Fat	Chol	Sod	Pro	Carb
Breakfast								
French Toast Dips; No Syrup	410	25	(55%)	6	0	380	6	40
Sunrise Swch; No Bacon/Saus.	370	21	(51%)	6	225	710	14	31
Breakfast Burrito	430	26	(54%)	12	460	810	22	29
Scrambled Eggs	160	11	(62%)	4	425	125	13	1
English Muffin w/Marg.	230	10	(39%)	2	0	330	5	30
Breakfast Quesadilla	300	14	(42%)	6	225	750	14	27
Bacon, 2 Strips	40	4	(90%)	2	10	125	3	0
Sausage, 1 Patty	200	18	(81%)	7	35	530	7	0
Sandwiches								
Famous Star Hamburger	610	38	(56%)	11	70	890	26	42
Super Star Hamburger	820	53	(58%)	20	120	1030	43	41
1/3 lb Classic Dbl. Cheeseburg.	660	42	(57%)	16	110	1060	34	37
Western Bacon Cheeseburger:	690	35	(46%)	16	90	1490	34	59
Double	970	57	(53%)	27	145	1810	56	58
Big Bacon Star	770	50	(58%)	16	135	990	43	40
Jr. Hamburger	300	12	(36%)	5	40	630	17	33
BBQ Charbroiled Chicken	310	6	(17%)	2	55	830	31	34
Charbroiled Chicken Club	550	29	(47%)	8	85	1160	35	37
Santa Fe Charbrld Chicken	530	30	(51%)	7	85	1230	30	36
Ranch Crispy Chicken	580	29	(45%)	6	60	1140	23	56
Bacon Swiss Crispy Chicken	670	36	(48%)	10	80	1480	28	57
Carl's Catch Fish	560	30	(48%)	7	60	1220	17	54
Great Stuff Potatoes: Plain	290	0	(0%)	0	0	40	6	68
Broccoli & Cheese	530	22	(37%)	5	15	930	11	76
Bacon & Cheese	630	29	(41%)	7	40	1720	20	76
Sour Cream & Chive	430	14	(29%)	3	10	160	8	70
Muffins/Desserts: Per Serving								
Blueberry Muffin	340	14	(37%)	2	40	340	5	49
Bran Muffin	370	13	(32%)	2	45	410	7	61
Chocolate Chip Cookie	370	19	(46%)	8	25	350	3	49
Chocolate Cake	300	10	(30%)	3	23	260	3	49
Choc. Caramel Crnch Moussie	320	16	(45%)	9	5	220	4	44
Cheese Danish	400	22	(49%)	5	15	390	5	49
Strawberry Swirl Cheesecake	300	17	(51%)	9	55	220	6	31
Side Orders								
Breadstick, 1 serv	35	<1	(7%)	0	0	60	1	7
Chicken Stars, 6 pieces	230	14	(55%)	3	85	450	13	11
CrissCut Fries, large	550	34	(56%)	9	0	1280	7	55
French Fries, regular	370	20	(49%)	7	0	240	4	44
Hash Brown Nuggets, 1 serv.	270	17	(57%)	4	0	410	3	27
Onion Rings, 1 serving	520	26	(45%)	6	0	840	8	63
Zucchini, 1 serving	380	23	(54%)	6	0	1040	7	38
Garden Fresh Salad								
Charbroiled Chicken, 1 serving								
No Dressing	260	9	(31%)	5	70	530	28	11
Garden Salad, 1 serving	50	3	(50%)	2	5	75	3	4

CARL'S JR CONT

	Cal	Fat	(%Fc)	S.Fat	Chol	Sod	Pro	Carb
Dressings: Blue Cheese	310	34	(99%)	6	25	360	2	1
Fat Free French	70	0	(0%)	0	0	760	0	18
Fat Free Italian	15	0	(0%)	0	0	800	0	4
House	220	22	(90%)	4	20	440	1	3
1000 Island	250	24	(86%)	4	20	540	<1	7
Sauces: BBQ	50	0	(0%)	0	0	270	<1	11
Honey	90	0	(0%)	0	0	5	0	23
Mustard	45	<1	(10%)	0	0	150	0	10
Salsa	10	0	(0%)	0	0	160	0	2
Sweet 'n Sour	50	0	(0%)	0	0	60	0	11
Shakes: Chocolate, small	390	7	(16%)	5	30	280	9	74
Strawberry, small	400	7	(16%)	5	30	240	9	77
Vanilla, small	330	8	(22%)	5	35	250	11	54

CHICK-FIL-A

	Cal	Fat	(%Fc)	S.Fat	Chol	Sod	Pro	Carb
Chick-fil-A Sandwiches								
Chicken	290	9	(27%)	2	50	870	24	29
Chicken Deluxe	300	9	(27%)	2	50	870	25	31
Chicken (no bun/pickles)	160	8	(44%)	2	45	690	21	1
Chargrilled Chicken:	280	3	(11%)	1	40	640	27	36
Deluxe	290	3	(10%)	1	40	640	28	38
No bun, no pickles	130	3	(23%)	1	30	630	27	0
Club (no dressing)	390	12	(28%)	5	70	980	33	38
Chick-n-Q	370	13	(32%)	3	20	1040	25	36
Chick. Salad (on whole wheat)	320	5	(12%)	2	10	810	25	42
Soup								
Hearty Breast of Chicken	110	1	(8%)	0	45	760	16	10
Strips, Nuggets								
Chick-n-Strips (4-count)	230	8	(30%)	2	20	380	29	10
Chick-Fil-A Nuggets (8-pack)	290	14	(52%)	3	60	770	28	12
Salads: Chick-n-Strips	290	9	(28%)	2	20	430	32	21
Chargrilled Chicken Garden	170	3	(18%)	1	25	650	26	10
Chicken Salad Plate	290	5	(14%)	0	35	570	21	40
Side Orders: Coleslaw (small)	130	6	(38%)	1	15	430	6	11
Carrot & Raisin Salad (small)	150	2	(13%)	0	6	650	5	28
Waffle Potato Fries (salted)	290	10	(31%)	4	5	960	1	49
(unsalted)	290	10	(31%)	4	5	80	1	49
Desserts/Beverages								
Icedream (small cup)	350	10	(26%)	3	70	390	16	50
Icedream (small cone)	140	4	(25%)	1	40	240	11	16
Lemon Pie (slice)	280	22	(71%)	6	5	550	1	19
Fudge Nut Brownie	350	16	(40%)	3	30	650	10	41
Cheesecake: with Topping	290	23	(72%)	10	10	550	14	9

CHURCH'S FRIED CHICKEN

	Cal	Fat (%Fc)	S.Fat	Chol	Sod	Pro	Carb
Fried Chicken: Breast	200	12 (54%)	na	65	510	19	4
Leg	140	9 (58%)	na	45	160	13	2
Thigh	230	16 (63%)	na	80	520	16	5
Wing	250	16 (58%)	na	60	540	19	8
Tender Strip	80	4 (45%)	na	15	140	6	5
Side Items: Apple Pie	280	12 (39%)	na	<5	340	2	41
Biscuit	250	16 (58%)	na	<5	640	2	26
Cajun Rice	130	7 (48%)	na	5	260	1	16
Cole Slaw	92	6 (59%)	na	0	230	4	8
Corn on the Cob	140	3 (19%)	na	0	15	4.5	24
French Fries	210	11 (47%)	na	0	60	3	29
Okra	210	16 (69%)	na	0	520	3	19
Potatoes & Gravy	90	3 (30%)	na	0	520	1	14

COUSINS SUBS

	Cal	Fat (%Fc)	S.Fat	Chol	Sod	Pro	Carb
Soup: Cheese, Regular	210	14 (60%)	5.5	18	1120	7	15
Large	330	22 (60%)	8.5	28	1760	11	23
Cheese Broccoli, Regular	170	11 (58%)	3.5	18	780	5.5	14
Large	260	17 (58%)	5.5	21	1220	8	22
Chicken Noodle, Regular	105	2.5 (21%)	1	18	920	6	13
Large	165	4 (21%)	1.5	28	1445	9.5	21
Clam Chowder, Regular	160	5.5 (30%)	2	13	640	8	19
Large	250	8 (30%)	3.5	21	1005	12	30
Cream of Potato, Regular	165	8 (44%)	2.5	4	650	4	20
Large	260	13 (44%)	4	7	1030	7	30
Red Beans & Rice, Regular	110	1 (8%)	0	0	675	4.5	23
Large	190	2 (9%)	0	0	1070	7	36
Tomato Basil, Regular	90	2.5 (25%)	1.5	4	605	2.5	13
Large	140	4 (25%)	2	7	950	4	21
Vegetable Beef, Regular	70	1.5 (19%)	0	9	890	4.5	12
Large	110	2 (16%)	0	14	1405	7	19
Chicken Soup: Large	290	17 (53%)	3.5	28	1690	11	23
w. Wild Rice, Regular	185	11 (53%)	2	18	1075	7	15
Chili Soup, Regular	220	9 (37%)	3.5	39	945	16	20
Large	345	14 (37%)	5.5	62	1485	25	32
Bread: Italian, 1 oz	65	2 (28%)	0.5	1	410	4	12
Wheat Bread, 1 oz	85	2 (21%)	0.5	1	450	5	11
Cold Italian Subs: Regular	620	40 (58%)	12	79	2010	35	30
Cousins Special	730	49 (60%)	15	111	2490	40	30
Genoa & Cheese	670	45 (60%)	15	75	2005	37	30
Cappocolla & Cheese/Genoa	570	34 (54%)	11	70	1850	35	30
Cold Subs (No extra mayonnaise)							
BLT	360	14 (35%)	5	18	1420	20	34
Cheese Sub	430	20 (42%)	14	57	1635	31	30
Club Sub	495	19 (35%)	9	143	2830	50	30
Cold Veggie	360	14 (35%)	7	36	1590	26	33

COUSINS SUBS CONT

	Cal	Fat	(%Fc)	S.Fat	Chol	Sod	Pro	Carb
Cold Subs (Cont)								
Ham Sub	310	8	(23%)	3	55	1440	29	30
Ham & Cheese	385	14	(33%)	6.5	77	1750	35	30
Roast Beef	360	9	(23%)	3.5	24	1570	41	30
Seafood with Crab	555	34	(55%)	11	35	1750	25	38
Tuna Sub	520	28	(48%)	7	65	1450	30	32
Turkey Sub	325	8.5	(24%)	3	72	2020	32	30
Hot Subs: Cheese Steak	470	17	(32%)	11	40	840	33	46
Double	550	26	(36%)	16	64	640	44	35
Chicken Breast (no Mayo)	320	6	(17%)	2	3	1390	37	30
Gyro: Regular	550	23	(38%)	8	36	650	28	57
w. Tzatziki Sauce	600	27	(41%)	10	56	760	29	58
Hot Veggie	380	11	(26%)	0	0	320	21	48
Italian Sausage	815	58	(64%)	19	35	5200	45	30
Meatball & Cheese	680	43	(57%)	18	104	3610	44	30
Pepperoni Melt (no mayo)	465	20	(39%)	9	101	1910	41	30
Philly Cheese Steak	510	23	(41%)	15	45	430	32	43
Steak Sub	425	12	(25%)	8	40	360	28	51
For mayonnaise on bread add: 235 Cals; 26g Fat (100%); 9g Sat.Fat; 30mg Cholesterol								
Mini Sub: Cousins Special	290	14	(43%)	6	6	680	13	26
Cheese (no mayonnaise)	230	11	(43%)	7.5	30	870	17	16
Ham (no mayonnaise)	170	4	(21%)	1.5	29	765	16	16
Ham & Cheese (no mayo)	205	7.5	(33%)	3.5	41	930	17	16
Meatball & Cheese	365	23	(57%)	10	55	1930	23	16
Seafood w. Crab	300	18	(54%)	6	19	935	13	21
Tuna	480	37	(69%)	10	56	670	14	22
Turkey (no mayonnaise)	170	4.5	(24%)	1.5	38	1080	17	16
For mayonnaise on bread add: 125 Cals; 14gFat (100%); 4.5g Sat.Fat; 16mg Cholesterol								
Kids Subs: Cheeseburger	290	17	(53%)	6	41	460	14	22
Hot Dog	275	16	(52%)	6	24	770	10	22
PBJ	360	12	(30%)	3	0	930	13	50
French Fries: Small	275	13	(43%)	5.5	11	240	3.5	38
Medium	400	17	(38%)	8	16	355	8.5	55
Large	525	25	(43%)	11	21	465	9	72
Chips: 1½ oz	230	15	(59%)	4	0	270	3	22
w. Sour Cream, 1½ oz	230	14	(55%)	4	0	270	3	22
Bacon Strips (3)	50	4	(72%)	1.5	8	145	3	1
Pepperoni, 6 slices	70	6	(77%)	3	25	180	4	0
Salads: Chef	195	8	(37%)	3.5	109	1000	24	6
Garden	135	6	(40%)	2.5	65	385	15	6
Italian	290	17	(53%)	6.5	106	1065	26	6
Seafood	175	6	(31%)	2.5	65	1045	21	12
Side	70	4	(51%)	2.5	39	200	8.5	0
Tuna	305	20	(59%)	4	85	465	26	6
Dessert								
Choc Chip Cookie	210	11	(47%)	4	20	190	2	25
Cranberry Walnut Cookie	190	8.5	(40%)	2.5	na	65	2.5	24

DAIRY QUEEN®/BRAZIER®

	Cal	Fat (%Fc)	S.Fat	Chol	Sod	Pro	Carb
Burgers							
DQ® Homestyle: Hamburger	290	12 (37%)	5	45	630	17	29
Cheeseburger	340	17 (45%)	8	55	850	20	29
Double Cheeseburger	540	31 (52%)	16	115	1130	35	30
Deluxe Double Hamburger	440	22 (45%)	10	90	680	30	29
Deluxe Dble Cheeseburger	540	31 (52%)	16	115	1130	36	31
Bacon Dble Cheeseburger	610	36 (53%)	18	130	1380	41	31
Ultimate Burger	670	43 (58%)	19	135	1210	40	29
Hot Dogs: Regular	240	14 (52%)	5	25	730	9	19
Cheese Dog	290	18 (56%)	8	40	950	12	20
Chili Dog	280	16 (51%)	6	35	870	12	21
Chili 'n' Cheese Dog	330	21 (57%)	4	45	1090	14	22
Sandwiches: Fish Fillet	370	16 (39%)	4	45	630	16	39
Fish Fillet w. Cheese	420	21 (45%)	6	60	850	19	40
Chicken Breast Fillet	430	20 (42%)	4	55	760	24	37
Grilled	310	10 (29%)	3	50	1040	24	30
with Cheese	480	25 (47%)	7	70	980	27	38
Chick. Strip Basket: w.Gravy	860	42 (44%)	11	55	1820	35	88
w. BBQ Sauce	810	37 (41%)	9	55	1590	33	88
French Fries: Small	210	10 (43%)	2	0	115	3	29
Regular	300	14 (42%)	3	0	160	4	40
Large	390	18 (42%)	4	0	200	5	52
Onion Rings	240	12 (45%)	3	0	135	4	29
Ice Cream, Desserts							
DQ® Vanilla Soft Serv., 1/2 cup	140	4 (26%)	3	15	70	22	3
DQ® Choc. Soft Serv., 1/2 cup	150	5 (30%)	35	15	75	22	4
Vanilla Cone: Small	230	7 (27%)	5	20	115	38	6
Regular	350	10 (26%)	7	30	170	57	8
Large	410	12 (26%)	8	40	200	65	10
Chocolate Cone: Small	240	8 (30%)	5	20	115	37	6
Regular	360	11 (27%)	8	30	180	56	9
Yogurt Cone: Regular	280	1 (5%)	<1	5	170	59	9
Chocolate Sundae: Small	290	7 (22%)	5	25	150	51	6
Regular	410	10 (22%)	6	30	210	73	9
Cup of Yogurt: Regular	230	0.5 (2%)	0	5	160	49	8
Yogurt Strawb. Sundae: Reg.	300	0.5 (1.5%)	0.5	5	180	66	9
Banana Split	510	12 (21%)	8	30	180	96	8
Misty Buster Bar®	450	28 (56%)	12	15	280	41	10
Butterfinger® Blizzard®: Small	520	18 (31%)	11	35	250	80	11
Regular	750	26 (31%)	16	50	360	115	16
Chocolate Malt: Small	650	16 (22%)	10	55	370	111	15
Regular	880	22 (22%)	14	70	500	153	19
Choc. Sand. Cookie Blizzard®:							
Small	520	18 (31%)	9	40	380	79	10
Regular	640	23 (32%)	11	45	500	97	12
Chocolate Shake: Small	560	15 (24%)	10	50	310	94	13
Regular	770	20 (23%)	13	70	420	130	17

DAIRY QUEEN®/BRAZIER®

	Cal	Fat (%Fc)	S.Fat	Chol	Sod	Pro	Carb
Ice Cream, Desserts (Cont)							
Dilly® Bar: Chocolate; Toffee	210	13 (56%)	7	10	75	21	3
Chocolate Mint	190	12 (57%)	9	15	100	20	3
Dipped Cone: Small	340	17 (45%)	9	20	130	42	6
Regular	510	25 (44%)	13	30	200	63	9
DQ® Caramel & Nut Bar	260	13 (45%)	0	15	90	32	5
DQ® Frozen Log Cake, 1/8 Cake	280	9 (29%)	6	15	220	43	5
8" Round Cake, 1/8 Cake	340	12 (32%)	7	25	250	53	7
10" Round Cake, 1/12 Cake	360	12 (30%)	8	25	260	55	7
Heart Cake, 1/10 Cake	270	9 (30%)	6	20	190	41	5
Sheet Cake, 1/20 Cake	350	12 (31%)	7	20	270	54	7
DQ® Fudge Bar	50	0 (0%)	0	0	70	13	4
DQ® Lemon Freez'r™, 1/2 cup	80	0 (0%)	0	0	10	20	0
DQ® Sandwich	150	5 (30%)	2	5	115	24	3
DQ® Treatzza Pizza™, 1/8 pizza:							
Strawberry/Banana	180	6 (30%)	3	5	140	29	3
Heath®	180	7 (35%)	4	5	160	28	3
M & M®	190	7 (33%)	4	5	160	29	3
Peanut Butter Fudge	220	10 (41%)	5	5	200	28	4
DQ® Vanilla Orange Bar	60	0 (0%)	0	0	40	17	2
Fudge Nut Bar™	410	25 (55%)	11	15	250	40	8
Heath® Blizzard®: Small	560	21 (34%)	14	45	380	82	10
Regular	820	33 (36%)	22	60	580	119	14
Heath® Breeze®: Small	470	10 (19%)	6	10	380	85	11
Regular	710	18 (23%)	11	20	580	123	15
Peanut Buster® Parfait	730	31 (38%)	17	35	400	99	16
Regular	950	36 (34%)	9	75	660	143	17
Queen's Choice®:							
Vanilla Big Scoop®	250	14 (50%)	9	55	100	27	4
Chocolate Big Scoop®	250	14 (50%)	9	55	95	28	4
Reeses® Peanut Butter Cup Blizzard®							
Small	590	24 (37%)	13	45	320	81	14
Regular	790	33 (38%)	17	55	430	105	19
Misty® Slush: Small	220	0 (0%)	0	0	20	56	0
Regular	290	0 (0%)	0	0	30	74	0
Choc. Chip Cookie Dough Blizzard®							
Small	660	24 (33%)	13	55	440	99	12
Starkiss®	80	0 (0%)	0	0	10	21	0
Strawberry Blizzard®: Small	400	11 (25%)	7	35	190	66	9
Regular	570	16 (25%)	10	50	260	95	12
Strawberry Breeze®: Small	320	0.5 (1%)	0.5	5	190	68	10
Regular	460	1 (1%)	1	10	270	99	13
Strawberry Misty® Cooler	190	0 (0%)	0	0	25	49	0
Strawberry Shortcake	430	14 (29%)	9	60	360	70	7

DEL TACO

	Cal	Fat	(%Fc)	S.Fat	Chol	Sod	Pro	Carb
Tacos: Regular	140	8	(51%)	3	16	100	6	10
Double Beef:	170	10	(53%)	3	25	150	8	12
Deluxe	205	13	(57%)	5	35	160	9	13
Soft Taco: Regular	145	6	(37%)	3	16	225	5	17
Double Beef	180	8	(40%)	3	25	275	7	18
Chicken Taco	185	13	(63%)	3	35	275	8	10
Chicken Soft Taco	200	11	(49%)	3	35	400	7	16
Kid's Meal - Taco	530	17	(29%)	6	16	375	8	87
Tostada: Regular	140	8	(51%)	3	15	335	6	12
Burritos: Red, Regular	340	12	(32%)	5	26	1035	15	46
Green, Regular	330	11	(30%)	3	22	1150	14	46
Chicken	265	10	(34%)	4	36	770	13	32
Deluxe	550	34	(56%)	10	83	980	21	40
Combination	415	17	(37%)	7	49	1035	21	46
Deluxe Combo	455	20	(40%)	9	59	1050	22	49
"The Works"	450	18	(36%)	6	27	1250	15	60
Macho Combo	775	31	(36%)	15	100	2180	38	87
Del Beef	440	20	(41%)	9	63	880	23	43
Macho Beef	895	41	(41%)	18	139	1970	49	84
Steak & Egg Burrito	500	25	(45%)	9	337	1070	30	41
Breakfast Burrito	256	11	(39%)	4	90	410	9	30
Salads: Taco	235	19	(73%)	6	31	270	9	9
Taco Deluxe	740	49	(60%)	16	83	1280	26	57
Chicken	255	19	(67%)	6	58	475	12	8
Burgers: Hamburger	230	8	(31%)	3	29	650	11	26
Del Burger	385	20	(47%)	6	42	1065	14	35
Cheeseburger	285	13	(41%)	6	42	850	14	26
Del Cheeseburger	440	25	(51%)	9	55	1270	18	35
Kid's Meal - Hamburger	620	20	(29%)	7	29	800	14	96
Quesadilla: Regular	485	27	(50%)	6	75	870	23	37
Chicken	545	31	(51%)	16	113	1150	30	38
Spicy Jack: Regular	475	27	(51%)	16	76	940	23	37
Chicken	540	30	(50%)	17	114	1215	31	38
Nachos: Regular	390	23	(53%)	4	2	505	6	39
Macho Nachos	1090	61	(50%)	13	46	1740	26	110
Side Dishes: Beans & Cheese	120	3	(22%)	2	9	890	7	17
French Fries (Small)	240	11	(41%)	4	0	135	3	32
Regular	400	19	(43%)	6	0	230	5	54
Large	570	26	(41%)	9	0	320	8	76
Nacho Fries	670	34	(45%)	11	2	925	10	80
Chili Cheese Fries	560	30	(48%)	13	38	845	15	58
Dressings: Sour Cream, 1 oz	60	6	(90%)	4	20	15	0	0
Guacamole, 1 oz	60	6	(90%)	0	0	130	1	2
Salsa - Side, 2 oz	14	0	(0%)	0	0	308	0	3
Hot Sauce - Pouch	2	0	(0%)	0	0	38	0	0
Salsa Dressing, 1 oz	35	3	(77%)	2	10	85	0	1
Nacho Cheese Sauce	100	8	(72%)	2	2	401	2	4

DENNY'S

	Cal	Fat (%Fc)	S.Fat	Chol	Sod	Pro	Carb
Breakfast: All American Slam	1030	87 (76%)	21	725	1925	48	24
w.Toast, 1 slice	1120	88 (71%)	21	725	2090	51	41
w.Bagel	1265	88 (63%)	21	725	2420	57	70
w.Biscuit, plain	1405	109 (70%)	26	725	2675	53	64
Big Country Biscuit w. Gravy	935	54 (52%)	17	50	2950	23	90
Country Scramble	795	50 (57%)	11	410	1820	20	67
w.Bacon, 4 slices	955	59 (56%)	16	445	2460	32	68
w.Sausage, 4 links	1150	82 (64%)	22	475	2765	36	67
Eggs Benedict	860	56 (59%)	23	525	1945	35	55
French Slam	1030	71 (62%)	20	777	1430	44	58
w.Toast, 1 slice	1120	71 (58%)	0	777	1595	47	75
w.Bagel	1265	72 (51%)	20	777	1925	53	104
w.Biscuit, plain	1405	93 (60%)	25	777	2180	49	98
Fruit Stack, no topping	515	9 (16%)	2	5	1820	12	96
Grand Slam	795	50 (57%)	14	460	2240	34	65
w.Syrup & Margarine	1030	60 (52%)	16	460	2385	34	101
Ham Scram	670	37 (50%)	11	415	1730	24	65
Ham Slam	730	39 (48%)	12	430	2205	35	66
Scram Slam	975	80 (74%)	18	700	1750	42	30
w.Toast, 1 slice	1065	81 (68%)	23	700	1915	45	47
w.Bagel	1210	81 (60%)	23	700	2245	51	76
w.Biscuit, plain	1350	102 (68%)	28	700	2500	82	70
Slim Slam (w.Syrup/Topping)	640	12 (17%)	3	34	1770	34	98
Southern Slam	1065	84 (71%)	23	484	2450	37	47
Sunshine Slam	540	25 (42%)	6	410	1445	20	64
w.Syrup & Margarine	775	35 (41%)	4	410	1590	20	10
w.Hashed Browns	760	39 (46%)	8	410	1870	22	84
Omelette: (no extras)							
Ham 'n Cheese	740	55 (67%)	10	660	1520	36	24
Ultimate	780	62 (72%)	14	640	1360	31	29
Veggie Cheese	720	53 (66%)	10	645	960	28	29
Cheddar Cheese	770	62 (72%)	20	675	1135	34	24
Farmer's Omelette	890	71 (72%)	20	670	1640	34	29
Steak & Eggs: (no extras)	885	66 (67%)	18	500	730	48	21
Sirloin	810	64 (71%)	18	476	950	37	21
T-Bone	1045	82 (71%)	26	530	1190	56	21
Pork Chops and Eggs	555	36 (58%)	9	469	970	33	21
Moons Over My Hammy	810	48 (53%)	8	430	2250	44	46
Belgian Waffles: Plain	300	21 (63%)	3	146	200	7	23
w. Syrup & Butter	540	31 (52%)	5	146	345	7	59
Supreme (no bacon/saus.)	430	23 (48%)	3	153	220	7	50
Pancakes: Plain (3)	490	7 (13%)	1	0	1820	12	95
w.Syrup & Butter	725	17 (21%)	3	0	1965	12	130
French Toast: w. Syrup & But.	725	37 (46%)	6	317	430	19	80
Fruity French Toast	400	22 (50%)	5	165	255	11	39

DENNY'S CONT

	Cal	Fat	(%Fc)	S.Fat	Chol	Sod	Pro	Carb
Breakfast Sides: Applesauce	60	0	(0%)	0	0	15	0	15
Bacon, 4 slices	160	9	(45%)	5	36	640	12	1
Bagel, 1 only	235	1	(4%)	0	0	495	9	46
Biscuit; Plain	375	22	(53%)	5	0	750	5	40
w.Sausage & Gravy	570	38	(60%)	10	24	1475	11	45
Cinnamon Roll	670	30	(40%)	0	20	400	10	88
Cream Cheese, 1 oz	100	10	(90%)	6	31	90	2	1
Blueberry, each	310	14	(41%)	0	0	190	4	42
Egg: 1 only	135	12	(80%)	3	205	60	6	1
Sunny Fresh Egg Substitute	95	7	(66%)	0	1	90	6	1
Grits, 4 oz	80	0	(0%)	0	0	520	2	18
Ham, 3 oz	95	3	(28%)	1	23	760	15	2
Hashed Browns, 4 oz	220	14	(57%)	2	0	420	2	20
Covered, 6 oz	320	23	(65%)	7	30	605	9	21
Covered & Smothered, 8 oz	360	26	(65%)	7	30	790	9	26
Muffins: English, each	125	1	(7%)	0	0	200	5	24
Blueberry, each	310	14	(41%)	0	0	190	4	42
Oatmeal, 4 oz	100	2	(18%)	0	0	175	5	18
Sausage, 4 links	355	32	(81%)	2	64	945	16	0
Syrup, 3 Tbsp	145	0	(0%)	0	0	25	0	36
Reduced Calorie	25	0	(0%)	0	0	95	0	6
Toppings: 3 oz	105	0	(0%)	0	0	15	0	26
Toast, 1 slice	90	1	(10%)	0	0	165	3	17
Whipped Margarine; 1/2 oz	90	10	(100%)	2	0	120	0	0
Whipped Cream, 2 oz	25	2	(72%)	0	7	5	0	2
Soup: Cheese	295	23	(10%)	13	19	895	6	13
Chicken Noodle	60	2	(30%)	0	10	640	2	8
Clam Chowder	215	11	(46%)	9	5	905	5	22
Cream of Broccoli	195	12	(55%)	9	0	820	4	15
Cream of Potato	220	12	(49%)	9	0	760	4	23
Split Pea	150	6	(36%)	2	5	820	8	18
Vegetable Beef	80	1	(11%)	1	5	820	6	11
Sandwiches: (no fries/sides)								
BLT	640	46	(65%)	8	55	1190	18	37
Bacon Swiss Burger	710	46	(58%)	11	125	965	47	27
Charleston Chicken	560	26	(42%)	5	66	1240	29	53
Chicken Melt	520	29	(50%)	5	40	1170	26	43
Club Sandwich	720	38	(47%)	7	75	1740	32	62
Delidinger	850	45	(48%)	6	80	3215	56	62
Deluxe Grilled Cheese	480	26	(49%)	2	1	1210	18	44
Denny Burger	510	28	(49%)	9	110	225	35	26
French Dip w. Horseradish	700	35	(45%)	6	120	2180	42	53
Fried Fish	910	58	(57%)	8	70	1780	29	74
Grilled Chicken	440	8	(16%)	2	67	1205	32	60
Ham & Swiss on Rye	535	31	(52%)	4	36	1710	23	40
Humdinger Hamburger	750	48	(58%)	11	127	945	49	30
Patty Melt	695	42	(54%)	10	110	1145	43	36
Prime Rib	660	37	(50%)	5	80	1745	33	47

DENNY'S CONT

	Cal	Fat (%Fc)	S.Fat	Chol	Sod	Pro	Carb
Sandwiches (Cont)							
Star Spangled Burger	750	48 (58%)	11	130	945	49	30
Super Bird	620	32 (46%)	5	60	1950	35	48
Tuna Melt Supreme	860	57 (60%)	9	64	1670	51	47
Turkey Breast	475	26 (49%)	3	57	1180	23	39
Veggie Burger	530	15 (25%)	2	2	1140	25	73
Veggie Cheese Melt	460	27 (53%)	3	1	1025	17	39
Salads: (no dressing/bread)							
Fried Chicken	505	31 (55%)	8	94	1175	38	30
Garden Chicken Delite	120	4 (30%)	1	67	600	28	14
Grilled Chicken Caesar	510	32 (56%)	7	84	1390	36	22
w. Dressing	655	47 (65%)	9	86	1730	37	23
Oriental Chicken w.Dressing	570	26 (41%)	5	67	1660	33	49
Side Garden	115	4 (31%)	1	0	150	3	16
Side Caesar w.Dressing	340	25 (66%)	5	7	725	8	20
Dressings: BBQ Sauce	50	1 (18%)	0	0	595	0	11
Bleu Cheese, 1 oz	125	12 (86%)	4	20	405	4	4
Caesar	140	15 (96%)	2	2	340	1	1
French: Regular	105	10 (86%)	2	7	275	0	3
Reduced Calorie	75	5 (60%)	1	0	265	0	8
Honey Mustard Fat-Free	40	0 (0%)	0	0	115	0	9
Oriental Dressing	105	8 (69%)	1	0	400	1	6
Ranch	100	11 (99%)	2	8	215	1	1
Sour Cream, 1 1/2 oz	90	9 (90%)	6	19	25	1	2
Thousand Island, 1 oz	105	10 (86%)	2	20	210	0	2
Horseradish Sauce, 1 oz	170	18 (95%)	3	45	230	1	3
Appetizers							
Buffalo Chicken Strips	735	42 (51%)	4	96	1675	48	43
Buffalo Wings (12)	855	54 (57%)	17	500	5550	92	1
Chicken Quesadilla	830	55 (60%)	23	181	1980	50	43
Chicken Strips (5)	720	33 (41%)	4	95	1665	47	56
Mozzarella Sticks w.Sce (8)	755	43 (51%)	24	48	5425	37	56
Onion Rings (7)	440	27 (55%)	7	7	1160	6	44
Sampler	1120	59 (47%)	19	70	3430	44	104
Entrees: Battered Cod w.Sce	730	47 (58%)	7	105	1335	30	48
Charleston Chicken	330	18 (49%)	4	65	990	25	14
Chicken Fried Steak	265	17 (58%)	8	27	670	15	14
Chicken Strip w. Dressing	635	25 (35%)	1	95	1510	47	55
Denny Cut Prime Rib, 8 oz							
(w.Sauce & Horseradish)	760	66 (78%)	27	181	1720	38	8
Grilled Alaskan Salmon	295	14 (43%)	2	102	260	43	1
Grilled Chicken Breast	130	4 (28%)	1	65	560	24	0
Porterhouse Steak	710	54 (61%)	24	160	710	56	0
Roast Turkey	700	27 (35%)	1	100	2345	47	63
Shrimp	560	32 (51%)	6	135	1110	19	49
T-Bone Steak Dinner	530	40 (68%)	18	120	535	42	0
Steak & Shrimp	645	42 (59%)	14	150	1140	36	31

DENNY'S CONT

	Cal	Fat (%Fc)	S.Fat	Chol	Sod	Pro	Carb
Sides: Broccoli in Butter Sauce	50	2 (36%)	2	2	5	3	7
Carrots in Honey Glaze	80	3 (34%)	1	0	220	1	12
Corn in Butter Sauce	120	4 (30%)	2	5	260	3	19
Cornbread Stuffing	180	9 (45%)	0	0	405	4	20
French Fries, unsalted	325	14 (39%)	3	0	130	5	44
seasoned	260	12 (42%)	3	0	555	5	35
Gravy, all types, average	15	0.5 (30%)	0	0	120	0	2
Green Beans w. Bacon	60	4 (60%)	2	5	390	1	6
Green Peas in Butter Sauce	100	2 (18%)	2	5	360	5	14
Potato: Baked, plain	185	0 (0%)	0	0	15	4	43
Mashed	105	1 (8%)	0	0	380	3	21
Rice Pilaf	110	2 (16%)	0	0	330	2	21
Lunch Baskets: no Fries							
Bacon Swiss Burger	710	46 (58%)	11	125	965	47	27
Charleston Chicken Ranch Melt	975	59 (54%)	10	95	2555	47	68
Chicken Strip (no sauce)	570	26 (41%)	4	70	1315	34	45
Delidinger	850	45 (48%)	6	80	3215	56	62
Deluxe Grilled Chicken	480	26 (49%)	2	1	1210	18	44
Denny Burger	510	28 (49%)	9	110	225	35	26
Five Star Philly	660	29 (40%)	8	97	725	41	55
Patty Melt	695	42 (54%)	10	110	1145	43	36
Super Bird	620	332 (46%)	5	60	1950	35	48
Dinner (no sides): Pot Roast	275	11 (36%)	4	140	1270	40	7
Chicken Strip	400	15 (34%)	0	55	985	28	38
Grilled Chopped Steak	640	44 (62%)	19	145	735	51	9
Junior Meals: Basic Breakfast	560	39 (63%)	9	230	1105	18	38
Jr Belgian Waffle	190	11 (52%)	2	75	100	3	20
Jr Burger, no fries	260	15 (52%)	4	40	115	14	16
Jr French Slam	460	35 (68%)	10	385	665	21	18
w. Syrup & Margarine	695	45 (58%)	12	385	810	21	54
Jr Fried Fish, no fries	465	34 (66%)	5	70	745	15	25
Jr Grand Slam	400	25 (56%)	7	230	1120	17	33
w. Syrup & Margarine	635	35 (50%)	9	230	1265	17	69
Jr Grilled Cheese, no fries	375	22 (53%)	3	1	810	12	35
Jr Shrimp Basket, no fries	290	16 (50%)	3	60	775	10	27
Desserts: Chocolate Cake	370	17 (41%)	4	29	375	4	53
Pies, 1/6 slice : Apple	430	20 (42%)	5	<5	390	3	59
Apple w/Equal	370	20 (49%)	5	<5	360	3	43
Cheesecake	580	28 (43%)	13	90	290	9	74
Cherry	540	21 (35%)	5	<5	430	5	83
Chocolate Pecan	790	37 (42%)	9	70	460	6	107
Coconut Cream	480	26 (49%)	16	15	440	5	58
Dutch Apple	440	19 (39%)	5	0	290	3	65
French Silk	650	43 (59%)	26	165	220	6	60
German Chocolate	580	33 (51%)	18	15	460	7	66

DENNY'S CONT

	Cal	Fat	(%Fc)	S.Fat	Chol	Sod	Pro	Carb
Pies (Cont): Key Lime	600	27	(41%)	15	35	300	10	79
Lemon Meringue	460	17	(33%)	4	95	310	5	71
Pecan	600	28	(42%)	4	50	430	5	81
Dessert Toppings: Blueberry	70	0	(0%)	0	0	10	0	17
Chocolate, 2 oz	320	25	(70%)	0	0	85	2	27
Fudge, 2 oz	200	10	(45%)	7	3	95	1	30
Strawberry, 2 oz	80	1	(11%)	0	0	10	1	17
Sundaes: Sgl Scoop, no top.	190	14	(66%)	5	37	40	3	14
Dble Scoop, no topping	375	27	(65%)	12	75	85	6	29
Banana Split	895	43	(43%)	19	75	175	15	121
Hot Fudge Cake	690	38	(50%)	11	60	485	9	83
Flavored Coffee: Average	70	1	(13%)	1	2	5	0	16

DOMINO'S

	Cal	Fat	(%Fc)	S.Fat	Chol	Sod	Pro	Carb
14" Hand Tossed: 2 Slices								
Beef	365	14	(35%)	6	26	745	16	44
Cheese	320	10	(28%)	4	18	620	14	44
Italian Sausage & Mushroom	365	13	(32%)	6	27	755	16	46
Pepperoni	375	15	(36%)	6	32	870	17	49
X-tra Cheese & Pepperoni	425	19	(40%)	8	39	910	19	45
Ham	335	11	(30%)	4.5	19	775	16	44
Veggie	345	11	(29%)	4	18	845	14	47
14" Thin Crust: Per Slice ($1/6$)								
Beef	300	15	(45%)	7	26	835	13	28
Cheese	255	11	(39%)	5	18	710	11	28
Pepperoni	310	16	(46%)	7	29	885	13	28
X-tra Cheese & Pepperoni	355	20	(55%)	9	38	1000	16	28
Ham	270	12	(40%)	5.5	25	865	13	28
Italian Sausage & Mushroom	300	15	(45%)	6	27	845	13	30
Veggie	280	12	(39%)	5	18	985	11	31
14" Deep Dish: Per 2 Slices								
Beef	505	24	(43%)	9	31	1105	20	55
Cheese	460	20	(39%)	7	23	980	18	55
Pepperoni	515	25	(44%)	9	35	1155	20	55
X-tra Cheese & Pepperoni	560	29	(46%)	11	44	1270	23	55
Ham	475	21	(40%)	7.5	30	1135	20	55
Italian Sausage & Mushroom	510	24	(42%)	8.5	32	1165	20	57
Veggie	485	21	(39%)	7	23	1205	18	59
12" Hand Tossed: Per 2 Slices								
Beef	405	16	(36%)	7	30	825	18	49
Cheese	350	11	(28%)	5	19	670	15	49
Pepperoni	410	16	(35%)	7	32	870	17	49
X-tra Cheese & Pepperoni	460	20	(39%)	9	42	1000	21	49
Ham	370	11	(27%)	5	26	835	17	49
Italian Sausage & Mushroom	365	13	(32%)	6	27	755	16	46
Veggie	370	12	(29%)	5	19	745	15	52

DOMINO'S CONT

	Cal	Fat (%Fc)	S.Fat	Chol	Sod	Pro	Carb
12" Thin Crust: Per Slice (1/4)							
Beef	325	17 (47%)	7	30	915	14	30
Cheese	270	12 (40%)	5	19	760	12	30
Pepperoni	335	17 (46%)	7	32	960	15	30
X-tra Cheese & Pepperoni	385	21 (49%)	9	42	1080	18	31
Ham	290	12 (37%)	5	26	920	15	30
Italian Sausage & Mushroom	330	16 (44%)	6	31	930	15	32
Veggie	300	13 (39%)	5	19	830	13	33
12" Deep Dish: Per 2 Slices							
Beef	525	26 (45%)	10	36	1155	21	52
Cheese	470	21 40%)	8	25	1000	18	52
Pepperoni	530	27 (46%)	10	38	1200	21	52
Ham	480	22 (41%)	8	32	1160	21	52
Italian Sausage & Mushroom	525	26 (45%)	10	36	1170	21	54
Veggie	490	23 (42%)	8	25	1070	19	54
6" Deep Dish: Per 2 Slices							
Beef	635	31 (44%)	12	39	2000	25	65
Cheese	590	27 41%)	10	31	1210	23	65
Pepperoni	640	32 (45%)	12	41	1370	25	66
Ham	610	28 (41%)	10	38	1370	25	66
Italian Sausage & Mushroom	440	31 (63%)	11	40	1345	25	67
Veggie	610	28 (41%)	10	31	1265	23	67
Toppings: Cheddar Cheese	55	4.5 (74%)	3	14	80	3	0.5
Bacon	80	6.5 (73%)	2	10	180	4	0
Green Peppers, Onions, Mushrooms, Fresh	3	0 (0%)	0	0	0.5	0	0.5
Canned Mushrooms	3	0 (0%)	0	0	65	0	0.5
Olives: Green	12	1 (75%)	0.2	0	245	0	0.5
Ripe	13	1 (69%)	0.2	0	65	0	0.5
Banana Peppers	3	0 (0%)	0	0	85	0	0.5
Pineapple Tidbits	9	0 (0%)	0	0	0	0	2
Anchovies	25	1 (36%)	0.2	9	395	2	0.5
Extra Cheese	45	4 (71%)	2	9	115	3	0
Sides: Breadstick, 1 stk	80	3 (34%)	0.5	0	160	2	11
Cheesy Bread, 1 piece	105	5 (43%)	2	6	180	3	11
Barbeque Wings, each	50	2 (36%)	0.5	26	175	6	2
Hot Wings, each	45	2 (40%)	0.5	26	355	5	<1
Garden Salad; Small; no dress.	20	0.3 (13%)	0	0	15	1	4
Large; no dressing	40	0.5 (11%)	0	0	25	2	8
Dressings: Blue Chse, 1 1/2 oz	220	24 (98%)	4	40	440	2	2
Creamy Caesar, 1 1/2 oz	200	22 (99%)	3	10	470	1	2
Honey French, 1 1/2 oz	210	18 (77%)	3	0	300	0	14
House Italian, 1 1/2 oz	220	24 (98%)	3	0	440	0	1
Lite Italian, 1 1/2 oz	20	1 (45%)	0	0	0	0	2
Ranch, 1 1/2 oz	260	29 (100%)	4	5	380	0	1
Fat Free Ranch, 1 1/2 oz	40	0 (0%)	0	0	560	0	10
1000 Island, 1 1/2 oz	200	20 (90%)	3	25	320	0	5

DUNKIN' DONUTS

	Cal	Fat	(%Fc)	S.Fat	Chol	Sod	Pro	Carb
Cake Donuts, each								
Blueberry	230	10	(39%)	3	0	240	4	30
Blueberry Crumb	260	11	(38%)	3	0	260	4	36
Cinnamon	300	19	(57%)	4	0	350	3	29
Coconut	320	20	(56%)	5	0	360	3	32
Old Fashioned	280	19	(61%)	4	0	350	7	24
Peanut	340	22	(58%)	4	0	360	5	32
Powdered	310	19	(55%)	3	0	350	3	30
Sugared	310	20	(58%)	4	0	380	4	28
Toasted Coconut	320	19	(53%)	5	0	360	3	33
Chocolate	215	14	(58%)	3	0	270	3	19
Chocolate Coconut	250	15	(54%)	5	0	270	3	25
Chocolate Glazed	250	13	(48%)	3	0	280	3	29
Double Chocolate	260	14	(43%)	3	0	280	3	30
Whole Wheat Glazed	230	11	(43%)	3	0	340	3	31
Yeast Donuts: each								
Apple Crumb	250	11	(40%)	3	0	270	4	34
Apple n' Spice	230	10	(39%)	3	0	250	4	31
Bavarian Kreme	250	11	(40%)	3	0	250	4	33
Boston Kreme	270	11	(37%)	3	0	260	4	38
Chocolate Frosted	210	8	(34%)	2	0	230	4	31
Chocolate Kreme Filled	320	16	(45%)	4	0	250	4	39
Glazed	160	7	(39%)	2	0	200	3	23
Jelly Filled	240	10	(37%)	3	0	260	4	32
Lemon	240	11	(41%)	3	0	250	4	31
Maple/Marble Frosted	210	8	(34%)	2	0	230	4	32
Strawberry	240	10	(37%)	3	0	250	4	32
Strawberry/Vanilla Frosted	220	8	(33%)	2	0	230	4	32
Sugar Raised	170	7	(37%)	2	0	220	4	23
Muffins: Apple n' Spice	330	10	(27%)	3	35	330	5	54
Lowfat	220	2	(8%)	0	0	380	3	54
Banana Nut	340	12	(32%)	3	35	210	6	53
Blueberry	310	10	(29%)	3	35	190	5	51
Lowfat	230	2	(8%)	0	0	370	3	51
Bran Lowfat	280	2	(6%)	0	0	440	4	59
Cherry	330	11	(30%)	3	35	210	5	53
Lowfat	230	2	(8%)	0	0	380	4	53
Chocolate Chip	400	16	(36%)	6	35	190	5	53
Corn	350	14	(36%)	0.5	50	310	6	51
Lowfat	250	2	(7%)	0	0	460	4	55
Cranberry Orange	310	11	(32%)	3	30	160	5	51
Lowfat	230	2	(8%)	0	0	380	3	53
English	130	1	(7%)	0.5	0	520	4	26
Honey Raisin Bran	330	10	(27%)	3	15	360	5	57
Lemon Poppy Seed	360	13	(32%)	3	40	440	6	57
Oat Bran	290	11	(34%)	1	0	330	4	44
French Roll: Baked	140	1	(6%)	0	0	220	3	27

DUNKIN' DONUTS CONT

	Cal	Fat (%Fc)	S.Fat	Chol	Sod	Pro	Carb
Cake Munchkins							
Butternut (3)	230	11 (43%)	4	0	210	2	30
Chocolate Glazed (3)	180	10 (50%)	2	0	240	2	22
Cinnamon (4)	240	13 (49%)	3	0	290	3	29
Coconut (3)	200	11 (49%)	4	0	220	2	22
Glazed Cake (3)	220	9 (37%)	2	0	220	2	32
Plain (4)	200	12 (54%)	3	0	290	3	21
Powdered Sugar (4)	240	13 (49%)	3	0	290	3	28
Toasted Coconut (3)	210	11 (47%)	3	0	220	2	26
Glazed Raised (4)	210	7 (30%)	2	0	170	3	36
Jelly (3)	170	5 (26%)	1	0	170	2	28
Lemon (3)	160	6 (24%)	1	0	160	2	23
Sugar Raised (6)	210	10 (43%)	3	0	250	4	26
Crullers/Sticks							
Dunkin' Donut	240	14 (52%)	3	0	370	4	26
Glazed	340	14 (37%)	3	0	320	3	49
Glazed Chocolate	410	24 (53%)	6	0	350	4	46
Jelly Stick	330	14 (38%)	3	0	350	3	48
Plain	260	14 (48%)	3	0	300	3	29
Powdered	290	15 (47%)	4	0	300	3	35
Sugar	270	14 (47%)	3	0	300	3	31
Fancies: Apple Fritter	300	13 (39%)	3	0	320	5	41
Bismark	310	14 (41%)	4	0	260	4	42
Blueberry Tart	300	10 (30%)	3	0	320	5	48
Bow Tie	250	10 (36%)	3	0	300	5	35
Cinnamon Raisin	330	13 (35%)	3	0	300	5	48
Coffee Roll	280	13 (42%)	3	0	300	5	35
Choc. Frosted	290	14 (43%)	3	0	300	5	38
Maple/Vanilla Frosted	300	13 (39%)	3	0	300	5	40
Glazed Fritter	290	13 (40%)	3	0	300	5	39
Eclair	290	12 (37%)	3	0	280	4	42
Strawberry Tart	310	10 (29%)	3	0	340	5	51
Apple Tart	290	10 (31%)	3	0	330	5	45
Apple Turnover	350	15 (39%)	4	0	340	5	49
Blueberry Turnover	370	15 (36%)	4	0	330	5	54
Lemon Tart	280	11 (35%)	3	0	340	5	43
Lemon Turnover	350	15 (39%)	4	0	360	5	48
Raspberry Tart	310	10 (29%)	3	0	350	5	51
Raspberry/Strawberry Turnover	380	15 (36%)	4	0	370	5	57
Cookies							
Chocolate Varieties	200	11 (49%)	6	30	150	2	26
Oatmeal Raisin Pecan	190	9 (43%)	5	25	150	2	27
Peanut Butter Varieties	210	12 (51%)	6	28	130	4	23
Bagels: Plain	200	0.5 (2%)	0	0	420	6	43
Onion	200	0.5 (2%)	0	0	400	5	41
Cinnamon Raisin	220	1.5 (6%)	0	0	320	5	46
Cream Cheese, 1 oz	100	10 (90%)	6	30	85	2	1

DUNKIN' DONUTS CONT

	Cal	Fat (%Fc)	S.Fat	Chol	Sod	Pro	Carb
Croissants: Plain	270	17 (57%)	4	5	260	4	27
Chocolate	370	23 (56%)	8	10	260	5	40
Almond	360	21 (53%)	5	10	300	6	38
Cheese	240	15 (56%)	3	5	260	6	28
Brownies							
Blondie w.Chocolate Chips	300	13 (39%)	3	25	150	4	41
Fudge	290	13 (40%)	3	35	85	5	37
Peanut Butter Blondie	330	18 (49%)	4	25	300	6	36
Breakfast Sandwiches							
Egg & Cheese	430	27 (57%)	9	280	640	16	30
Egg, Sausage & Cheese	630	49 (70%)	15	320	1180	24	30
Egg, Bacon & Cheese	500	34 (61%)	12	290	930	20	30
Egg, Ham & Cheese	530	29 (49%)	9	295	1080	23	30
Lunch Sandwiches							
Broccoli & Cheese	370	21 (51%)	6	20	680	10	36
Ham & Cheese	710	32 (41%)	13	85	1840	33	29
Roast Beef & Cheese	490	27 (50%)	8	30	680	31	28
Tuna Salad	540	30 (50%)	6	50	1140	30	39
Chicken Salad	540	31 (52%)	7	75	710	27	37
Seafod Salad	480	26 (49%)	6	50	1020	16	45
Soup							
Chicken Noodle	80	1.5 (17%)	0	15	890	6	12
Minestrone	100	1 (9%)	0	0	900	5	16
Beef Barley	90	0.5 (5%)	0	10	970	7	15
Harvest Vegetable	80	2 (23%)	0	0	1120	4	12
Chile Con Carne w.Beans	300	15 (45%)	0	45	690	17	25
Chile	170	6 (32%)	2.5	20	860	8	20
New England Clam Chowder	200	10 (45%)	3	30	1050	10	16
Beef Noodle	90	1 (10%)	0	20	980	8	12
Cream of Broccoli	200	11 (50%)	6	25	1050	8	17
Manhattan Clam Chowder	70	0.5 (6%)	0	5	890	5	11
Cream of Potato	190	9 (47%)	5	25	770	6	19
Split Pea w.Ham	190	9 (43%)	3	15	830	8	20
Coffee: No Cream or Sugar							
Decaf (10 oz)	0	0 (0%)	0	0	0	0	0
Hazelnut (10 oz)	5	0 (0%)	0	0	10	0	1
Other varieties (10 oz)	5	0 (0%)	0	0	5	0	1
Cream, 1 oz	60	5 (75%)	3	20	10	1	1

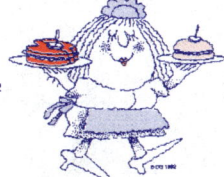

EL POLLO LOCO

	Cal	Fat (%Fc)	S.Fat	Chol	Sod	Pro	Carb
Chicken: Breast	160	6 (34%)	2	110	390	26	0
Leg	90	5 (50%)	2	75	150	11	0
Thigh	180	12 (60%)	4	130	230	16	0
Wing	110	6 (49%)	2	80	220	12	0
Tortillas							
Corn, each, 6"	70	1 (13%)	0	0	35	1	14
Flour, each, 6"	90	3 (30%)	0	0	225	3	13
Side Dishes: Per Serving							
Coleslaw	205	16 (70%)	3	11	360	2	12
Corn on the Cob, 5 1/2"	145	2 (12%)	0	0	20	5	33
French Fries	320	14 (39%)	3	0	330	5	44
Pinto Beans	185	4 (19%)	0	0	740	11	29
Potato Salad	255	14 (49%)	2	15	530	3	30
Smokey Black Beans	255	13 (46%)	5	11	610	6	29
Spanish Rice	130	3 (21%)	1	0	400	2	24
Specialities: (no dressing)							
Flame Broiled Chicken Salad	170	5 (26%)	0	56	765	27	11
Garden Salad	30	0 (0%)	0	0	20	3	6
Chicken (no Tostada/Cream)	330	14 (38%)	5	80	1280	35	26
Steak (no Tostada/Sr.Cream)	525	31 (53%)	14	100	1205	40	26
Tostada Shell	440	27 (55%)	4	0	610	7	42
Burritos							
Bean, Rice & Cheese	480	15 (28%)	5	15	1250	16	72
Classic/Spicy Hot Chicken	560	22 (35%)	7	117	1500	30	61
Grilled Steak	705	32 (41%)	13	77	1690	39	68
Loco Grande Chicken	630	26 (37%)	7	129	1650	33	67
Smokey Black Bean	570	22 (35%)	8	22	1340	16	78
Whole Wheat Chicken	590	26 (40%)	9	146	1200	31	60
Tacos: Chicken Soft	225	12 (48%)	4	66	585	16	15
Chicken Al Carbon	265	12 (41%)	2	28	225	10	30
Steak Al Carbon	400	22 (49%)	7	46	470	20	30
Pollo Bowl	505	13 (23%)	2	56	2070	37	69
Taquito	370	17 (41%)	4	25	690	15	43
Condiments							
Guacamole, 1 3/4 oz	50	3 (54%)	0	0	280	0	5
Lite Sour Cream, 1 oz	45	3 (60%)	0	12	25	2	2
Salsa; Jalapeno Hot Sauce	5	0 (0%)	0	0	100	0	1
Dressings							
Bleu Cheese	300	32 (96%)	6	50	590	2	2
Light Italian	25	1 (36%)	1	0	990	0	3
Ranch	350	39 (100%)	6	5	500	1	2
Thousand Island	270	27 (90%)	4	30	460	1	9
Desserts							
Flan	220	2 (8%)	2	5	140	6	46
Churro	150	8 (48%)	2	4	160	2	18

FAZOLI'S

	Cal	Fat (%Fc)	S.Fat	Chol	Sod	Pro	Carb
Soup							
Minestrone Soup	90	1 (10%)	<1	0	1040	5	16
Bean & Pasta Soup	170	7 (37%)	1	4	1080	7	20
Bread							
Breadstick	130	4 (28%)	<1	0	330	3	20
Breadstick/dry	100	0.5 (4%)	<1	0	200	3	20
Dinners: Per Serving							
Spaghetti: w.Tomato Sauce	340	7 (19%)	1	2	175	11	62
w.Meat Sauce	370	8 (19%)	2	20	160	19	60
w.Meatballs	580	25 (39%)	6	59	870	24	67
Baked Spaghetti Parmesan	560	21 (34%)	10	51	590	32	65
Ravioli: w.Tomato Sauce	330	15 (41%)	1	27	710	16	36
w.Meat Sauce	360	16 (40%)	2	45	700	22	34
Fettucine: Alfredo	400	13 (29%)	5	20	710	12	58
Broccoli	430	13 (27%)	5	20	730	13	62
Shrimp: Pasta	550	19 (31%)	<1	242	1120	37	58
& Scallop	520	14 (24%)	5	181	1090	36	63
Chicken Parmesan	480	14 (26%)	5	132	370	55	34
Baked Ziti: Regular	330	13 (35%)	5	30	350	20	38
Large	570	20 (32%)	8	109	520	32	68
Lasagna: Regular	530	24 (41%)	10	120	1150	33	47
Broccoli	570	27 (43%)	10	120	1440	34	50
Meatball Sub	650	30 (42%)	10	87	1530	28	62
Sampler Platter	610	20 (30%)	4	74	900	27	80
Pizza: Per Serving							
Cheese	360	11 (27%)	6	33	620	10	45
Pepperoni	430	17 (36%)	7	33	910	12	45
Combination	480	21 (39%)	9	44	1040	13	47
Salads: No Dressing							
Italian Chef Salad	390	30 (69%)	5	65	1310	22	10
Pasta Salad	400	20 (45%)	0	14	1030	9	46
Garden Salad	30	0 (0%)	0	0	20	2	5
Dressings: Per 1 oz							
Honey French	160	14 (79%)	2	0	230	0	11
House Italian	140	14 (90%)	<1	0	230	0	3
Reduced Calorie	70	4 (51%)	1	0	110	0	2
Ranch	180	20 (100%)	3	8	250	0	1
1000 Island	140	14 (90%)	2	15	230	0	4
Desserts: Per Serving							
Lemon Ice	140	0 (0%)	0	0	10	0	36
Cheesecake; Plain	270	21 (70%)	14	88	210	7	16
Choc.Choc. Chip	300	22 (66%)	14	83	200	8	22
Strawberry Topping	40	0 (0%)	0	0	1	0	10

GODFATHER'S PIZZA

	Cal	Fat	(%Fc)	S.Fat	Chol	Sod	Pro	Carb
Original Crust: Per Slice								
Cheese Pizza: Mini, 1/4 pizza	140	4	(26%)	na	15	160	6	20
Small, 1/6 pizza	240	7	(26%)	na	25	290	10	32
Medium, 1/8 pizza	240	7	(26%)	na	20	285	10	35
Large, 1/10 pizza	270	8	(27%)	na	30	330	12	37
Combo Pizza: Mini, 1/4 pizza	165	5	(27%)	na	15	290	8	21
Small, 1/6 pizza	300	11	(33%)	na	35	575	15	34
Medium, 1/8 pizza	320	12	(34%)	na	40	570	16	37
Large, 1/10 pizza	330	12	(33%)	na	40	620	16	39
Golden Crust: Per Slice								
Cheese Pizza: Small, 1/6 pizza	215	8	(33%)	na	20	260	8	27
Medium, 1/8 pizza	230	9	(31%)	na	20	270	8	28
large, 1/10 pizza	260	11	(38%)	na	25	315	8	31
Combo Pizza: Small, 1/6 pizza	270	12	(40%)	na	30	540	13	29
Medium, 1/8 pizza	280	13	(42%)	na	30	525	13	30
Large, 1/10 pizza	320	15	(42%)	na	35	600	14	33

GOLDEN CORRAL

	Cal	Fat	(%Fc)	S.Fat	Chol	Sod	Pro	Carb
Chicken								
Grilled	170	5	(26%)	na	100	520	32	0
Fried	370	19	(46%)	na	85	570	37	14
Shrimp, fried	250	12	(43%)	na	90	470	12	24
Steak: Ribeye, 6 oz	450	35	(70%)	na	120	220	34	0
Sirloin, 5 oz	230	14	(55%)	na	90	270	27	0
Chopped, 4 oz	320	23	(65%)	na	100	160	28	0
Tips w.Onions	290	13	(40%)	na	120	260	30	8
Baked Potato	225	2	(8%)	na	0	60	5	46
Texas Toast	170	6	(32%)	na	0	230	5	26

HAAGEN-DAZS

	Cal	Fat	(%Fc)	S.Fat	Chol	Sod	Pro	Carb
Ice Cream: Per 1/2 Cup								
Belgian Chocolate Chocolate	330	21	(57%)	12	85	60	29	5
Brownies a la Mode	280	18	(58%)	11	100	115	4	26
Butter Pecan	320	24	(68%)	11	105	140	5	20
Capppucino Commotion	310	21	(61%)	12	100	105	5	25
Caramel Cone Explosion	310	20	(58%)	12	95	130	5	27
Chocolate	270	18	(60%)	11	115	75	5	22
Chocolate Chocolate Chip	300	20	(60%)	12	100	70	5	26
Chocolate Chocolate Mint	300	20	(60%)	11	95	65	25	5
Coffee	270	18	(60%)	11	120	85	5	21
Coffee Chip	290	19	(59%)	12	100	75	25	5
Cookie Dough Dynamo	300	19	(57%)	12	95	140	4	29
Cookies & Cream	270	17	(57%)	11	110	115	5	23

HAAGEN-DAZS CONT

	Cal	Fat (%Fc)	S.Fat	Chol	Sod	Pro	Carb
Ice Cream: Per 1/2 Cup (Cont)							
Deep Chocolate Peanut Butter	370	25 (61%)	11	85	100	27	8
Macadamia Brittle	300	20 (60%)	11	110	120	4	25
Macadamia Nut	320	24 (68%)	12	110	115	20	5
Midnight Cookies & Cream	300	18 (54%)	11	90	140	5	29
Pralines & Cream	290	18 (56%)	9	95	180	4	27
Rum Raisin	270	17 (57%)	10	110	75	4	22
Strawberry	250	16 (58%)	10	95	80	4	23
Strawberry Cheesecake Craze	280	17 (55%)	9	100	140	4	27
Swiss Chocolate Almond	300	20 (60%)	11	100	65	6	23
Vanilla	270	18 (60%)	11	120	85	5	21
Vanilla Chocolate Chip	290	19 (59%)	12	100	75	5	24
Vanilla Fudge	280	18 (58%)	11	105	105	5	25
Vanilla Swiss Almond	310	21 (61%)	11	105	80	6	23
Ice Cream Sandwich							
Vanilla	260	13 (45%)	8	65	125	4	32
Vanilla & Chocolate	260	13 (45%)	8	65	120	4	31
Ice Cream Bars: Single Pack							
Chocolate & Dark Chocolate	400	27 (60%)	18	85	90	5	33
Coffee & Almond Crunch	360	26 (65%)	15	100	85	5	27
Vanilla & Almonds	370	27 (66%)	14	90	80	6	26
Vanilla & Dark Chocolate	390	27 (62%)	18	85	65	5	33
Vanilla & Milk Chocolate	330	24 (65%)	14	90	75	5	24
Multi Pack: 1 Bar							
Chocolate & Dark Chocolate	320	22 (62%)	15	70	70	4	27
Coffee & Almond Crunch	290	21 (65%)	12	80	70	4	22
Vanilla & Almonds	300	22 (66%)	12	70	65	5	21
Vanilla & Dark Chocolate	320	22 (62%)	15	70	50	4	27
Vanilla & Milk Chocolate	280	20 (64%)	12	75	65	4	20
Uncoated Ice Cream Bars							
Chocolate	200	13 (59%)	8	85	55	4	16
Coffee; Vanilla	190	13 (62%)	8	85	65	3	15
Ice Cream Cordials: Per 1/2 Cup							
Baileys Irish Cream	270	17 (57%)	10	115	85	5	23
DiSaronno Amaretto	260	15 (52%)	9	95	80	4	26
Sorbet: Per 1/2 Cup							
Banana Strawberry; Peach	140	0 (0%)	0	0	5	0	34
Chocolate	130	0 (0%)	0	0	80	2	30
Mango; Raspberry; Lemon	120	0 (0%)	0	0	0	0	30
Strawberry	130	0 (0%)	0	0	0	0	33
Sorbet & Cream: Per 1/2 Cup							
Orange; Raspberry	190	9 (43%)	5	60	45	2	24
Sorbet Soft Serving: Per 1/2 Cup							
Mango; Raspberry	100	0 (0%)	0	0	0	0	25
Sorbet Bars							
Chocolate	80	0 (0%)	0	0	50	1	20
Wild Berry	90	0 (0%)	0	0	5	0	22

HAAGEN-DAZS CONT

	Cal	Fat	(%Fc)	S.Fat	Chol	Sod	Pro	Carb
Frozen Yogurt: Per 1/2 Cup								
Chocolate; Coffee	140	0	(0%)	0	<5	45	6	29
Vanilla; Cherry Vanilla	140	0	(0%)	0	<5	45	6	29
Vanilla Fudge	160	0	(0%)	0	<5	100	6	34
Vanilla Raspberry Swirl	130	0	(0%)	0	<5	30	4	28
Soft Serving: Per 1/2 Cup								
Coffee	140	4	(26%)	2.5	35	75	5	20
Nonfat Chocolate	110	0	(0%)	0	0	65	4	23
Nonfat Chocolate Mousse	80	0	(0%)	0	0	65	5	24
Nonfat Vanilla	110	0	(0%)	0	<5	70	5	22
Nonfat Vanilla Mousse	70	0	(0%)	0	0	65	4	23
Sorbet 'N Yogurt Bars: Each								
Banana & Strawberry	90	0	(0%)	0	0	15	2	20
Chocolate & Cherry	100	0	(0%)	0	0	40	3	21
Raspberry & Vanilla	90	0	(0%)	0	0	15	2	20

HARDEES

	Cal	Fat	(%Fc)	S.Fat	Chol	Sod	Pro	Carb
Breakfast Items								
Biscuits: Rise 'N' Shine	390	21	(48%)	6	0	1000	6	44
Apple Cinnamon 'N' Raisin	200	8	(36%)	2	0	350	2	30
Sausage	510	31	(55%)	10	25	1360	14	44
Sausage & Egg	630	40	(57%)	22	285	1480	23	45
Bacon & Egg	570	33	(52%)	11	275	1400	22	45
Bacon, Egg & Cheese	610	37	(55%)	13	280	1630	24	45
Ham	400	20	(45%)	6	15	1340	9	47
Ham, Egg & Cheese	540	30	(50%)	11	285	1660	20	48
Jelly	440	21	(43%)	6	0	1000	6	57
Country Ham	430	22	(46%)	6	25	1930	15	45
Ultimate Omelet	570	33	(52%)	12	290	1370	22	45
Big Country: Sausage	1000	66	(59%)	38	570	2310	41	62
Bacon	820	49	(54%)	15	535	1870	33	62
Frisco Brfast Sandwich (Ham)	500	25	(45%)	9	290	1370	24	46
Hash Rounds	230	14	(55%)	3	0	560	3	24
Biscuit 'N' Gravy	510	28	(49%)	9	15	1500	10	55
Pancakes: Three Pancakes	280	2	(6%)	1	15	890	8	56
w/1 Sausage Pattie	430	16	(33%)	6	40	1290	16	56
w/2 Bacon Strips	350	9	(23%)	3	25	1130	13	56
Orange Juice, regular	140	0	(0%)	0	0	5	2	34
Hamburgers & Sandwiches								
Hamburger	270	11	(37%)	3	35	670	14	29
Cheeseburger	310	14	(41%)	6	40	890	16	30
Mushroom 'N' Swiss	490	25	(46%)	12	80	1100	28	39
Cravin' Bacon Cheeseburger	690	46	(60%)	15	95	1150	30	38
1/4 Pound Dble Cheeseburger	470	27	(52%)	11	80	1290	27	31
Frisco Burger	720	46	(57%)	16	95	1340	33	43

HARDEES CONT

	Cal	Fat (%Fc)	S.Fat	Chol	Sod	Pro	Carb
Hamburgers (Cont)							
Roast Beef; Regular	320	16 (45%)	6	43	820	17	26
Big	460	24 (47%)	9	70	1280	26	35
The Boss	570	33 (52%)	12	85	910	27	42
The Works	530	30 (51%)	12	80	1030	25	41
Mesquite Bacon Chsburger	370	18 (44%)	7	45	970	19	32
Chicken Fillet Sandwich	480	18 (34%)	3	55	1280	26	54
Grilled Chicken Sandwich	350	11 (28%)	2	65	950	25	38
Hot Ham 'N' Cheese	310	12 (35%)	6	50	1410	16	34
Fisherman's Fillet	560	27 (43%)	7	65	1330	26	54
Fried Chicken: Breast, each	370	15 (36%)	4	75	1190	29	29
Wing, each	200	8 (36%)	2	30	740	10	23
Thigh, each	330	15 (41%)	4	60	1000	19	30
Leg, each	170	7 (37%)	2	45	570	13	15
French Fries: Small	240	10 (37%)	3	0	100	4	33
Medium	350	15 (39%)	4	0	150	5	49
Large	430	18 (38%)	5	0	190	6	59
Mashed Potatoes, 4oz	70	0.5 (6%)	0.5	0	330	2	14
Gravy, 1.5oz	20	0.5 (22%)	0	0	260	1	3
Baked Beans, 5 oz	170	1 (5%)	0	0	600	8	32
Salads; Dressings							
ColeSlaw	240	20 (75%)	3	10	340	2	13
Side Salad; no dressing	25	0.5 (18%)	0	0	45	1	4
Garden Salad; no dressing	220	13 (53%)	9	40	350	12	11
Grilled Chicken Salad; no drssng	150	3 (18%)	1	60	610	20	11
Fat Free French Dressing	70	0 (0%)	0	0	580	0	17
Ranch Dressing	290	29 (90%)	4	25	510	1	6
Thousand Island Dressing	250	23 (83%)	3	35	540	1	9
Shakes; Desserts: Vanilla	350	5 (13%)	3	20	300	12	65
Chocolate	370	5 (12%)	3	30	270	13	67
Strawberry	420	4 (9%)	3	20	270	11	83
Peach	390	4 (9%)	3	25	290	10	77
Cool Twist: Vanilla Cone	170	22 (11%)	1	10	130	4	34
Chocolate Cone	180	2 (1%)	1	5	110	5	34
Vanilla/Chocolate Cone	180	2 (0%)	1	10	120	4	34
Sundae: Hot Fudge	290	6 (19%)	3	20	310	7	51
Strawberry	210	2 (9%)	1	10	140	5	43
Big Cookie	280	12 (39%)	4	15	150	4	41
Peach Cobbler: Small	310	7 (20%)	1	0	360	2	60

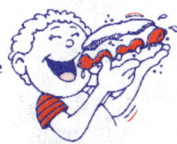

HARVEYS

	Cal	Fat	(%Fc)	S.Fat	Chol	Sod	Pro	Carb
Breakfast Items: Per Serving								
Pancakes	90	1	(10%)	na	8	na	2	17
Sausage	170	14	(75%)	na	12	na	9	3
Toast, plain	250	3	(11%)	na	1	na	8	48
Burgers								
Hamburger: Regular	360	14	(35%)	na	17	na	12	40
Double	530	26	(44%)	na	34	na	31	44
Super	480	19	(36%)	na	112	na	37	38
Cheeseburger	420	18	(39%)	na	30	na	22	41
Chicken Fingers, 1 serving	240	12	(45%)	na	57	na	15	18
Sandwiches: Chicken	420	16	(34%)	na	110	na	19	46
Western	350	10	(26%)	na	265	na	15	58
French Fries	480	24	(45%)	na	5	na	10	56
Hash Browns	150	9	(55%)	na	2	na	2	15
Hot Dog	330	15	(41%)	na	50	na	12	32
Onion Rings	290	14	(44%)	na	5	na	4	36
Muffins: Blueberry	260	6	(21%)	na	1	na	4	45
Bran	300	13	(39%)	na	1	na	5	42
Apple Turnover, each	180	7	(35%)	na	7	na	1	28
Drinks: Apple Juice	80	2	(23%)	na	0	na	2	20
Orange Juice	80	1	(12%)	na	0	na	1	18
Shakes: Chocolate	320	11	(31%)	na	36	na	12	74
Strawberry; Vanilla	300	10	(30%)	na	36	na	11	69

IHOP - INTL. HOUSE OF PANCAKES

	Cal	Fat	(%Fc)	S.Fat	Chol	Sod	Pro	Carb
Pancakes: (Syrup/Butter extra)								
Buttermilk, 1 (2 oz)	105	3	(25%)	1	30	460	3	17
Short Stack, 3	315	9	(25%)	3	90	1380	9	51
Full Stack, 5	525	15	(25%)	5	150	2300	15	85
Buckwheat, 1 (2½ oz)	135	5	(33%)	1	60	370	4	19
Country Griddle, 1 (2¼ oz)	135	4	(26%)	1	38	500	4	22
Harvest Grain 'N Nut, 1	160	8	(45%)	1.5	38	390	4.5	18
Crepes (Egg Pancakes), 1 (2 oz)	100	5	(45%)	1	66	210	2	12
Syrup: 1 Tbsp	50	0	(0%)	0	0	0	0	12
Whipped Butter, 1 Tbsp	70	7	(90%)	4.5	20	70	0	0
Waffles (Plain):								
Regular, 1 (4 oz)	300	15	(45%)	3.5	70	470	6	37
Belgian: Regular, 1 (6 oz)	410	20	(44%)	11	145	880	4	49
Harvest Grain 'N Nut, 1	450	28	(56%)	12	145	870	10	40

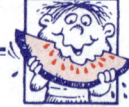

I CAN'T BELIEVE IT'S YOGURT

	Cal	Fat (%Fc)	S.Fat	Chol	Sod	Pro	Carb
Per Medium Serving							
Original Frozen Yogurt							
Awesome Amaretto	285	6.5 (21%)	4.5	22	230	7	51
Cookies 'N Cream	265	4.5 (15%)	1	11	200	7	55
French Vanilla	265	6.5 (22%)	4.5	44	200	7	46
Peanut Butter Bliss	310	13 (38%)	5	11	210	6	46
Nonfat Frozen Yogurt							
Per Medium Serving							
Chocolicious	220	0 (0%)	0	0	155	7	46
Coffee Break	200	0 (0%)	0	0	155	7	44
Eggnog Eggstravaganza	240	0 (0%)	0	11	145	7	53
German Chocolate Cake	220	0 (0%)	0	0	175	7	51
Go Bananas!	220	0 (0%)	0	0	130	7	46
Key Lime Pie	220	0 (0%)	0	0	145	7	48
New Orleans Praline	220	0 (0%)	0	0	200	7	51
New York Cheesecake	220	0 (0%)	0	0	155	7	48
Not Just Plain Vanilla	200	0 (0%)	0	0	155	7	44
Peppermint Stick	220	0 (0%)	0	0	145	7	51
Strictly Strawberry	240	0 (0%)	0	0	155	5	53
The Great Pumpkin	220	0 (0%)	0	0	155	7	51
Nonfat (w/NutraSweet)							
Chocolicious	220	0 (0%)	0	0	155	7	46
All Other Flavors	200	0 (0%)	0	0	165	7	42
Hard Scooped Frozen Yogurt							
Per Medium Serving							
Amaretto Cherry Crunch	375	11 (27%)	4.5	55	210	11	59
Chocolate	330	9 (24%)	6.5	22	300	11	55
Chocolate Cherry Cheesecake	395	11 (25%)	6.5	55	240	11	70
Choc. Chip Cookie Dough	395	11 (25%)	6.5	88	265	11	66
Chocolate Mint Chip	395	15 (34%)	11	55	210	11	59
Chunky Choc. Brownie	395	13 (29%)	6.5	22	300	11	62
Cookies 'N Cream	375	11 (27%)	6.5	55	265	11	62
Macadamia Mania	395	13 (30%)	9	55	330	11	66
Peanut Butter Cup	440	18 (37%)	9	55	300	13	59
Pralines 'N Cream	395	11 (25%)	6.5	55	285	11	68
Rocky Road	395	13 (30%)	6.5	22	275	11	59
Rum Raisin	375	9 (22%)	4.5	55	210	11	68
Tin Roof Fudge	395	13 (30%)	6.5	55	240	13	62
Classic Vanilla	350	9 (23%)	4.5	88	255	13	57
Yoglace' Desserts							
Belgian Chocolate	130	0 (0%)	0	0	100	7	31
Lemon Spritzer; Swiss Vanilla	100	0 (0%)	0	11	65	5	26
Margarita	110	0 (0%)	0	11	65	5	29

JACK IN THE BOX

	Cal	Fat	(%Fc)	S.Fat	Chol	Sod	Pro	Carb
Breakfast								
Breakfast Jack	300	12	(36%)	5	185	890	18	30
Pancake Platter	400	12	(27%)	3	30	980	13	59
Sausage Croissant	670	48	(64%)	19	250	940	21	39
Scrambled Egg Pocket	430	21	(44%)	8	355	1060	29	31
Sourdough Breakfast Sandwich	380	20	(47%)	7	235	1120	21	31
Supreme Croissant	570	36	(57%)	15	245	1240	21	39
Ultimate Breakfast Sandwich	620	35	(51%)	11	455	1800	36	39
Hash Browns	160	11	(62%)	3	0	310	1	14
Country Crock Spread	25	3	(100%)	0.5	0	40	0	0
Grape Jelly, 1 packet	40	0	(0%)	0	0	5	0	9
Pancake Syrup, 1 packet	120	0	(0%)	0	0	5	0	30
Burgers								
Hamburger	280	11	(35%)	4	25	470	13	31
Cheeseburger	320	15	(42%)	6	35	670	16	32
Double	450	24	(48%)	12	75	970	24	35
Ultimate	1030	79	(69%)	26	205	1200	50	30
Jumbo Jack	560	32	(51%)	10	65	740	26	41
W. Cheese	650	40	(55%)	14	90	1150	31	42
Grilled Sourdough Burger	670	43	(58%)	16	110	1180	32	39
1/4 lb. Burger	510	27	(48%)	10	65	1080	26	39
Sandwiches								
Chicken Caesar	520	26	(45%)	6	55	1050	27	44
Chicken Fajita Pita	290	8	(25%)	3	35	700	24	29
Chicken Sandwich	400	18	(40%)	4	45	1290	20	38
Chicken Supreme	620	36	(52%)	11	75	1520	25	48
Grilled Chicken Fillet	430	19	(40%)	5	65	1070	29	36
Spicy Crispy Chicken	560	27	(43%)	5	50	1020	24	55
Finger Foods								
Egg Rolls - 3 piece	440	24	(49%)	7	30	960	3	54
5 piece	750	41	(49%)	12	50	1640	5	92
Chicken Strips - 4 piece	290	13	(40%)	3	50	700	25	18
6 piece	450	20	(40%)	5	80	1100	39	28
Stuffed Jalapenos - 7 piece	420	27	(58%)	12	55	1620	15	29
10 piece	600	39	(58%)	16	75	2320	22	41
Bacon/Cheddar Pot. Wedges	800	58	(65%)	16	55	1470	20	49
Mexican Food: Taco	190	11	(52%)	4	20	410	7	15
Monster	280	17	(55%)	6	30	760	12	22
Guacamole	50	4	(72%)	0	60	95	<1	3
Salsa	10	0	(0%)	0	0	200	0	2
Teriyaki Bowls: Chicken	580	1.5	(2%)	0.5	30	1220	28	115
Soy Sauce	5	0	(0%)	0	0	480	<1	<1
Salads: No Dressing								
Garden Chicken	200	9	(40%)	4	65	420	23	8
Side	70	4	(51%)	3	10	80	4	3

JACK IN THE BOX CONT

	Cal	Fat (%Fc)	S.Fat	Chol	Sod	Pro	Carb
Dressing							
Blue Cheese	210	18 (77%)	4	15	750	1	11
Buttermilk House	290	30 (93%)	11	20	560	1	6
Low Calorie Italian	25	1.5 (54%)	0	0	670	0	2
Thousand Island	250	24 (86%)	4	20	570	1	10
Croutons	50	2 (36%)	0.5	0	105	1	8
Sides							
Seasoned Curly Fries	360	20 (50%)	5	0	1070	5	39
French Fries: Small	220	11 (45%)	3	0	120	3	28
Regular	350	17 (44%)	4	0	190	4	45
Jumbo Fries	400	19 (43%)	5	0	220	5	51
Super Scoop	590	29 (44%)	7	0	330	8	76
Onion Rings	380	23 (54%)	6	0	450	5	38
Condiments							
Cheese: American, 1 slice	45	3.5 (70%)	2.5	10	200	2	0
Swiss-style, 1 slice	40	3 (67%)	2	10	190	3	0
Packet: Hot Sauce	5	0 (0%)	0	0	110	<1	1
Ketchup	10	0 (0%)	0	0	100	0	3
Mayonnaise	150	17 (100%)	2.5	15	120	0	0
Mustard	5	0 (0%)	0	0	55	0	0
Chinese Hot Mustard	10	0 (0%)	0	0	50	0	1
Dipping Sauce: Tartar	150	15 (90%)	1	10	200	0	2
Barbeque	45	0 (0%)	0	0	300	1	11
Buttermilk House	130	13 (90%)	5	10	240	<1	3
Sweet & Sour	40	0 (0%)	0	0	160	<1	11
Sour Cream	60	6 (90%)	4	20	30	1	1
Desserts: Carrot Cake	370	15 (36%)	3	30	310	3	58
Cheesecake	310	18 (52%)	9	65	210	8	29
Choc Chip Cookie Dough	360	18 (45%)	8	45	200	7	44
Hot Apple Turnover	350	19 (49%)	4	0	460	3	48
Drinks							
Shake: Vanilla, regular	350	7 (18%)	4	30	180	9	62
Chocolate, regular	390	6 (14%)	5	25	210	9	74
Strawberry	330	7 (19%)	4	30	180	9	60
Ice Cream Shake: Choc, reg.	630	27 (39%)	16	85	330	11	85
Cappuccino, regular	630	29 (41%)	17	90	320	11	80
Strawberry, regular	640	28 (39%)	15	85	300	10	85
Vanilla, regular	610	31 (46%)	18	95	320	12	73
Orange Juice	80	0 (0%)	0	0	0	1	20
Lowfat Milk (2%)	120	5 (38%)	3	20	120	8	12
Coca Cola, small	190	0 (0%)	0	0	20	0	51
Ramblin Root Beer	240	0 (0%)	0	0	45	0	61
Sprite, small	190	0 (0%)	0	0	60	0	48
Dr Pepper	190	0 (0%)	0	0	25	0	49

KENNY ROGERS ROASTERS

	Cal	Fat	(%Fc)	S.Fat	Chol	Sod	Pro	Carb
Chicken								
1/4 White Meat: w. Skin	250	11	(39%)	3	136	600	35	1
no Skin or Wing	140	2	(13%)	0.5	92	420	31	<1
1/4 Dark Meat: w. Skin	270	17	(57%)	4	165	520	29	<1
no Skin	170	7	(37%)	2	130	455	25	<1
1/2 Chicken: w. Skin	515	28	(49%)	7	300	1130	65	2
no Skin or Wing	315	10	(29%)	3	220	880	56	<1
Turkey: Sliced Breast	160	2	(11%)	0.5	78	590	34	0
Sandwiches; Pitas; Pies								
Turkey Sandwich	385	12	(28%)	2	88	920	39	30
BBQ Chicken Pita	400	7	(16%)	1	112	1310	33	51
Chicken Caesar Pita	600	35	(52%)	3	122	830	36	34
Roasted Chicken Pita	685	35	(46%)	3	159	1620	47	42
Chicken Pot Pie	710	33	(42%)	11	69	1500	26	78
Soup								
Chicken Noodle, 1 cup	55	1	(16%)	0.5	13	560	4	7
1 bowl	90	2	(20%)	0.5	22	930	7	12
Salads: (no dressing)								
Chicken Caesar	285	9	(28%)	3	122	700	34	18
Pasta Salad	230	12	(47%)	2	40	300	6	28
Roasted Chicken	290	10	(31%)	2	218	570	35	19
Side Salad	25	0	(0%)	0	0	15	1	5
Sour Cream & Dill Pasta	230	16	(63%)	3	16	430	4	20
Tomato Cucumber	125	2	(14%)	1	0	790	1	10
Side Dishes: Per Serving								
Cinnamon Apples	200	5	(22%)	3	13	5	0	41
Cole Slaw	225	16	(64%)	3	13	290	1	18
Corn: Muffin	175	8	(41%)	1	0	210	2	24
On the Cob	70	0.5	(6%)	0.5	0	10	2	14
Sweet Corn Niblets	115	0.5	(3%)	0.5	0	385	3	26
Cornbread Stuffing	320	19	(53%)	3	5	765	7	34
Creamy Parmesan Spinach	120	6	(45%)	3	12	550	10	10
Honey Baked Beans	150	1	(6%)	0.5	0	790	6	32
Italian Green Beans	115	8	(63%)	1	0	375	2	10
Macaroni & Cheese	200	6	(27%)	3	26	660	6	24
Potatoes: Baked Sweet	260	0	(0%)	0	0	25	4	62
Garlic Parsley	260	12	(42%)	5	16	870	3	37
Real Mashed	295	14	(43%)	3	2	480	4	39
Potato Salad	390	27	(62%)	3	0	630	3	34
Rice Pilaf	175	5	(26%)	0.5	0	145	3	43
Steamed Vegetables	50	0	(0%)	0	0	60	3	8
Zucchini & Squash Santa Fe	70	5	(64%)	0.5	0	210	<1	8

K F C

	Cal	Fat (%Fc)	S.Fat	Chol	Sod	Pro	Carb
Original Recipe							
Breast	400	24 (54%)	6	135	1120	29	16
Drumstick	140	9 (58%)	2	75	420	13	4
Thigh	250	18 (65%)	4.5	95	750	16	6
Wing	140	10 (64%)	2.5	55	415	9	5
Extra Tasty Crispy							
Breast	470	28 (54%)	7	80	930	31	25
Drumstick	190	11 (52%)	3	60	260	13	8
Thigh	370	25 (61%)	6	70	540	19	18
Wing	200	13 (58%)	4	45	290	10	10
Hot & Spicy							
Breast	530	35 (58%)	8	110	1110	32	23
Drumstick	190	11 (52%)	3	50	300	13	10
Thigh	370	27 (66%)	7	90	570	18	13
Wing	210	15 (64%)	4	50	340	10	9
Tender Roast							
Breast: with Skin	250	11 (40%)	3	151	830	37	1
No skin	170	4.5 (21%)	1	112	800	31	1
Drumstick: with Skin	100	4.5 (36%)	1	85	270	15	<1
No Skin	70	2.5 (26%)	<1	63	260	11	<1
Thigh: with Skin	210	12 (51%)	4	120	500	18	1.5
No Skin	105	6 (51%)	2	84	310	13	<1
Wing: with Skin	120	8 (36%)	2	74	330	12	1
Snackables							
Colonel's Crispy Strips, 3 pces	260	16 (55%)	4	40	660	20	10
Chunky Chicken Pot Pie	770	42 (49%)	13	70	2160	29	69
Hot Wings, 6 pieces	470	33 (63%)	8	150	1230	27	18
Kentucky Nuggets (6)	285	18 (57%)	4	66	865	16	15
Sandwich							
Chicken	500	22 (40%)	5	52	1210	29	46
BBQ Flavored Chicken	255	8 (28%)	1	57	780	17	28
Side Dishes: Per Serving							
BBQ Baked Beans	190	3 (14%)	1	5	760	6	33
Buttermilk Biscuit	180	10 (50%)	2.5	0	560	4	20
Coleslaw	180	9 (45%)	1.5	5	280	2	21
Corn on the Cob	190	3 (14%)	0.5	0	20	5	34
Corn Bread	230	13 (50%)	2	42	190	3	25
Garden Rice	120	1.5 (11%)	0	0	890	3	23
Green Beans	45	1.5 (30%)	0.5	5	730	1	7
Macaroni & Cheese	180	8 (40%)	3	10	860	7	21
Mean Greens	70	3 (39%)	1	10	650	4	11
Potato:							
Potato Salad	230	14 (55%)	2	15	540	4	23
Mashed Potatoes w. Gravy	120	6 (45%)	1	<1	440	1	17
Potato Wedges	280	13 (42%)	4	5	750	5	28
Red Beans & Rice	130	3 (21%)	1	5	360	5	21

KRYSTAL

	Cal	Fat	(%Fc)	S.Fat	Chol	Sod	Pro	Carb
Breakfast								
Biscuit: Biscuit	245	12	(44%)	2	2	440	3	31
Bacon	310	17	(49%)	5	14	730	8	32
Country Ham	335	17	(46%)	4	23	1150	14	31
Egg	330	19	(52%)	4	134	480	8	32
Gravy	420	26	(56%)	7	23	980	7	40
Sausage	440	30	(61%)	8	49	670	10	31
Bacon, Egg & Cheese	420	26	(56%)	8	153	900	14	33
Pancakes	250	12	(43%)	2	0	210	5	31
Sunriser	260	17	(59%)	5	162	540	14	17
Sandwiches								
Krystal	160	7	(39%)	2	22	30	10	16
Double	280	14	(45%)	4	43	585	18	24
Cheese	190	10	(48%)	4	29	450	11	16
Double Cheese	340	19	(50%)	8	57	815	21	25
Big K	540	35	(58%)	14	93	1280	29	29
Bacon Cheeseburger	520	34	(59%)	14	89	1080	26	29
Burger Plus	415	26	(56%)	10	63	620	20	28
w. Cheese	475	31	(59%)	13	77	870	23	28
Crispy Crunchy Chicken	470	24	(46%)	7	56	950	16	48
Plain Pup	160	9	(50%)	5	20	470	6	12
Chili Pup	180	10	(50%)	6	24	600	7	13
Chili Cheese Pup	210	13	(56%)	7	31	640	9	14
Corn Pup	215	14	(59%)	6	24	710	6	17
Side Items								
Chili: Regular	220	8	(33%)	3	19	855	11	27
Large	330	12	(33%)	5	28	1285	16	41
French Fries: Small	260	13	(45%)	5	9	115	3	33
Regular	360	18	(45%)	6	12	160	4	45
Large	460	23	(45%)	8	16	205	5	59
Krys Kross Fries:	490	29	(53%)	11	31	605	5	52
w. Cheese	515	31	(54%)	12	31	805	5	54
Chili Cheese	625	39	(56%)	16	61	1110	12	57
Shakes/Desserts								
Chocolate Shake	275	10	(33%)	5	32	180	8	44
Apple Pie	300	1	(30%)	4	0	420	3	49
Lemon Meringue Pie	340	9	(24%)	3	50	190	7	57
Pecan Pie	450	23	(46%)	6	55	290	5	56
Donut: Plain	150	9	(54%)	2	5	135	2	17
w. Choc Icing	210	11	(47%)	3	5	135	2	27
w. Vanilla Icing	200	9	(40%)	2	5	135	2	29

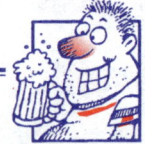

LONG JOHN SILVER

	Cal	Fat	(%Fc)	S.Fat	Chol	Sod	Pro	Carb
Flavorbaked								
Fish, 1 piece	120	3.5	(26%)	1	45	430	20	2
Chicken	150	4	(24%)	1	75	810	26	1
Sandwiches								
Batter-Dipped Fish (no sauce)	320	13	(37%)	4	30	800	17	40
Ultimate Fish	430	21	(44%)	7	35	1340	18	44
Flavorbaked Fish	320	14	(39%)	7	55	930	23	28
Flavorbaked Chicken	290	10	(31%)	2	60	970	24	27
Popcorn Items								
Fish	290	14	(43%)	4	20	1090	13	27
Chicken	250	14	(50%)	4	35	590	15	17
Shrimp	280	15	(48%)	4	85	920	11	27
Fish; Shrimp; Chicken								
Battered Fish, 1 piece	170	11	(58%)	3	30	470	11	12
Battered Chicken, 1 piece	120	6	(45%)	2	15	400	8	11
Battered Shrimp, 1 piece	35	2.5	(64%)	0.5	10	95	1	2
Clams	300	17	(51%)	4	40	670	11	31
Wraps								
Chicken: South of the Border								
Regular, 11 oz	700	32	(40%)	7	20	1690	18	81
Large, 22 oz	1370	64	(40%)	13	35	3370	36	162
Cajun/Caesar/Classic/Ranch								
Aver., regular, 11 oz	730	36	(45%)	7	25	1830	18	82
Large, 22 oz	1450	72	(45%)	14	50	3650	36	165
Fish: South of the Border								
Regular, 11.5 oz	700	32	(40%)	7	25	1640	18	84
Large, 23 oz	1380	64	(40%)	14	45	3280	35	167
Cajun/Caesar/Classic/Ranch								
Aver., regular, 11.5 oz	730	36	(45%)	8	25	1780	18	85
Large, 23 oz	1450	72	(45%)	15	58	3550	35	170
Popcorn Shrimp:								
Regular, 11 oz	700	32	(40%)	9	40	1660	16	84
Large, 22 oz	1380	64	(40%)	17	85	3310	32	170
Cajun/Caesar/Classic/Ranch								
Average, regular, 11 oz	730	36	(45%)	9	45	1810	16	86
Large, 22 oz	1450	72	(45%)	18	95	3600	32	172
Side Items: Fries	250	15	(54%)	3	0	500	3	28
Cheese Sticks	160	9	(50%)	4	10	360	6	12
Hushpuppy, 1 piece	60	2.5	(37%)	0	0	25	1	9
Corn Cobbette:	140	8	(51%)	2	0	0	3	19
no Butter	80	0.5	(6%)	0	0	0	3	19
Green Beans	30	0.5	(15%)	0	<5	310	2	5
Rice Pilaf	140	3	(19%)	1	0	210	3	26
Coleslaw	140	6	(39%)	na	0	260	1	20
Side Salad, no dressing	25	0	(0%)	0	0	15	1	4
Ocean Chef Salad, no dressing	100	2	(18%)	0	40	730	12	12
Baked Potato	210	0	(0%)	0	0	10	4	49

LONG JOHN SILVER CONT

	Cal	Fat	(%Fc)	S.Fat	Chol	Sod	Pro	Carb
Desserts								
Pineapple Cream Cheesecake	310	17	(49%)	9	5	105	4	36
Chocolate Cream Pie	280	17	(55%)	8	15	125	4	29
Double Lemon Pie	350	18	(46%)	10	40	180	6	41
Key Lime Cream Cheese Pie	310	19	(55%)	11	20	140	4	33
Apple Crumb Cheesecake	300	15	(45%)	6	25	160	3	38
Condiments: Ketchup	10	0	(0%)	0	0	110	0	2
Shrimp Sauce	15	0	(0%)	0	0	180	0	3
Tartar Sauce	35	1.5	(39%)	na	0	35	0	5
Honey Mustard Sauce	20	0	(0%)	0	0	60	0	5
Malt Vinegar	0	0	(0%)	0	0	15	0	0
Sweet 'n Sour Sauce	20	0	(0%)	0	0	45	0	5
Margarine	35	4	(100%)	0	0	35	0	0
Sour Cream	60	6	(90%)	4	15	<1	1	1
Dressings: Ranch	170	18	(95%)	3	5	260	0	1
Fat Free Ranch	50	0	(0%)	0	0	380	2	13
Fat Free French	50	0	(0%)	0	0	360	0	14
Italian	130	14	(97%)	2	0	280	0	2
Thousand Island	110	10	(82%)	2	15	280	0	5

MRS WINNER'S CHICKEN

	Cal	Fat	(%Fc)	S.Fat	Chol	Sod	Pro	Carb
Chicken: Baked Fillet	120	2	(15%)	na	35	360	10	<1
Breaded Chicken Sandwich	205	10	(44%)	na	35	1000	19	12
Chicken Fillet Sandwich	380	7	(17%)	na	30	540	12	45
Chicken Salad	585	8	(12%)	na	5	875	9	39
Chicken Salad Sandwich	315	6	(17%)	na	<5	600	10	33
Biscuit	245	5	(18%)	na	<1	500	4	45
Cole Slaw	190	16	(76%)	na	<5	560	1	9
Potato Fries	225	9	(36%)	na	<5	220	6	27
Seafood Salad	555	9	(15%)	na	5	760	5	41
Steak Sandwich	540	11	(18%)	na	20	650	11	43

MRS FIELDS COOKIES

See Cookies Section ~ Page 86
(Only Calorie & Fat Estimates Available)

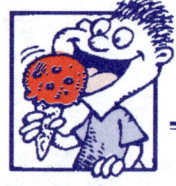

LITTLE CAESARS

	Cal	Fat (%Fc)	S.Fat	Chol	Sod	Pro	Carb
Medium Pizza: Per Slice							
Cheese Pizza! Pizza!	200	7 (31%)	4	17	280	11	24
Pepperoni Pizza! Pizza!	220	9 (37%)	4	17	360	12	24
Cheese Pan! Pan!	180	6 (30%)	3	15	380	9	22
Pepperoni Pan! Pan!	200	8 (36%)	4	15	450	11	22
Baby Pan! Pan!, 1 serving	620	24 (35%)	12	47	1470	33	67
Hot Oven-Baked Mealsa Sandwiches							
Cheeser	820	39 (43%)	20	58	2240	40	75
Mealsa	1040	56 (48%)	24	130	3300	55	75
Pepperoni	900	47 (47%)	23	58	2430	43	74
Supreme	890	46 (47%)	21	70	2370	41	77
Veggie	670	24 (32%)	14	58	1535	33	79
Deli-Style Cold Sandwiches							
Ham & Cheese	730	35 (43%)	13	54	1600	30	71
Italian	740	37 (45%)	12	62	1830	29	71
Veggie	650	29 (40%)	9	29	1195	22	74
Sides							
Crazy Bread	105	3 (26%)	<1	<1	115	3	16
Crazy Sauce	75	0.5 (6%)	0	0	380	5	14
Salads (No Dressing)							
Antipasto Salad	180	12 (60%)	2	19	540	12	7
Caesar Salad	140	5 (32%)	3	11	370	9	14
Greek Salad	170	10 (53%)	<1	37	655	9	12
Tossed Salad	120	3 (25%)	<1	0	170	5	19
Salads Dressings: Per Pkt							
Blue Cheese	160	14 (80%)	2	17	600	0	8
Caesar	255	27 (95%)	4	13	405	0	3
French	165	16 (87%)	2	0	555	0	6
Greek	270	30 (100%)	8	9	200	0	<1
Italian: Regular	200	21 (95%)	3	12	470	0	3
Fat-Free	15	0 (0%)	0	0	420	0	3
Ranch	220	22 (90%)	3	18	340	0	5
1000 Island	185	17 (82%)	3	30	540	0	6

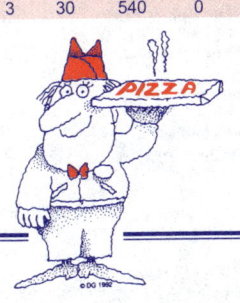

McDONALD'S

	Cal	Fat	(%Fc)	S.Fat	Chol	Sod	Pro	Carb
Sandwiches/Burgers								
Arch Deluxe™	570	31	(49%)	11	90	1110	29	43
with Bacon	610	34	(50%)	12	100	1250	33	43
Big Mac®	530	28	(48%)	10	80	880	25	47
Fish Fillet Deluxe™	510	20	(35%)	4.5	50	1120	24	59
Crispy Chicken Deluxe™	530	26	(44%)	4	60	1140	27	47
Grilled Chicken Deluxe	330	6	(16%)	1	50	970	27	42
Hamburger	270	10	(33%)	3.5	30	530	12	34
Cheeseburger	320	14	(39%)	6	45	770	15	35
Quarter Pounder®	430	2	(44%)	8	70	730	23	37
with Cheese	530	30	(51%)	13	95	1200	28	38
French Fries								
Small, 2.4 oz	210	10	(43%)	1.5	0	135	3	26
Large, 5.2 oz	450	22	(44%)	4	0	290	6	57
Super Size, 6.2 oz	540	26	(43%)	4.5	0	350	8	68
Chicken McNuggets/Sauces								
Chick McNuggets®-4 Pces	190	11	(52%)	2.5	40	340	12	10
6 Pieces	290	17	(53%)	3.5	60	510	18	15
9 Pieces	430	26	(54%)	5	90	770	27	23
Hot Mustard Sauce(1 pkg), 1 oz	60	3.5	(0%)	0	5	240	1	7
Barbeque Sauce(1 pkg), 1 oz	45	0	(0%)	0	0	250	0	10
Sweet 'N' Sour Sce(1 pkg), 1 oz	50	0	(0%)	0	0	140	0	11
Honey(1 pkg), 1/2 oz	45	0	(0%)	0	0	0	0	12
Honey Mustard(1 pkg), 1/2 oz	50	4.5	(81%)	0.5	10	85	0	3
Light Mayonnaise (1 pkg)	40	4	(90%)	0.5	5	85	0	<1
Salads/Salad Dressings								
Grilled Chicken Salad Deluxe	110	1	(8%)	0	45	240	21	5
Garden Salad, 6 1/4 oz	35	0	(0%)	0	0	20	2	7
Croutons(1 pkg)	50	1.5	(27%)	0	0	80	2	7
Ranch(1 pkg), 2 oz	230	21	(82%)	3	20	550	1	10
Caesar (1 pkg), 2 oz	160	14	(79%)	3	20	450	2	7
Fat-Free Herb (1 pkg), 2 oz	50	2	(0%)	0	0	330	0	11
Red French Reduced Cal, 2 oz	160	8	(34%)	1	0	490	0	23
Breakfast Menu								
Biscuit, 2.7 oz	260	13	(45%)	3	0	840	4	32
Egg McMuffin®	290	12	(37%)	4.5	235	710	17	27
Sausage McMuffin®	360	23	(58%)	8	45	740	13	26
with Egg	440	28	(57%)	10	255	810	19	27
English Muffin, 2 oz	140	2	(13%)	0	0	210	4	25
Sausage Biscuit	430	29	(60%)	9	35	1130	10	32
with Egg	510	35	(62%)	10	245	1210	16	33
Bacon, Egg & Cheese Biscuit	440	26	(53%)	8	235	1310	17	33
Sausage, 1 1/2 oz	170	16	(85%)	5	35	290	6	0
Scrambled Eggs (2)	160	11	(62%)	3.5	425	170	13	1

McDONALD'S CONT

	Cal	Fat (%Fc)	S.Fat	Chol	Sod	Pro	Carb
Breakfast (Cont)							
Hash Browns, 2 oz	130	8 (55%)	1.5	0	330	1	14
Hotcakes, Plain, 5.3 oz	310	7 (20%)	1.5	15	610	9	53
w. Marg. 2 pats & Syrup	580	16 (23%)	3	15	760	9	100
Breakfast Burrito	320	20 (56%)	7	195	600	13	23
Muffins/Danish							
Lowfat Apple Bran Muffin, 4 oz	300	3 (9%)	0.5	0	380	6	61
Apple Danish, 3.7 oz	360	16 (40%)	5	40	290	5	51
Cheese Danish, 3.7 oz	410	22 (48%)	8	70	340	7	47
Cinnamon Roll, 3.4 oz	400	20 (45%)	5	75	340	7	47
Raspberry Danish, 3.7 oz	400	16 (36%)	5	45	300	5	58
Desserts; Shakes							
Vanilla Lowfat IcecreamCone	120	0.5 (3%)	0	5	95	4	23
Lowfat Icecream Sundae:							
Strawberry Sundae, 6.3 oz	240	1 (3%)	0.5	5	130	6	51
Hot Caramel Sundae, 6.3 oz	310	3 (8%)	2	5	210	7	62
Hot Fudge Sundae, 6.3 oz	290	5 (16%)	4.5	5	200	8	53
Nuts(Sundae/Topping), 1/4 oz	40	3.5 (79%)	0	0	0	2	2
Baked Apple Pie, 2 3/4 oz	260	13 (45%)	3.5	0	200	3	34
McDonaldland Cookies, 1 pkg	180	5 (25%)	1	0	190	3	32
Choc Chip Cookie, 2 3/4 oz	170	10 (53%)	6	20	120	2	22
Shakes (Lowfat)							
Choc./Vanilla, small, 14 floz	340	5 (13%)	3.5	25	270	12	60
Strawberry, small, 14 floz	340	5 (13%)	3.5	25	200	12	61
Drinks							
1% Lowfat Milk, 8 fl.oz ctn	100	2.5 (23%)	1.5	10	115	8	13
Orange Juice, 6 fl.oz	80	0 (0%)	0	0	20	1	20
Coca-Cola Classic:							
Child, 12 fl.oz	110	0 (0%)	0	0	10	0	29
Small, 16 fl.oz	150	0 (0%)	0	0	15	0	40
Medium, 21 fl.oz	210	0 (0%)	0	0	20	0	58
Large, 32 fl. oz	310	0 (0%)	0	0	30	0	86
Diet Coke: Child, 12 fl.oz	0	0 (0%)	0	0	0	0	0
Small, 16 fl.oz	0	0 (0%)	0	0	30	0	0
Medium, 21 fl.oz	0	0 (0%)	0	0	40	0	0
Large, 32 fl.oz	0	0 (0%)	0	0	60	0	0
Sprite: Child, 12 fl.oz	110	0 (0%)	0	0	40	0	28
Small, 16 fl.oz	150	0 (0%)	0	0	55	0	39
Medium, 21 fl.oz	210	0 (0%)	0	0	80	0	56
Large, 32 fl.oz	310	0 (0%)	0	0	115	0	83
Hi-C Orange Drink:Child, 12 fl.oz	120	0 (0%)	0	0	20	0	32
Small, 16 fl.oz	160	0 (0%)	0	0	30	0	44
Medium, 21 fl.oz	240	0 (0%)	0	0	40	0	64
Large, 32 fl. oz	350	0 (0%)	0	0	60	0	94

NATHAN'S FAMOUS

	Cal	Fat	(%Fc)	S.Fat	Chol	Sod	Pro	Carb
Breaded Chicken Sandwich	510	25	(44%)	4	56	930	23	48
Charbroiled Chicken S'wich	290	6	(19%)	1	53	860	35	24
Cheese Steak Sandwich	485	26	(48%)	10	73	580	26	37
Chicken Platter (2)	1095	66	(54%)	14	212	1420	54	72
4 pieces	1790	109	(55%)	23	425	2370	102	99
Chicken Salad	155	4	(23%)	1	49	345	35	9
Double Burger	670	41	(55%)	18	154	460	44	32
Fillet of Fish Platter	1455	74	(46%)	10	147	1840	60	137
Fillet of Fish S'wich	405	15	(33%)	2	32	715	20	46
Frank Nuggets (7)	360	24	(60%)	6	46	740	9	25
Frankfurter	310	19	(55%)	8	45	820	13	22
French Fries	515	26	(45%)	0	0	60	8	62
Fried Clam Platter	1025	51	(45%)	7	49	1825	23	119
Fried Shrimp Platter	795	34	(38%)	5	83	1435	22	100
Hamburger	435	23	(48%)	10	77	280	25	32
Pastrami Sandwich	325	12	(33%)	4	48	1015	21	34
Super Burger	535	32	(54%)	9	86	525	27	34
Turkey Sandwich	270	2	(7%)	0	27	1460	28	34

OLIVE GARDEN

	Cal	Fat	(%Fc)	S.Fat	Chol	Sod	Pro	Carb
Baked Lasagna	330	18	(49%)	na	na	1030	na	na
Breadstick w. margarine	70	2	(26%)	na	0	365	na	na
no margarine	30	0	(0%)	na	0	365	na	na
Eggplant Parmigiana	220	14	(57%)	na	45	720	na	na
Fettucine Alfredo	790	50	(57%)	na	160	820	na	na
Garden Salad	230	15	(59%)	na	4	560	na	na
Pasta & Fagioli	140	5	(32%)	na	15	470	na	na
Salad Dressing, 1 Tbsp	60	7	(100%)	na	2	230	na	na
Spaghetti w. Marinara Sce	315	8	(23%)	na	tr	768	na	na
Spaghetti w. Tomato Sce	400	9	(20%)	na	75	1196	na	na
Veal Marsala	330	29	(79%)	na	100	460	na	na
Veal Parmigiana	590	40	(61%)	na	150	1120	na	na
Veal Piccata	230	16	(63%)	na	45	150	na	na
Venetian Grilled Chicken	320	12	(34%)	na	140	500	na	na

PAPA JOHN'S PIZZA

	Cal	Fat	(%Fc)	S.Fat	Chol	Sod	Pro	Carb
14" Pizza: Per Slice: Cheese	290	9	(28%)	3	18	540	14	37
Garden	300	11	(33%)	4	20	570	14	36
Meats	410	18	(40%)	7	35	1040	21	42
Pepperoni	310	13	(38%)	5	25	570	15	35
Works	370	17	(41%)	6	29	840	18	37
Side Items: Breadstick, 1 stick	170	3	(16%)	0	0	270	6	27
Cheese BreadSticks, (2)	160	6	(34%)	2	10	290	7	20
Garlic Sauce	75	9	(100%)	2	0	115	0	2

PERKINS

	Cal	Fat (%Fc)	S.Fat	Chol	Sod	Pro	Carb
Entrees: Chicken Dinner	620	13 (18%)	na	136	1360	60	60
Fish Dinner	470	7 (13%)	na	133	1390	33	60
Fruit Cup	50	0.5 (6%)	na	0	10	1	12
'Lite & Healthy'	105	2 (18%)	na	0	495	3.5	15
Omelette: Country Club	930	79 (76%)	na	1154	1135	47	6
Deli Ham & Cheese	960	79 (74%)	na	864	1830	53	8
'Denver' w/Fruit Cup	235	6.5 (25%)	na	154	795	23	22
'Everything'	695	54 (69%)	na	814	870	45	9
Granny's Country	940	82 (78%)	na	810	785	43	7
w. 9oz Hash Browns	1245	90 (64%)	na	810	870	48	57
Ham & Cheese	645	51 (72%)	na	743	830	41	2.5
Mushroom & Cheese	685	60 (78%)	na	744	925	32	5
Seafood, w. Fruit Cup	270	5.5 (19%)	na	197	595	29	28
Hash Browns, 3oz	100	2.5 (23%)	na	na	30	1.5	17
Pita Stir-fry:	310	9 (27%)	na	26	750	44	41
w. Coleslaw	440	18 (36%)	na	36	880	45	54
& Pasta Salad	625	33 (47%)	na	37	1395	49	63
w. Pasta Salad	490	24 (44%)	na	27	1270	48	50
Salads: Chef's, Mini	215	11 (46%)	na	55	645	23	7
Muffins: Apple	545	24 (40%)	na	95	730	9	76
Banana Nut	585	29 (45%)	na	92	700	9	75
Blueberry	505	23 (41%)	na	88	670	7	71
Bran	475	17 (32%)	na	0	570	9	83
Carrot	560	23 (37%)	na	81	780	7	88
Choc Choc Chip	545	26 (43%)	na	83	630	10	73
Corn	680	17 (22%)	na	33	1550	12	121
Cranberry Nut	560	28 (45%)	na	88	670	9	71
Oat Bran:	515	16 (28%)	na	0	590	10	87
Plain	585	26 (40%)	na	104	795	9	81
98% fat-free	495	1 (2%)	na	5	800	12	111
Pancakes: Buttermilk, (3)	440	12 (24%)	na	24	990	13	70
Harvest Grain:							
w. Low-Cal Syrup (5)	475	3.5 (6%)	na	0	1640	11	93
Short Stack(3)	270	2 (7%)	na	0	1020	7	56
Syrup, low cal: 1.5 oz	25	0 (0%)	na	na	0	0	7
Pies: Per Slice: Apple Pie	520	26 (45%)	na	0	460	3	72
made w. Equal	420	24 (51%)	na	0	370	3	55
Cherry Pie	570	26 (41%)	na	0	700	4	84
made w. Equal	425	24 (51%)	na	0	510	4	55
Coconut Cream Pie	440	33 (68%)	na	5	490	6	56
French Silk Pie	550	37 (60%)	na	53	480	4	59
Lemon Meringue Pie	395	16 (36%)	na	0	530	2	63
Peanut Butter Brownie	455	35 (69%)	na	29	435	9	44
Pecan Pie	670	26 (35%)	na	17	670	7	106

PETER PIPER PIZZA

Per Slice	Cal	Fat	(%Fc)	S.Fat	Chol	Sod	Pro	Carb
Bacon: 1/8 large	330	12	(33%)	na	27	440	17	39
1/8 medium	250	9	(32%)	na	20	330	13	29
1/4 Express Lunch	180	7	(35%)	na	16	240	10	21
Beef: 1/8 large	295	8	(24%)	na	20	480	16	39
1/8 medium	220	6	(25%)	na	15	360	12	29
1/4 Express Lunch	165	5	(27%)	na	13	260	9	21
Black Olive: 1/8 large	280	7	(22%)	na	18	480	14	40
1/8 medium	210	5	(21%)	na	13	360	11	30
1/4 Express Lunch	160	4	(22%)	na	12	260	8	21
Cheese: 1/8 large	270	6	(20%)	na	18	270	14	39
1/8 medium	200	5	(22%)	na	13	200	11	29
1/4 Express Lunch	150	4	(24%)	na	12	150	8	21
Extra Cheddar: 1/8 large	300	9	(27%)	na	27	330	16	39
1/8 medium	225	7	(28%)	na	19	235	12	29
1/4 Express Lunch	180	6	(30%)	na	19	195	10	21
Extra Mozzarella: 1/8 lge	320	10	(28%)	na	31	350	18	39
1/8 medium	235	7	(27%)	na	22	250	13	29
1/4 Express Lunch	175	6	(31%)	na	18	185	10	21
Green Pepper: 1/8 large	270	6	(20%)	na	18	270	14	39
1/8 medium	205	5	(22%)	na	13	200	11	30
1/4 Express Lunch	155	4	(23%)	na	12	150	8	21
Ham: 1/8 large	275	6	(20%)	na	21	330	15	39
1/8 medium	210	5	(21%)	na	15	245	11	29
1/4 Express Lunch	155	4	(23%)	na	14	190	9	21
Jalapeno: 1/8 large	270	6	(20%)	na	18	335	14	39
1/8 medium	205	5	(22%)	na	13	245	10	30
1/4 Express Lunch	150	4	(24%)	na	12	200	8	21
Mushroom: 1/8 large	205	5	(22%)	na	13	200	11	30
1/8 medium	180	4	(20%)	na	12	180	9	26
1/4 Express Lunch	155	4	(23%)	na	12	150	8	21
Onion: 1/8 large	270	6	(20%)	na	18	270	14	39
1/8 medium	205	5	(22%)	na	13	200	10	30
1/4 Express Lunch	155	4	(23%)	na	12	150	8	21
Pepperoni: 1/8 large	310	9	(26%)	na	24	555	15	39
1/8 medium	230	7	(26%)	na	18	430	12	29
1/4 Express Lunch	170	6	(32%)	na	15	290	9	21
Pineapple; Tomato: 1/8 large	275	6	(20%)	na	18	270	14	40
1/8 medium	205	5	(22%)	na	13	200	10	30
1/4 Express Lunch	155	4	(23%)	na	12	150	8	22
Salami: 1/8 large	290	8	(25%)	na	23	340	15	39
1/8 medium	215	6	(25%)	na	17	255	11	29
1/4 Express Lunch	165	6	(27%)	na	15	200	9	21
Sausage: 1/8 large	300	8	(24%)	na	21	520	16	39
1/8 medium	225	6	(24%)	na	15	375	12	29
1/4 Express Lunch	180	6	(30%)	na	14	360	10	21

PIZZA HUT

	Cal	Fat	(%Fc)	S.Fat	Chol	Sod	Pro	Carb
Medium Size Pizza: Per Slice								
Stuffed Crust: Cheese	420	15	(32%)	7	47	1080	22	48
Beef Topping	440	16	(33%)	7	45	1345	24	49
Ham	400	13	(29%)	6	40	1130	21	48
Pepperoni	420	16	(34%)	7	44	1180	22	48
Italian Sausage	460	19	(37%)	8	54	1240	23	48
Pork Topping	455	19	(38%)	8	47	1270	23	49
Meat Lover's	500	22	(40%)	9	60	1485	26	49
Veggie Lover's	400	13	(29%)	6	35	1090	20	50
Pepperoni Lover's	490	21	(39%)	10	64	1410	26	49
Supreme	470	19	(36%)	8	50	1405	25	50
Super Supreme	460	18	(35%)	8	49	1435	24	50
Stuffed Crust with Pepperoni								
Cheese	455	18	(36%)	8	56	1255	24	49
Beef Topping	475	20	(38%)	9	54	1520	26	49
Ham	430	17	(36%)	7	49	1300	23	48
Pepperoni	460	20	(39%)	8	53	1355	23	48
Italian Sausage	495	23	(42%)	9	63	1415	25	49
Pork Topping	495	22	(40%)	9	56	1445	25	49
Meat Lover's	540	26	(43%)	11	69	1655	28	49
Veggie Lover's	435	17	(35%)	7	44	1260	22	50
Pepperoni Lover's	530	25	(42%)	11	73	1585	27	49
Supreme	505	23	(41%)	9	59	1580	26	50
Super Supreme	500	22	(40%)	9	58	1610	26	50
Thin 'n Crispy: Cheese	200	8	(36%)	4	35	570	11	21
Beef Topping	220	9	(37%)	4	33	835	12	21
Ham	175	6	(31%)	3	28	620	10	21
Pepperoni	205	9	(40%)	4	32	670	10	21
Italian Sausage	240	12	(45%)	5	42	730	12	21
Pork Topping	240	11	(41%)	5	35	760	12	21
Meat Lover's	285	15	(47%)	6	48	970	15	21
Veggie Lover's	180	6	(30%)	3	23	580	9	23
Pepperoni Lover's	270	14	(47%)	7	52	900	14	22
Supreme	250	12	(43%)	5	38	895	13	22
Super Supreme	240	11	(41%)	5	37	925	13	22
Hand Tossed: Cheese	230	7	(27%)	4	35	650	13	28
Beef	250	9	(32%)	4	33	920	15	28
Ham	205	5	(22%)	3	28	700	12	27
Pepperoni	235	8	(31%)	4	32	755	13	28
Italian Sausage	270	11	(37%)	5	42	815	14	28
Pork Topping	270	11	(37%)	5	35	845	14	28
Meat Lover's	315	14	(40%)	6	48	1060	17	28
Veggie Lover's	210	5	(20%)	3	23	660	11	30
Pepperoni Lover's	300	13	(39%)	7	52	990	17	29
Supreme	280	11	(35%)	5	38	980	16	29
Super Supreme	270	10	(33%)	5	37	1010	15	29

PIZZA HUT CONT

	Cal	Fat (%Fc)	S.Fat	Chol	Sod	Pro	Carb
Pan Pizza: Cheese	240	8 (30%)	4	35	540	13	28
Beef	260	10 (35%)	5	33	805	14	29
Ham	220	7 (29%)	3	28	590	12	28
Pepperoni	245	10 (37%)	4	32	640	12	28
Italian Sausage	280	13 (42%)	5	42	700	13	28
Pork Topping	280	12 (39%)	5	35	730	14	29
Meat Lover's	325	16 (44%)	7	48	945	16	29
Pepperoni Lover's	310	15 (44%)	7	52	870	16	29
Veggie Lover's	220	7 (29%)	3	23	550	10	30
Supreme	290	13 (40%)	5	38	865	15	29
Super Supreme	280	12 (39%)	5	37	895	15	30
Personal Pan Pizza							
Pepperoni	585	22 (34%)	10	73	1480	28	69
Supreme	675	28 (37%)	12	85	1935	34	73
Entrees/Sandwiches							
Cavatini Pizza	550	16 (26%)	6	40	1460	22	79
Cavatini Supreme Pizza	590	19 (29%)	7	48	1650	24	81
Spaghetti w.Meatless Sauce	560	6 (10%)	<1	5	1285	18	107
Spaghetti w.Meat Sauce	630	14 (20%)	4	26	1370	23	103
Ham & Cheese Sandwich	445	24 (48%)	9	80	1960	31	27
Supreme Sandwich	520	32 (55%)	12	87	2260	32	27
Sides: Buffalo Wings, (12)	565	35 (56%)	9	150	2350	61	2
Wings Dip 'n Blue Cheese	220	24 (98%)	4	40	440	2	2
Wings Dip 'n Ranch	260	29 (100%)	4	5	380	0	1
Breadsticks (5)	770	25 (29%)	5	6	1085	22	114
Breadsticks Dipping Sce, 3 oz	70	2 (26%)	<1	2	550	2	11
Garlic Dipping Sauce	150	17 (100%)	3	0	220	0	0

PIZZERIA UNO

	Cal	Fat (%Fc)	S.Fat	Chol	Sod	Pro	Carb
Thin Crust Pizza: 9" individual							
Vegetarian: w. Cheese	850	22 (23%)	12	55	1660	46	127
No Cheese	620	5 (7%)	1	0	1100	20	124
Soup: Tomato Garden Veg.	125	1 (7%)	0	0	900	2.5	25
Light Lunch w. Soup	745	6 (7%)	1	0	2000	23	150
Entrees: Veggie Burger Meal	610	15 (22%)	1	0	1800	15	104
Tomato Basil Chicken	570	8 (13%)	1.5	55	1280	42	83
Zesty Pasta Marinara	380	3.5 (8%)	0.5	0	800	13	75
Salads: Special House	90	1 (10%)	0	0	860	4	17
Light Lunch w. Salad	710	6 (7%)	1	0	1960	24	141
Pasta Green Salad	410	9 (13%)	1	0	700	14	69
Veggie Dip Platter	460	11 (22%)	2	0	770	14	77

POPEYE'S

	Cal	Fat	(%Fc)	S.Fat	Chol	Sod	Pro	Carb
Apple Pie	290	16	(50%)	na	10	820	3	37
Biscuit	250	15	(54%)	na	3	430	4	26
Cajun Rice, 4 oz	150	5	(30%)	na	25	1260	10	17
Chicken Breast: Mild, Fried	270	16	(53%)	na	60	660	23	9
Spicy, Fried	270	16	(53%)	na	60	590	23	9
Chicken Leg: Mild/Spicy, Fried	120	7	(52%)	na	40	240	10	4
Chicken Thigh: Mild, Fried	300	23	(69%)	na	70	620	15	9
Spicy, Fried	300	23	(69%)	na	70	450	15	9
Chicken Wing: Mild/Spicy	160	11	(62%)	na	40	290	9	7
Coleslaw, 4 oz	150	11	(66%)	na	3	270	1	14
Corn on the Cob	130	3	(21%)	na	0	20	4	21
French Fries, 3 oz	240	12	(45%)	na	10	610	3.5	31
Nuggets, 1 serving	410	32	(70%)	na	55	660	17	18
Onion Rings, 3 oz	310	19	(55%)	na	25	210	5	31
Potatoes & Gravy	100	6	(54%)	na	3	460	5	11
Red Beans & Rice, 6 oz	270	17	(57%)	na	10	680	8	30
Shrimp	250	16	(58%)	na	110	650	15	13

QUINCY'S STEAKHOUSE

	Cal	Fat	(%Fc)	S.Fat	Chol	Sod	Pro	Carb
Breakfast: Per Serving								
Escalloped Apples	120	2	(15%)	0	0	20	0	26
Bacon	35	3	(77%)	1	5	100	2	0
Corned Beef Hash	210	15	(64%)	8	45	795	10	11
Scrambled Eggs	95	7	(66%)	2	215	270	7	1
Country Ham	90	6	(60%)	2	35	1100	9	1
Oatmeal	175	2	(10%)	0	0	285	4	18
Pancakes	95	3	(28%)	1	30	250	3	12
Syrup	75	0	(0%)	0	0	15	0	20
Sausage Gravy	70	6	(77%)	2	10	150	2	3
Sausage Links	225	22	(88%)	8	20	390	7	0
Sausage Patties	230	23	(90%)	9	45	350	7	0
Steak Fingers	360	25	(62%)	11	50	690	16	18
Soup: Chili with Beans	235	11	(42%)	2	15	920	13	21
Clam Chowder	180	9	(45%)	1	0	835	3	21
Cream of Broccoli	170	10	(53%)	1	0	770	2	18
Vegetable Beef	90	2	(20%)	1	0	325	5	14
Steaks: Chopped, 8 oz	500	42	(76%)	20	89	350	31	0
Country Style Steak w. Gravy	530	25	(42%)	7	54	1160	32	44
Cowboy Steak, 14 oz	580	33	(51%)	15	176	1310	61	9
Filet w. Bacon	340	17	(45%)	7	125	310	48	2
N.Y.Strip Steak, 10 oz	450	26	(52%)	13	148	155	53	1
Porterhouse Steak	680	46	(61%)	23	154	345	67	0
Ribeye, 10 oz	450	29	(58%)	13	116	155	48	0
Sirloin: Large	370	20	(49%)	9	119	390	46	2
Regular	285	16	(50%)	7	71	320	34	0

QUINCY'S STEAKHOUSE

	Cal	Fat (%Fc)	S.Fat	Chol	Sod	Pro	Carb
Steaks (Cont)							
Sirloin Junior	195	10 (46%)	5	69	200	25	0
Sirloin Tips	205	8 (35%)	3	63	790	27	4
Smothered Strip Steak	620	41 (59%)	16	148	240	55	12
T-Bone, 13 oz	520	35 (60%)	18	118	265	51	0
Entrees							
Grilled Chicken, regular	125	2 (14%)	0.5	55	540	25	1
Homestyle Chicken Filet	220	9 (37%)	2	25	680	13	21
Grilled Salmon	230	4 (16%)	1	109	110	46	1
Sth Breaded Shrimp	545	31 (51%)	6	135	820	19	47
Steak & Shrimp	680	39 (52%)	12	170	820	48	33
Roasted Herb Chicken	875	65 (67%)	17	340	1240	70	4
Roasted BBQ Chicken	940	65 (62%)	17	340	1550	70	21
Grilled Trout	300	12 (36%)	3	115	520	41	2
Sandwiches: no Mayo/Extras							
Bacon Cheeseburger	665	41 (55%)	17	87	1000	37	33
Grilled Chicken Sandwich	325	4 (11%)	1	55	1185	33	39
Philly Cheese Steak	590	30 (46%)	11	87	1685	37	38
Smothered Steak	430	15 (31%)	6	69	850	34	36
Spicy BBQ Chicken	370	5 (12%)	1	55	1610	34	45
Breads: Banana Nut	165	7 (38%)	1	5	195	2	22
Biscuit	270	15 (50%)	4	11	610	5	29
Cornbread	140	5 (32%)	1	0	340	3	19
Yeast Roll	160	4 (23%)	<1	0	285	1	29
Sides: Baked Potatoes	370	0 (0%)	0	0	25	8	86
Corn on the Cob	140	1 (6%)	0	0	540	5	33
Rice Pilaf	105	2 (17%)	0	0	270	2	20
Salad Dressings: Bleu Cheese	155	16 (93%)	3	10	165	2	2
French:	125	12 (86%)	1	0	500	0	4
Light	85	4 (42%)	0	0	285	2	13
Honey Mustard	100	6 (54%)	1	0	220	2	10
Italian:	135	14 (93%)	2	0	230	0	3
Light	20	2 (90%)	0	0	485	2	2
Light Creamy Italian	65	4 (55%)	0	0	485	2	8
Light Thousand Island	65	4 (55%)	0	20	340	2	8
Parmesan Peppercorn	150	14 (84%)	0	0	280	1	4
Ranch	110	11 (90%)	2	10	195	1	1
Desserts: Banana Pudding	240	12 (45%)	9	10	240	3	30
Brownie Pudding Cake	310	5 (15%)	<1	0	395	4	66
Chocolate Chip Cookie	60	3 (45%)	1	5	35	1	8
Apple Cobbler	255	8 (28%)	2	5	285	1	49
Cherry Cobbler	410	8 (18%)	2	5	185	1	55
Peach Cobbler	305	8 (24%)	1	5	190	1	50
Frozen Yogurt	135	2 (13%)	1	5	85	5	25
Sugar Cookie	60	3 (45%)	1	5	30	<1	8
Toppings: Caramel	105	1 (8%)	<1	0	120	0	24
Fudge	105	4 (34%)	1	0	75	1	15
Pineapple	70	0 (0%)	0	0	20	0	20

RALLY'S

	Cal	Fat (%Fc)	S.Fat	Chol	Sod	Pro	Carb
Specialities							
Rallyburger	435	22 (46%)	na	63	1175	20	35
with Cheese	490	27 (50%)	na	78	1375	23	35
Big Bufford	745	46 (56%)	na	151	1860	41	35
Chicken Fillet Sandwich	400	15 (34%)	na	42	790	21	43
Chili w.Cheese & Onion, 7 oz	360	22 (55%)	na	74	1140	23	20
13 oz	670	41 (55%)	na	137	2125	43	37
Super Barbecue Bacon	595	31 (47%)	na	88	1710	29	49
Super Double Cheeseburger	760	48 (57%)	na	154	1735	41	37
French Fries, Regular	210	11 (47%)	na	7	295	3	26
Large	320	16 (45%)	na	10	440	5	39
X-Large	425	21 (44%)	na	13	585	7	52
Shakes							
Vanilla, small	320	11 (31%)	na	38	200	9	49
Other flavors, small	410	12 (26%)	na	38	260	10	73

RAX

(na) ~ Data not available

	Cal	Fat (%Fc)	S.Fat	Chol	Sod	Pro	Carb
Sandwiches							
Regular Rax	340	22 (59%)	na	54	710	16	31
Deluxe	520	35 (60%)	na	69	785	18	34
BBC (Beef Bacon & Cheddar)	715	51 (64%)	na	102	1455	28	36
Grilled Chicken	525	33 (56%)	na	69	995	24	32
Jr. Deluxe	370	25 (61%)	na	42	510	11	25
Barbeque Beef	400	20 (45%)	na	40	1030	13	43
Mushroom Melt	600	37 (56%)	na	104	1690	30	35
Turkey Bacon Club	680	46 (61%)	na	76	1900	29	37
Turkey	485	32 (60%)	na	50	1285	17	32
Cheddar Melt	345	23 (60%)	na	41	540	10	26
Philly Melt	540	32 (54%)	na	78	1295	28	35
Potatoes							
Plain	210	0 (0%)	0	0	10	0	50
Cheese/Broccoli	280	6 (19%)	na	4	620	7	50
Cheese	270	6 (20%)	na	4	620	7	47
Cheese/Bacon	400	19 (51%)	14	82	875	7	50
Butter	305	11 (32%)	9	0	30	0	50
Sour Cream Topping	260	4 (14%)	3	0	30	4	50
Soups							
Cream of Broccoli	170	10 (53%)	1	0	770	2	18
Chili w. Beans	235	11 (42%)	2	15	920	13	21
Salads							
Grilled Chicken Caesar	160	5 (28%)	3	50	1150	23	6
Caesar Side Salad	40	2 (45%)	1	5	330	2	3
Side Salad	40	4 (90%)	1	0	90	0	2
Gourmet Garden	220	9 (37%)	3	5	840	23	12

RED LOBSTER

	Cal	Fat	(%Fc)	S.Fat	Chol	Sod	Pro	Carb
Fish: Per Lunch Portion (5oz raw wt.)								
(For **Dinner Portion** of 10 oz, double the figures.)								
Prepared with No Added Fat								
Add extra for butter sauce. (1 tsp = 30 cals; 3g fat (90%); 30mg sodium)								
Catfish	170	10	(53%)	3	85	50	20	0
Cod (Atlantic)	100	1	(9%)	0	70	200	23	0
Flounder	100	1	(9%)	0	70	95	21	1
Grouper	110	1	(8%)	0	65	70	26	0
Haddock	110	1	(8%)	0	85	180	24	2
Halibut	110	1	(8%)	0	60	105	25	1
Lemon Sole	120	1	(7%)	0	65	90	27	1
Mackerel	190	12	(57%)	4	100	250	20	1
Monkfish	110	1	(8%)	0	80	95	24	0
Norwegian Salmon	230	12	(47%)	3	80	60	27	3
Ocean Perch (Atlantic)	130	4	(28%)	1	75	190	24	1
Pollock	120	1	(7%)	0	90	90	28	1
Rainbow Trout	170	9	(48%)	3	90	90	23	0
Red Rockfish	90	1	(10%)	0	85	95	21	0
Red Snapper	110	1	(8%)	0	70	140	25	0
Sockeye Salmon	160	4	(22%)	1	50	60	28	3
Swordfish	100	4	(36%)	1	100	140	17	0
Tilefish	100	2	(18%)	1	80	60	20	0
Yellowfin Tuna	180	6	(30%)	2	70	70	32	0
Shellfish								
King Crab Legs 16 oz	170	2	(11%)	0	100	900	32	6
Snow Crab Legs, 16 oz	150	2	(12%)	1	130	1630	33	1
Calamari, breaded, fried, 5 oz	360	21	(52%)	6	140	1150	13	30
Langostino, 5 oz	120	1	(8%)	0	210	410	26	2
Maine Lobster, 18 oz	240	8	(30%)	2	310	550	36	5
Rock Lobster, 1 tail, 13 oz	230	3	(12%)	1	200	1090	49	2
Calico Scallops, 5 oz	180	2	(10%)	0	115	260	32	8
Deep Sea Scallops, 5 oz	130	2	(14%)	0	50	260	26	2
Shrimp, 8-12 pcs., 7 oz	120	2	(15%)	0	230	110	25	0
Steaks/Chicken								
Sirloin, 8 oz	350	15	(39%)	na	150	110	51	0
Strip Steak, 7 oz	690	64	(83%)	na	140	70	29	0
Hamburger, 1/3 lb	320	23	(65%)	na	105	70	27	0
Filet Mignon, 8 oz	350	16	(41%)	na	140	105	47	0
Rib Eye Steak, 12 oz	980	82	(75%)	na	220	150	56	0
Skinless Chicken Breast, 4 oz	140	3	(19%)	na	70	60	26	0

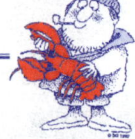

ROUND TABLE PIZZA

	Cal	Fat (%Fc)	S.Fat	Chol	Sod	Pro	Carb
Per Slice: Large (Thin = 1/16 whole. Pan = 1/12 whole)							
Alfredo Contempo: Thin	170	6.5 (34%)	4	25	210	9	17
Pan	220	7.5 (31%)	4	25	240	12	27
Bacon Super Deli: Thin	200	13 (58%)	5	25	360	9	16
Pan	260	14 (48%)	5	25	380	12	26
Cheese: Thin	160	6 (34%)	4	20	240	7	16
Pan	210	7 (30%)	5	20	250	10	26
Chicken & Garlic Gourmet:							
Thin	170	7 (37%)	4	25	280	9	17
Pan	230	8 (31%)	4	25	310	11	27
Classic Pesto: Thin	170	8 (42%)	4	15	210	7	18
Pan	230	9 (35%)	4	15	240	9	27
Garden Pesto: Thin	170	8 (42%)	4	15	200	7	18
Pan	230	8.5 (33%)	4	15	230	9	28
Gourmet Veggie: Thin	160	6.5 (37%)	3	15	200	7	18
Pan	220	7.5 (31%)	4	20	230	9	28
Guinevere's Garden Delight:							
Thin	150	5.5 (33%)	3	15	250	7	18
Pan	200	6 (27%)	4	15	250	9	27
Italian Garlic Supreme:							
Thin	200	10 (47%)	4	25	220	8	17
Pan	250	11 (40%)	4	25	240	10	27
King Arthur's Supreme:							
Thin	200	10 (45%)	3	25	340	9	18
Pan	240	9 (33%)	4	25	320	10	27
Pepperoni: Thin	170	8 (42%)	3	20	240	8	17
Pan	220	8 (33%)	4	20	240	9	26
Salute Chicken & Garlic:							
Thin	150	5.5 (33%)	3	20	250	8	18
Pan	200	6 (27%)	3	20	270	9	28
Salute Veggie: Thin	140	5 (32%)	2	10	170	6	19
Pan	190	5 (24%)	3	10	190	8	28
Western BBQ Chicken Supreme:							
Thin	170	5.5 (29%)	4	25	330	8	17
Pan	220	6.5 (27%)	4	30	360	11	27
Zesty Santa Fe Chicken:							
Thin	180	8 (40%)	4	25	310	9	17
Pan	240	9 (34%)	5	30	360	11	27
Sandwiches							
Chicken Club	800	38 (43%)	14	115	1510	39	72
Ham & Honey Mustard	760	33 (39%)	13	95	1630	36	76
Turkey Pesto	830	40 (43%)	14	85	1200	42	71
Turkey Santa Fe	840	44 (47%)	16	95	1360	39	72
Vegetarian	670	29 (39%)	10	55	990	25	75

ROY ROGERS

	Cal	Fat (%Fc)	S.Fat	Chol	Sod	Pro	Carb
Breakfast Items: Biscuit	390	21 (48%)	6	0	1000	6	44
Cinnamon 'N' Raisin Biscuit	370	18 (44%)	5	0	450	3	48
Sausage Biscuit	510	31 (55%)	10	25	1360	14	44
Sausage & Egg Biscuit	560	35 (56%)	11	170	1400	18	44
Bacon Biscuit	420	23 (49%)	7	5	1140	9	44
Bacon & Egg Biscuit	470	26 (50%)	8	150	1190	14	44
Ham & Egg Biscuit	460	23 (45%)	7	165	1395	14	48
Ham & Cheese Biscuit	450	24 (48%)	8	25	1570	11	48
Ham, Egg & Cheese Biscuit	500	27 (49%)	10	170	1620	16	48
Sourdough Ham, Egg & Cheese	480	24 (45%)	9	185	1440	20	45
Big Country Breakfast Platter							
with Bacon	740	43 (52%)	13	305	1800	25	61
with Sausage	920	60 (59%)	19	340	2230	33	61
with Ham	710	39 (49%)	11	330	2210	24	67
3 Pancakes	280	2 (6%)	1	15	890	8	56
with 1 Sausage	430	16 (33%)	6	40	1290	16	56
with 2 Bacon	350	9 (23%)	3	25	1130	13	56
Plain Bagel	300	2 (6%)	0.5	0	520	10	60
Cinnamon Raisin Bagel	300	1 (3%)	0.5	0	490	10	63
Hashrounds	230	14 (55%)	3	0	560	3	24
Burgers, Sandwiches							
Hamburger	260	9 (31%)	4	20	460	11	33
Cheeseburger	300	13 (39%)	7	25	690	13	34
1/4 lb Hamburger	430	18 (38%)	8	25	450	25	41
1/4 lb Cheeseburger	470	22 (42%)	10	30	680	27	42
Sourdough Bacon Chseburger	730	46 (57%)	18	65	1470	35	43
Sourdough Grilled Chicken	500	21 (38%)	6	45	1530	30	46
Bacon Cheeseburger	490	28 (51%)	13	35	800	30	29
Sandwiches: Roast Beef	260	4 (14%)	1	60	700	24	30
Chicken Fillet	500	24 (43%)	5	20	1050	19	49
Grilled Chicken	340	11 (29%)	2	30	910	25	32
Fisherman's Fillet (seasonal)	490	21 (39%)	5	15	1040	21	56
Chicken: Fried: Breast	370	15 (36%)	4	75	1190	29	29
Wing	200	8 (36%)	2	30	740	10	23
Thigh	330	15 (41%)	4	60	1000	19	30
Leg	170	7 (37%)	2	45	570	13	15
1/4 Roy's Roaster: White Meat	500	29 (52%)	9	240	1450	56	3
No Skin	190	6 (28%)	2	100	700	32	2
Dark Meat	490	34 (62%)	10	225	1120	43	2
No Skin	190	10 (47%)	3	110	400	24	1
Nuggets: 6 piece	290	18 (56%)	4	15	610	12	20
9 piece	460	29 (57%)	6	25	970	20	32
Salads: Grilled Chicken	120	4 (30%)	1	60	520	18	2
Garden	190	14 (66%)	9	40	280	12	3
Fries: Regular	350	15 (39%)	4	0	150	5	49
Large	430	18 (38%)	5	0	190	6	59

Continued Next Page

ROY ROGERS CONT

	Cal	Fat	(%Fc)	S.Fat	Chol	Sod	Pro	Carb
Baked Potato	130	1	(7%)	0	0	65	3	27
w. Margarine	240	13	(49%)	2	0	220	3	27
w. Margarine & Sour Cream	300	19	(57%)	6	15	230	4	28
Mashed Potatoes, 5 oz	95	0.3	(2%)	0	0	320	2	20
Gravy, 1.5 oz	20	0.5	(22%)	0	0	260	0.2	3
Baked Beans, 5 oz	160	2	(11%)	1	10	560	6	30
Cornbread	310	17	(49%)	3	30	260	4	35
Coleslaw, 5 oz	295	25	(78%)	4	15	430	2	16
Desserts								
Vanilla Frozen Yogurt Cone	180	4	(20%)	3	15	80	5	29
Sundae: Hot Fudge	320	10	(28%)	5	25	260	8	50
Strawberry	260	6	(21%)	3	15	95	6	44
Strawberry Shortcake	480	21	(39%)	5	40	330	8	39

SHAKEY'S

	Cal	Fat	(%Fc)	S.Fat	Chol	Sod	Pro	Carb
Pizzas (12"):1 Slice (1/10 Pizza)								
Cheese only: Thin Crust	135	5	(33%)	na	15	320	8	13
Thick Crust	170	5	(26%)	na	15	420	7	22
Homestyle Pan	305	14	(41%)	na	20	590	14	31
Onion/Olives/Mushrooms:								
Thin Crust	125	5	(36%)	na	10	315	7	14
Thick Crust	160	4	(22%)	na	15	420	9	22
Homestyle Pan	320	15	(42%)	na	20	650	15	32
Sausage Pepperoni: Thin Crust	165	8	(44%)	na	15	395	9	13
Thick Crust	205	8	(35%)	na	20	425	11	22
Homestyle Pan	375	20	(48%)	na	25	680	17	31
Sausage Mushroom:								
Thin Crust	140	6	(39%)	na	15	335	8	13
Thick Crust	180	6	(30%)	na	15	420	10	22
Homestyle Pan	340	17	(45%)	na	25	680	16	31
Pepperoni: Thin Crust	150	7	(42%)	na	15	400	8	13
Thick Crust	185	6	(29%)	na	15	420	10	22
Homestyle Pan	345	15	(39%)	na	25	740	16	31
Shakey's Special:								
Thin Crust	170	9	(48%)	na	15	475	13	13
Thick Crust	210	8	(34%)	na	20	420	13	22
Homestyle Pan	385	21	(49%)	na	30	880	18	32
Other Items								
Spagh. w.Meat Sce/Garlic Brd.	940	33	(32%)	na	na	1900	26	134
Potato Wedges, 15 pieces	950	36	(34%)	na	na	3700	17	120
Shakey's Super Hot Hero	810	44	(49%)	na	na	2690	36	67
Hot Ham & Cheese S/wich	550	21	(34%)	na	na	2135	36	56
5-Piece Fried Chicken & Pot.	1700	90	(48%)	na	na	5330	97	130
3-Piece Chicken & Pot.	945	56	(53%)	na	na	2290	57	51

7-ELEVEN

	Cal	Fat (%Fc)	S.Fat	Chol	Sod	Pro	Carb
Microwave Sandwiches							
Oscar Mayer:							
Big Bite w. Bun	300	19 (57%)	8	30	800	10	22
1/4 Pound Big Bite	480	36 (66%)	15	60	1370	16	23
Mesquite Jalapeno Bite	380	26 (60%)	10	0	1100	15	23
Spicy Bite	380	25 (60%)	10	55	1140	16	22
Croissants							
Egg, Cheese & Bacon	410	28 (60%)	10	155	880	16	26
Egg, Ham & Cheese	350	22 (57%)	7	155	950	17	25
English Muffin with							
Egg/Cheese/Canad.Bacon	270	25 (85%)	7	240	940	18	21
Biscuit: Saus./Egg/Cheese	560	41 (66%)	14	170	1330	16	36
Burritos							
Ramona: Beef & Bean	290	9 (27%)	4	76	290	16	37
Potato & Beef	340	14 (37%)	6	33	280	13	41
Bean & Cheese	340	13 (34%)	6	34	300	15	41
Reynoldos Jumbo Burritos:							
Beef & Bean	630	20 (28%)	5	10	1470	25	88
Beef & Potato	550	16 (26%)	5	15	1650	19	82
Bean & Cheese	680	25 (33%)	10	22	1335	25	88
Red Hot	600	20 (30%)	5	15	1810	22	82
Green	640	22 (31%)	7	22	1680	23	85
Chimichanga							
Don Miguel: Chicken	270	8 (27%)	1.5	20	580	11	37
Shredded Beef	260	9 (31%)	2	20	610	11	35
Hot & Spicy Beef	280	9 (29%)	2	15	580	10	39
Fountain Drinks							
(Figures Assume 1/4 Ice)							
Coca-Cola/Pepsi/Dr.Pepper/7Up:							
Gulp, 16 oz	150	0 (0%)	0	0	15	0	38
Big Gulp, 32 oz	300	0 (0%)	0	0	30	0	75
Super Gulp, 44 oz	410	0 (0%)	0	0	40	0	102
Double Gulp, 64 oz	600	0 (0%)	0	0	60	0	150
Diet Coke/Diet Pepsi:							
(Negligible Calories/Fat)							
Slurpees							
Average All Flavors:							
16 oz size	200	0 (0%)	0	0	15	0	50
22 oz size	275	0 (0%)	0	0	20	0	69
32 oz size	400	0 (0%)	0	0	30	0	100
44 oz size	550	0 (0%)	0	0	40	0	138

SHONEY'S

	Cal	Fat	(%Fc)	S.Fat	Chol	Sod	Pro	Carb
Main Menu								
All-American Burger	500	33	(59%)	na	86	600	25	27
Bacon Burger	590	40	(61%)	na	86	800	28	29
Baked Fish	170	1	(5%)	<1	83	1640	34	2
Baked Ham Sandwich	290	10	(31%)	na	42	1265	19	28
Baked Potato, 10 oz	265	0	(0%)	0	0	15	6	61
Charbroiled Chicken S'wich	450	17	(34%)	na	90	1000	43	28
Chicken Fillet Sandwich	465	21	(41%)	na	51	585	30	39
Country Fried Sandwich	590	26	(40%)	na	29	1500	25	67
Fish 'N Chips w. Fries	640	35	(49%)	na	103	875	32	50
French Fries, 4 oz	250	10	(36%)	na	0	365	4	39
Fried Fish, Light	300	14	(42%)	na	65	535	19	22
Grilled Bacon & Cheese S'wich	440	28	(57%)	na	36	1200	18	28
Grilled Cheese S'wich	300	17	(51%)	na	36	880	12	25
Half O'Pound	435	34	(70%)	na	123	280	32	0
Hawaiian Chicken	260	7	(24%)	na	85	595	43	7
Italian Feast	500	20	(36%)	na	74	370	38	44
Lasagna	300	10	(30%)	na	26	870	8	45
Mushroom Swiss Burger	615	42	(61%)	na	106	1135	32	29
Old-Fashioned Burger	470	28	(54%)	na	82	680	25	26
Patty Melt	640	42	(59%)	na	171	825	39	30
Philly Steak S'wich	675	44	(59%)	na	103	1245	32	37
Reuben Sandwich	595	35	(53%)	na	138	3875	33	32
Seafood Platter	566	28	(45%)	na	127	895	33	46
Shoney Burger	500	36	(65%)	na	79	785	23	22
Shrimper's Feast	385	22	(51%)	na	125	215	17	30
Large	575	33	(52%)	na	188	325	25	45
Slim Jim Sandwich	485	24	(45%)	na	57	1620	27	40
Spaghetti	495	16	(29%)	na	55	390	24	63
Steak 'N Shrimp (Charbroiled)	360	23	(57%)	na	141	200	37	1
Steak 'N Shrimp (Fried)	510	33	(58%)	na	150	250	37	15
Turkey Club/Whole Wheat	635	33	(47%)	na	100	1290	44	44
Children's Menu								
All-American Jnr Burger	235	11	(42%)	na	30	545	14	20
Kid's: Chicken Dinner	245	13	(48%)	na	40	150	21	11
Fish 'N Chips w. Fries	335	17	(46%)	na	41	460	13	33
Fried Shrimp	195	12	(55%)	na	70	635	10	12
Spaghetti	250	8	(29%)	na	27	195	13	32
Desserts: Apple Pie	490	23	(42%)	na	35	575	6	67
Carrot Cake	500	26	(47%)	na	37	475	9	56
Strawberry Pie	332	17	(46%)	na	0	250	2	45
Walnut Brownie	575	34	(53%)	na	35	435	10	61
Icecream/Sundaes								
Hot Fudge Cake	525	20	(34%)	na	27	485	7	82
Hot Fudge Sundae	450	22	(44%)	na	60	225	7	60
Strawberry Sundae	380	19	(45%)	na	70	145	6	48

SKIPPER'S

	Cal	Fat	(%Fc)	S.Fat	Chol	Sod	Pro	Carb
Chowder: Per Serving								
Smoked Salmon	165	7	(38%)	na	na	75	13	14
Clam: 1 cup	100	3.5	(32%)	na	12	525	3	14
Entrees: Per Serving								
Chicken: Tenderloin Strips								
w. Fries, 5 pcs	795	38	(43%)	na	77	800	44	69
'Lite Catch', 3 pcs	305	15	(44%)	na	58	675	26	17
Chicken: Strips, Create A Catch	80	4	(45%)	na	15	150	8	4
Strips, Fish, Fries	805	40	(45%)	na	100	860	80	72
Strips, Shrimp, Fries	800	39	(44%)	na	97	1035	36	77
Clam: Strips w. Fries	1005	70	(63%)	na	14	570	22	90
Strips, Fish, Fries	870	54	(56%)	na	61	670	25	81
Cod: 3 pcs. w. Fries	665	32	(43%)	na	38	1055	27	68
4 pcs. w. Fries	760	36	(43%)	na	50	1390	34	74
5 pcs. w. Fries	855	41	(43%)	na	62	1725	42	80
Fish Meal: 1 fillet w/Fries	560	28	(45%)	na	55	410	17	51
2 fillets w. Fries	735	38	(47%)	na	108	765	28	71
2 pces w. Salad, Lite Catch	410	23	(51%)	na	120	940	25	27
3 fillets, w. Fries	910	48	(48%)	na	160	1120	39	82
3 fillets + Salad, small	410	23	(51%)	na	119	940	25	27
'Create a Catch'	175	10	(51%)	na	53	360	11	11
Fish, Oysters, Fries	885	44	(45%)	na	80	810	25	95
Oyster w. Fries, 'Basket'	1040	51	(44%)	na	52	855	28	118
Salmon, baked	270	11	(37%)	na	70	505	39	1
Shrimp, Fish, Fries:	730	37	(46%)	na	105	945	24	77
Jumbo, w. Fries, Basket	710	35	(45%)	na	73	910	20	79
Original, Fries, Basket	725	36	(45%)	na	102	1120	20	82
Skipper's Platter Basket	1040	63	(55%)	na	111	1200	32	97
Sandwiches								
Chicken, 'Create a Catch'	605	32	(48%)	na	82	975	31	44
Fish: 'Create a Catch', regular	525	33	(57%)	na	86	1190	19	43
Double	700	73	(94%)	na	139	1550	30	54
French Fries	385	18	(42%)	na	2	50	6	50
Potato, baked	145	0	(0%)	0	0	5	4	32
Salads: Coleslaw	290	27	(84%)	na	50	330	2	10
Green, small, Lite Catch	60	3	(46%)	na	13	225	3	6
Shrimp & Seafood	170	3	(16%)	na	80	660	23	15
Side	25	0	(0%)	0	0	10	0	4
Salad Dressings & Sauces								
Blue Cheese	220	23	(93%)	na	8	240	1	4
Italian Gourmet	140	15	(96%)	na	0	200	0	2
Low Cal	15	1	(53%)	<1	0	680	0	2
Ranch House	190	20	(96%)	na	0	300	1	2
Thousand Island	160	14	(79%)	na	6	415	0	8
Barbeque Sauce, 1Tbsp	25	1	(36%)	<1	0	225	0	5
Cocktail Sauce, 1 Tbsp	20	0	(0%)	0	0	215	0	5
Tartar Sauce, 1Tbsp	65	7	(97%)	na	4	100	0	0
Root Beer Float	300	10	(30%)	na	10	65	3	33

SIZZLER

	Cal	Fat (%Fc)	S.Fat	Chol	Sod	Pro	Carb
Hot Entrees							
Hamburger	625	33 (47%)	12	142	335	45	36
Dakota Ranch Steak: 6 oz	315	20 (57%)	8	100	255	30	0
8 oz	420	27 (58%)	11	135	340	37	0
9 1/2 oz	500	32 (58%)	13	160	400	47	0
Hibachi Chicken Breast w. Pineapple	195	3 (14%)	1	65	685	28	13
Lemon-Herb Chicken Breast	140	3 (19%)	1	65	380	27	0
Malibu Chick. Patty, each	310	19 (55%)	3	75	590	23	11
Salmon	250	12 (44%)	2	41	230	32	0
Santa Fe Chick. Breast	150	3 (18%)	1	65	350	30	0
Shrimp, Broiled	150	6 (36%)	0	218	375	23	0
Fried, 4 only	225	2 (8%)	0	118	705	18	35
Mini	150	1 (6%)	0	80	480	13	24
Shrimp Scampi	145	3 (19%)	1	150	385	27	0
Swordfish	315	14 (40%)	3	89	330	45	0
Accompaniments							
Cheese Toast, 1 pce	275	21 (69%)	5	5	495	6	16
French Fries	360	12 (30%)	6	0	245	5	45
Potato, Baked, Flesh Only	105	0 (0%)	0	0	5	2	24
Rice Pilaf	260	5 (18%)	1	0	865	4	47
Condiments: Per 1 1/2 oz							
Sauces: Butlery Dipping	330	37 (100%)	7	0	0	0	0
Cocktail	40	0 (0%)	0	0	395	0	8
Hibachi	60	0 (0%)	0	0	710	0	11
Malibu	285	31 (99%)	6	28	355	0	0
Marinara, 1 oz	15	0 (0%)	0	0	90	0	3
Nacho Cheese, 2 oz	120	10 (75%)	5	30	600	5	3
Sour Dressing	90	9 (91%)	8	0	45	0	0
Tartar	170	17 (90%)	3	14	455	0	6
Margarine, Whipped, 1 1/2 T.	105	12 (100%)	2	0	145	0	0
Hot Bar							
Broccoli Cheese Soup, 4 oz	140	9 (58%)	2	8	355	3	10
Chicken Noodle Soup, 4 oz	30	1 (29%)	0	7	495	2	4
Chicken Wings, 1 oz	75	4 (49%)	1	20	135	4	4
Clam Chowder, 4 oz	120	6 (46%)	0	6	510	3	11
Focaccia Bread, 2 pces	110	7 (58%)	1	0	135	2	9
Meatballs, 4 balls	155	11 (63%)	5	30	460	9	5
Minestrone Soup, 4 oz	35	0 (0%)	0	0	445	1	7
Pasta, Fettucine, 2 oz	80	1 (11%)	0	5	5	3	15
Pasta, Spaghetti, 2 oz	80	0 (0%)	0	0	0	3	16
Potato Skins, 2 oz	160	8 (45%)	1	0	465	2	22
Refried Beans, 1/4 cup	60	1 (15%)	2	5	270	4	11
Saltine Crackers, 2 crackers	25	1 (36%)	0	2	75	1	4
Taco Filling, 2 oz	105	9 (79%)	4	16	230	2	3
Taco Shells, each	50	2 (36%)	0	0	20	1	7

SIZZLER CONT

	Cal	Fat	(%Fc)	S.Fat	Chol	Sod	Pro	Carb
Salads & Toppings								
Prepared Salads - Per 2 oz								
Carrot & Raisin	130	10	(69%)	2	10	105	1	10
Chinese Chicken	55	2	(33%)	0	10	120	4	6
Mediterranean Minted Fruit	30	0	(0%)	0	0	10	1	7
Mexican Fiesta	55	1	(17%)	0	0	100	2	10
Old Fashioned Potato	85	5	(53%)	1	10	230	1	10
Red Herb Potato	120	9	(67%)	1	10	270	1	9
Seafood Louis Pasta	65	2	(28%)	0	15	140	3	9
Seafood	55	3	(48%)	1	7	255	3	4
Spicy Jicama	15	0	(0%)	0	0	30	0	4
Teriyaki Beef	50	2	(37%)	1	7	135	4	5
Tuna Pasta	135	10	(68%)	1	10	190	6	6
Sides								
Cottage Cheese, 2 oz	50	1	(18%)	1	5	230	8	2
Eggs, 1 oz	45	3	(61%)	1	120	35	4	0
Garbanzo Beans, 1/4 cup	65	1	(14%)	0	0	255	3	11
Turkey Ham, 1 oz	60	5	(73%)	2	19	375	4	0
Kidney Beans, 1/4 cup	50	0	(0%)	0	0	220	3	10
Olives, 1 oz	60	6	(87%)	1	0	180	1	1
Peas, 1/4 cup	30	0	(0%)	0	0	35	2	6
Peaches, 1/4 cup	35	0	(0%)	0	0	5	0	9
Real Bacon Bits, 1 Tbsp	30	2	(67%)	0	0	165	2	2
Dressings & Condiments: Per 1 oz								
Dressing; Blue Cheese	110	12	(98%)	4	8	170	1	1
Honey Mustard	160	16	(90%)	2	10	110	0	4
Italian, Lite	15	0	(0%)	0	0	350	0	2
Japanese Rice Vinegar, Fat Free	10	0	(0%)	0	0	180	0	2
Parmesan Italian	100	10	(90%)	2	0	450	0	2
Ranch	120	12	(90%)	2	10	240	0	2
Ranch, Reduced-Calorie	90	8	(80%)	2	10	270	0	4
Thousand Island	145	15	(94%)	2	10	125	0	3
Guacamole	40	4	(86%)	1	0	425	0	2
Salsa	10	0	(0%)	0	0	155	0	2
Sour Dressing, 2 Tbsp	60	6	(90%)	5	0	30	0	0
Dessert Bar								
Choc/Van. Soft Serv., 4 oz	135	4	(26%)	4	0	100	1	24
Chocolate Syrup, 1 oz	90	0	(0%)	0	0	15	0	21
Strawberry Topping, 1 oz	70	0	(0%)	0	0	5	0	18
Whipped Topping, 1 Tbsp	10	1	(75%)	1	0	0	0	1

SOUPLANTATION

	Cal	Fat (%Fc)	S.Fat	Chol	Sod	Pro	Carb
Soups: Per 1 Cup							
Low Fat: Chicken Tortilla	100	3 (27%)	1	20	990	12	5
Chicken/Turkey Noodle	160	3 (17%)	2	20	480	15	17
Sweet Tomato Onion	110	3 (25%)	1	0	450	2	12
Vegetable Medley	90	1 (10%)	0	0	520	2	14
Regular: Albondigas Buenas	190	9 (43%)	4	15	720	12	17
Chesapeake Corn Chowder	310	13 (38%)	5	20	720	12	43
Chicken Fajitas & Black Bean	280	7 (23%)	2	20	980	22	33
Chicken Jambalaya	160	7 (39%)	2	30	980	12	13
Chunky Potato Cheese	210	10 (43%)	6	30	480	10	19
Cream of Broccoli/Chicken	250	18 (65%)	8	30	890	11	14
Cream of Mushroom	290	21 (65%)	8	30	820	10	15
Irish Potato Leek	290	17 (53%)	8	40	870	11	24
Minestrone w. Italian Sausage	210	11 (47%)	4	20	890	13	14
Navy Bean w.Ham	340	10 (26%)	4	40	980	35	30
New England Clam Chowder	330	20 (55%)	10	80	630	18	21
New Orleans Style Jambalaya	160	8 (45%)	3	30	900	8	14
Shrimp Bisque	300	19 (57%)	8	70	880	11	20
Split Pea Ham; Turk. Cassoulet	350	10 (26%)	4	40	980	36	32
Turkey Vegetable	270	12 (40%)	4	40	990	22	16
Vegetarian Harvest	190	8 (38%)	2	0	990	5	23
Chili: Arizona /Texas Red	230	8 (31%)	4	20	680	14	30
Yucatan Chili	280	10 (32%)	4	40	890	28	31
House Chili	230	3 (12%)	2	15	560	15	26
Santa Fe Black Bean Chili	190	3 (14%)	0	0	580	9	26
Fresh Tossed Salads: Per 1 Cup							
Antipasto Salad; BBQ Aver.	140	10 (64%)	3	15	350	5	6
Caribbean Krab Salad	120	7 (68%)	1	110	180	5	10
Classic Caesar Salad	190	14 (66%)	2	10	280	5	10
Ensalada Azteca	130	9 (62%)	3	15	230	6	7
Greek Salad	120	9 (68%)	3	10	320	3	4
Mandarin Spinach w. Walnuts	170	11 (58%)	1	0	150	3	14
Roma Tomato, Mozzarella & Basil	120	9 (68%)	2	10	180	4	7
Shrimp & Krab Louis; Spinach	180	12 (60%)	4	190	340	10	6
Sonoma w. Artichokes	160	12 (68%)	2	0	640	2	8
Spinach & Pasta w.Raspb. Vin.	180	6 (40%)	0	0	620	6	22
Won Ton Chicken Salad	150	8 (48%)	1	10	220	6	12
Prepared Salads: Per 1/2 Cup							
Artichoke Rice	160	8 (45%)	1	3	780	3	21
Aunt Doris' Red Pepper Slaw	70	0 (0%)	0	0	480	18	18
Baja Bean & Cilantro	180	3 (15%)	0	0	190	9	29
BBQ Potato	160	8 (45%)	1	5	270	2	20
Carrot Raisin	90	3 (30%)	0	5	80	1	17
Chinese Krab	160	8 (45%)	1	3	260	5	19
Confetti Pasta w. Cheddar & Dill	160	9 (45%)	2	10	380	5	16
Cucumber Tomato w.Chile Lime	20	0 (0%)	0	0	20	1	4

205

SOUPLANTATION CONT

	Cal	Fat (%Fc)	S.Fat	Chol	Sod	Pro	Carb
Salads (Cont): Per ½ Cup							
Dijon Potato w. Garlic Dill Vin.	140	7 (51%)	1	0	260	3	16
German Potato; Gemeilli Pasta	130	3 (21%)	0	5	380	5	20
Greek Couscous w.Feta Cheese	170	9 (42%)	1	4	480	6	19
Mazatian Krab & Pasta	160	9 (45%)	1	2	480	4	15
Mandarin Krab Salad	150	3 (18%)	0	2	280	5	26
Mandarin w.Broccoli/Almonds	120	3 (23%)	0	0	380	3	19
Marinated Summer Vegetables	80	0 (0%)	0	0	210	1	19
Mediterranean Harvest	120	3 (23%)	1	2	180	3	17
Mediterranean Krab & Rotini	170	10 (53%)	1	2	380	4	15
Moroccan Marinated Vegetables	90	3 (30%)	0	0	230	2	9
Old Fashioned Macaroni w.Ham	180	11 (55%)	2	10	360	4	15
Oriental Ginger Slaw w.Krab	70	3 (39%)	0	2	80	2	8
Pesto Kashi	170	10 (53%)	2	5	310	5	17
Pesto Pasta	160	7 (39%)	1	2	320	4	18
Picnic Potato	150	7 (42%)	1	80	320	3	19
Pineapple Coconut Slaw	150	10 (60%)	3	15	190	1	14
Poppyseed Coleslaw	120	9 (68%)	1	10	130	1	9
Rst. Potato w. Chipotle Chile	140	6 (39%)	1	0	250	3	18
Shrimp & Tortellini a la Russe	120	6 (45%)	2	20	230	6	9
Southern Dill Potato	120	3 (23%)	2	5	300	4	20
Spicy Southwestern Pasta	130	3 (21%)	0	0	350	5	21
Spinach Krab	230	12 (47%)	2	15	550	5	25
Summer Barley w.Black Beans	110	3 (25%)	0	0	280	4	19
Thai Noodle w. Peanut Sce	170	8 (42%)	1	0	310	5	17
Three Bean Marinade	170	6 (32%)	1	0	320	4	27
Tortellini Salad w.Basil	170	10 (53%)	2	2	260	4	14
Tumbleweed Tortellini	140	9 (58%)	1	2	330	4	11
Tuna Tarragon	240	14 (53%)	2	10	480	6	21
Turkey Chutney Pasta	230	9 (35%)	2	30	310	14	21
Zesty Tortellini	190	15 (71%)	2	10	460	4	18
Dressing & Croutons: 2 Tbsp							
Parmesan & Garlic Crout. (10)	40	3 (68%)	1	2	160	2	2
Blue Cheese Dressing	140	14 (90%)	2.5	10	230	1	3
Blush Vinaigrette	120	12 (90%)	2	0	320	0	3
Creamy Cucumber Dressing	80	7 (79%)	1	0	290	0	4
Garden French Tomato	40	1.5 (34%)	0	0	270	0	7
Honey Mustard Dressing	150	13 (78%)	2	10	230	0	8
Fat Free	45	0 (0%)	0	10	160	0	10
Parmesan Pepper Cream	160	17 (97%)	2.5	5	330	1	2
Ranch House Dressing	130	13 (90%)	2	10	180	1	1
Fat Free	50	0 (0%)	0	0	180	1	2
Raspberry Vinaigrette	120	13 (98%)	2	0	150	0	3
Thousand Island Dressing	110	11 (90%)	1.5	5	250	0	3
Zesty Italian Dressing	160	18 (100%)	2.5	0	280	0	1
Fat Free	20	0 (0%)	0	0	340	0	5

SOUPLANTATION CONT

	Cal	Fat	(%Fc)	S.Fat	Chol	Sod	Pro	Carb
Pasta: Plain or Spinach, 1 cup	360	3	(7%)	0	0	180	10	62
Sauces: Per 1/2 Cup								
Alfredo: Camberetto/Vongole	220	12	(49%)	7	45	360	14	13
Traditional Style	180	11	(55%)	6	10	320	8	11
Italian Bruschetta	30	0	(0%)	0	0	250	1	4
Pesto Cream & Garlic	220	16	(65%)	6	25	480	8	12
Vegetarian Marinara Sauce	80	3	(34%)	0	0	580	2	12
Salsa Alla: Bolognese	140	8	(51%)	2	10	750	5	13
Carne Polpetta	100	5	(45%)	2	5	620	4	11
Sicilian	80	3	(34%)	0	0	630	2	12
Muffins: Per Muffin								
96% Fat Free: All types	80	0.5	(5%)	0	0	110	2	17
Regular: Apple Raisin	150	7	(42%)	1	10	190	2	22
Apricot/Banana/Cherry Nut	150	7	(42%)	1	10	190	2	22
Carrot Pineapple w.Oat Bran	150	6	(36%)	1	10	230	3	23
Chili Corn	140	3	(19%)	1	10	320	3	27
Chocolate Varieties	170	8	(42%)	2	10	190	3	22
Georgia Peach Poppyseed	150	6	(36%)	1	10	210	2	20
Lemon Poppyseed Surprise	130	5	(35%)	1	10	190	2	19
Mandarin Almond w. Oat Bran	140	7	(45%)	1	10	210	3	20
Nutty Peanut Butter	170	8	(42%)	1	10	210	4	21
Peanut Butter Choc. Chip	190	9	(43%)	2	10	230	5	23
Pumpkin Raisin	150	6	(36%)	1	10	210	2	25
Strawberry Buttermilk	140	6	(39%)	1	10	210	2	21
Wild Maine Blueberry	140	5	(32%)	1	10	180	2	22
Large	310	12	(35%)	2	20	380	5	40
Zucchini Nut	150	7	(42%)	1	10	190	2	22
Breads: Buttermilk Corn	140	2	(13%)	0	10	270	3	27
Indian Grain	200	1.5	(7%)	0	15	260	11	35
Sourdough	150	0.5	(3%)	0	0	240	9	27
Focaccia: Garlic Parmesan	100	3	(27%)	0	0	170	2	15
Pizza /Tomarillo	140	6	(39%)	2	10	270	5	16
Desserts: Per 1/2 Cup								
Apple Medley	70	0	(0%)	0	0	5	1	18
Banana Royale	80	0	(0%)	0	0	5	1	20
Chocolate Chip Cookie, small	70	3	(39%)	1	5	90	1	10
Chocolate Pudding	140	4	(26%)	0	10	220	4	23
Ghirardelli Chocolate Frozen	95	0	(0%)	0	0	80	3	21
Jello, flavored	80	0	(0%)	0	0	40	1	20
Rice Pudding	110	2	(16%)	1	10	50	3	20
Tapioca Pudding	140	3	(19%)	0	10	160	4	24
Tropical Fruit Salad	75	0	(0%)	0	0	5	1	19
Vanilla Pudding	140	3	(19%)	0	10	160	4	24
Vanilla Soft Serving	140	4	(26%)	3	20	70	3	22
Toppings: Choc. Syrup, 2 Tbsp	70	0	(0%)	0	10	15	0	18
Candy Sprinkles, 1 Tbsp	70	2	(26%)	0	0	0	0	11
Granola Topping, 2 Tbsp	110	4	(33%)	2	0	14	2	16

SONIC DRIVE-IN

(na) ~ Data not available

	Cal	Fat (%Fc)	S.Fat	Chol	Sod	Pro	Carb
Hamburgers							
#1. Hamburger	410	27 (59%)	na	58	450	20	23
with Cheese	480	32 (60%)	na	76	710	24	24
#2. Hamburger	325	16 (44%)	na	50	550	20	23
with Cheese	395	21 (48%)	na	67	820	24	24
Bacon Cheeseburger	550	39 (64%)	na	87	840	28	23
Hickory Burger	315	16 (46%)	na	50	460	20	23
Jalapeno Burger	640	41 (58%)	na	136	1360	44	22
Super Sonic w. Mayonnaise	730	52 (64%)	na	144	1025	44	24
with Mustard	645	41 (57%)	na	136	1130	44	24
Mini Burger	245	12 (44%)	na	36	510	14	20
Mini Cheeseburger	280	14 (45%)	na	45	645	17	20
Sandwiches: Steak (breaded)	630	42 (60%)	na	50	1050	19	46
Chicken (breaded)	455	25 (49%)	na	42	755	23	36
Grilled Chicken, no dressing	215	4 (17%)	na	63	715	21	23
Fish	280	7 (23%)	na	6	655	17	38
B-L-T	325	19 (52%)	na	9	600	8	27
Grilled Cheese	290	17 (53%)	na	36	840	12	25
Coneys/Local Flavors							
Chili Pie	330	23 (63%)	na	28	315	12	20
Regular Hot Dog	260	15 (52%)	na	23	240	8	21
Regular Cheese Coney	360	23 (58%)	na	40	340	14	23
Extra-Long Cheese Coney	635	39 (55%)	na	65	630	24	45
Corn Dog	280	15 (48%)	na	35	700	7	30
Sides: French Fries; Reg.	235	8 (31%)	na	8	50	3	37
Large	315	11 (31%)	na	11	70	5	50
w. Cheese, large	420	20 (43%)	na	38	470	11	51
Onion Rings, regular	405	27 (60%)	na	na	370	5	38
Onion Rings, large	580	38 (59%)	na	na	530	8	54
Tater Tots	150	7 (42%)	na	10	330	2	19
Tater Tots, w. Cheese	220	13 (53%)	na	28	570	6	19

SUB STATION II

	Cal	Fat (%Fc)	S.Fat	Chol	Sod	Pro	Carb
Sandwiches: Ham: & Cheese	505	30 (53%)	na	na	1160	18	40
Turkey & Cheese	510	30 (53%)	na	na	1140	19	40
Salami, Pepperoni, Turkey Bologna, Ham, Cheese	635	42 (60%)	na	na	1590	23	40
Roast Beef & Cheese	520	31 (54%)	na	na	1045	24	39
Turkey & Cheese	525	31 (53%)	na	na	1150	21	40

STEAK 'N SHAKE

	Cal	Fat (%Fc)	S.Fat	Chol	Sod	Pro	Carb
Steakburgers & Sandwiches							
Steakburger	275	7 (23%)	na	60	425	18	33
with Cheese	355	13 (33%)	na	80	660	23	33
Super	375	12 (29%)	na	100	445	30	33
Super with Cheese	450	18 (36%)	na	120	680	35	33
Triple	475	17 (32%)	na	160	470	43	33
Triple with Cheese	625	30 (43%)	na	180	935	52	34
Ham Sandwich	450	22 (44%)	na	na	1860	29	37
Grilled Cheese Sandwich	250	13 (47%)	na	20	610	9	24
Grilled Chicken Sandwich	510	22 (39%)	na	85	1150	26	53
Other Items: French Fries	210	10 (43%)	na	10	300	3	28
Chili & Oyster Crackers	335	14 (38%)	na	na	1160	16	37
Chili Mac & 4 Saltines	310	12 (35%)	na	na	1300	15	34
Chili 3 Ways & 4 Saltines	410	16 (35%)	na	na	1730	19	45
Baked Beans	175	4 (21%)	na	0	655	9	27
Lett./Tom/ Salad/1 oz 1000 Isl.	170	15 (79%)	na	15	225	1	7
Chef Salad	315	18 (51%)	na	120	1580	41	6
Cottage Cheese, 1/2 cup	95	4 (38%)	na	20	200	12	3
Desserts: Apple Danish	390	24 (55%)	na	30	350	6	35
Brownie	260	12 (42%)	na	10	165	3	39
Cheesecake	370	11 (27%)	na	60	295	7	61
with Strawberries	385	11 (26%)	na	60	295	7	65
Pies: Apple	405	18 (40%)	na	40	480	4	61
Cherry	335	14 (38%)	na	30	270	6	48
Apple, A La Mode	550	25 (41%)	na	80	525	4	76
Cherry, A La Mode	475	22 (42%)	na	70	315	6	63
Sundaes: Brownie Fudge	645	35 (49%)	na	30	260	7	81
Hot Fudge Nut	530	34 (58%)	na	60	120	5	51
Strawberry	330	22 (60%)	na	50	80	2	29
Vanilla Ice Cream	215	12 (50%)	na	40	70	1	23
Shakes & Drinks							
Floats: Coca-Cola	515	17 (30%)	na	0	230	16	76
Orange	500	17 (31%)	na	0	225	16	74
Lemon	555	19 (31%)	na	0	250	18	82
Root Beer	530	17 (29%)	na	0	240	17	78
Freezes: Lemon	550	25 (41%)	na	0	215	15	69
Orange	515	24 (42%)	na	0	200	14	63
Hot Chocolate	685	19 (25%)	na	50	670	17	129
Shakes: Chocolate	610	38 (56%)	na	100	180	13	57
Strawberry	650	40 (55%)	na	100	190	16	62
Vanilla	620	38 (55%)	na	100	180	13	58

(Cholesterol Figures - Estimates only)

SUBWAY

	Cal	Fat	(%Fc)	S.Fat	Chol	Sod	Pro	Carb
6" Subs: Cheese & Condiments Not Included								
BLT	330	10	(27%)	na	16	960	14	44
Chicken Taco Sub	435	16	(33%)	na	52	1275	25	49
Cold Cut Trio	380	13	(31%)	na	64	1410	20	46
Ham	300	5	(15%)	na	28	1320	19	45
Ham & Cheese	340	8	(21%)	na	38	1525	21	45
Meatball	420	16	(34%)	na	33	1045	19	51
Pizza Sub	465	22	(43%)	na	50	1620	19	48
Roast Beef	305	5	(15%)	na	20	940	20	45
Rst Chicken Breast	350	6	(15%)	na	48	980	27	47
Steak & Cheese	440	13	(27%)	na	80	1320	32	47
Subway Club	310	5	(15%)	na	26	1350	21	46
Subway Melt	380	12	(28%)	na	42	1750	23	46
w. Light Mayonnaise	350	10	(26%)	na	32	885	20	45
Subway Seafood & Crab	430	19	(40%)	na	34	860	20	44
w. Light Mayonnaise	370	12	(29%)	na	34	920	20	45
Tuna	540	32	(53%)	na	36	890	19	44
w. Light Mayonnaise	390	15	(35%)	na	32	940	19	46
Turkey Breast	290	4	(12%)	na	19	1405	18	46
& Ham	295	5	(15%)	na	24	1360	18	46
Veggie Delite	240	3	(11%)	na	0	590	9	44

Note: Figures based on White Bread. For Wheat Bread add 15 cals, 1g fat, 3g carbohydrate, 11mg sodium.

Sandwiches								
Bologna	290	12	(37%)	na	20	745	10	38
Ham	235	4	(15%)	na	14	775	11	37
Roast Beef	245	4	(15%)	na	13	640	13	38
Tuna	355	18	(46%)	na	18	560	11	37
W. Light Mayonnaise	280	9	(29%)	na	16	580	11	38
Turkey Breast	235	4	(15%)	na	12	945	12	38

Salads: Note: Values do not include Dressing, Cheese or Condiments unless indicated.

	Cal	Fat	(%Fc)	S.Fat	Chol	Sod	Pro	Carb
BLT	140	8	(51%)	na	16	670	7	10
Bread Bowl	330	4	(11%)	na	0	760	12	63
Chicken Taco	250	14	(50%)	na	52	990	18	15
Classic Italian BMT	460	22	(43%)	na	56	1665	21	45
Cold Cut Trio	190	11	(52%)	na	64	1130	13	11
Ham	120	3	(23%)	na	28	1035	12	11
Meatball	235	14	(54%)	na	33	760	12	16
Pizza w. Cheese	320	23	(65%)	na	60	1540	14	13
Roast Beef	120	3	(23%)	na	20	655	12	11
Roast Chicken Breast	160	4	(23%)	na	48	695	20	13
Seafood & Crab:	240	17	(64%)	na	34	575	13	10
w. Light Mayonnaise	160	8	(46%)	na	32	600	13	11
Steak and Cheese	250	11	(40%)	na	80	1035	24	13
Subway Club	125	3	(22%)	na	26	1070	12	12
Subway Melt w. Cheese	235	18	(69%)	13	52	1665	18	12
Tuna Salad	355	30	(76%)	na	36	600	12	10
w. Light Mayonnaise	205	13	(58%)	na	32	660	12	11

SUBWAY CONT

	Cal	Fat (%Fc)	S.Fat	Chol	Sod	Pro	Carb
Salads: (Cont)							
Turkey Breast and Ham	110	3 (25%)	na	24	1075	11	11
Turkey Breast Salad	100	2 (18%)	na	19	1120	11	12
Veggie Delite Salad	50	1 (20%)	na	0	310	2	10
Fixin's & Dressings							
Bacon, 2 slices	45	4 (80%)	na	8	180	2	0
Cheese, 2 triangles	40	3 (67%)	na	10	200	2	0
Creamy Italian, 1 pkg	260	24 (83%)	na	16	530	0	8
Fat-Free Italian, 1 pkg	20	0 (0%)	na	0	610	0	4
French, 1 pkg	260	20 (69%)	na	0	400	0	20
Fat-Free, 1 pkg	60	0 (0%)	na	0	340	0	16
Thousand Island, 1 pkg	260	24 (83%)	0	28	430	0	8
Ranch, 1 pkg	350	36 (93%)	0	4	470	0	4
Fat-Free, 1 pkg	50	0 (0%)	0	0	710	0	12
Mayonnaise, 1 tsp	37	4 (97%)	0	3	25	0	0
Light Mayonnaise, 1 tsp	18	2 (100%)	0	2	35	0	0
Mustard, 2 tsp	8	0 (0%)	0	0	0	1	1
Olive Oil Blend, 1 tsp	45	5 (100%)	0	0	0	0	0
Cookies: Chocolate Chip	210	10 (43%)	na	10	140	2	29
Choc Chip M & M	210	10 (43%)	na	15	140	2	29
Chocolate Chunk	210	10 (43%)	na	10	140	2	29
Double Choc Brazil Nut	230	12 (49%)	na	10	115	3	27
Oatmeal Raisin	200	8 (36%)	na	15	160	3	29
Peanut Butter	220	12 (49%)	na	0	180	3	26
Sugar Cookie	230	12 (47%)	na	20	180	2	28
White Choc Macadamia	230	12 (47%)	na	10	140	2	28

Note: Figures are for small cookies. For large cookies, add 87 cals, 4g fat, 6mg cholesterol, 60mg sodium, 1g protein, 12g carbohydrate.

SWEET TOMATOES

SAME MENU & FIGURES AS SOUPLANTATION

TACO BELL

	Cal	Fat (%Fc)	S.Fat	Chol	Sod	Pro	Carb
Tacos: Taco, regular	170	10 (53%)	4	30	280	10	11
Taco Supreme	230	13 (53%)	6	45	290	11	13
Soft Taco, regular	210	9 (39%)	4	30	530	12	20
Supreme	260	13 (45%)	7	45	550	13	22
BLT	330	22 (60%)	8	40	610	11	22
Chicken	250	11 (40%)	4	45	380	15	23
Light Chicken	180	5 (25%)	1	30	660	13	21
Kid's Chicken Soft Taco	190	7 (33%)	3	35	590	12	20
Kid's Soft Taco Roll-Up	280	15 (48%)	8	50	790	16	20
Big Border Taco	280	16 (51%)	7	55	610	16	17
Supreme	320	20 (56%)	9	65	620	17	19

TACO BELL CONT

	Cal	Fat (%Fc)	S.Fat	Chol	Sod	Pro	Carb
Tacos (Cont)							
Double Decker Taco	340	14 (37%)	5	30	700	16	37
Supreme	380	18 (43%)	7	45	720	16	39
Tostada	300	14 (42%)	5	15	700	11	31
Burritos							
Breakfast: Country	260	14 (48%)	5	195	700	8	26
Double Bacon & Egg B'fast	470	26 (50%)	9	400	1250	18	39
Fiesta Breakfast	270	15 (50%)	6	25	590	9	25
Grande Breakfast	410	21 (46%)	7	205	1060	13	43
Bean	370	11 (27%)	4	10	1150	13	54
Burrito Supreme	430	18 (38%)	8	45	1230	19	50
Bacon Cheeseburger	550	29 (47%)	11	85	1370	29	43
Big Beef Supreme	510	22 (39%)	10	70	1470	26	51
Chicken:	400	16 (36%)	5	55	720	19	45
Light	300	7 (21%)	2	30	1000	18	40
Light Supreme	410	12 (26%)	3	55	1390	26	52
Supreme	550	26 (43%)	9	95	730	30	50
Club	540	31 (52%)	10	75	1210	22	43
Chili Cheese	320	12 (34%)	5	35	890	14	37
7-Layer Burrito	530	22 (37%)	8	25	1280	16	65
Speciality Items							
Big Beef Meximelt	290	16 (50%)	8	50	860	16	21
Mexican Pizza	570	36 (57%)	11	50	1050	21	41
Mexican Rice	190	9 (43%)	4	15	430	6	21
Nachos:	310	18 (52%)	4	5	540	2	34
Big Beef Nachos Supreme	430	24 (50%)	7	40	720	12	43
BellGrande	740	39 (47%)	10	40	1200	16	83
Pintos 'N Cheese	180	8 (40%)	4	15	690	9	18
Quesadilla: Cheese	370	20 (49%)	12	55	720	16	32
Chicken	420	22 (47%)	12	85	1020	24	33
Breakfast: Cheese	390	22 (51%)	10	280	940	15	32
w. Bacon	460	28 55%)	12	295	1130	20	33
w. Sausage	440	26 (53%)	12	290	1010	17	33
Sandwiches							
Breakfast S/wich w. Bacon	610	46 (68%)	13	165	1060	19	30
Breakfast S/wich w. Sausage	680	53 (70%)	16	180	1110	20	30
3-Cheese Melt	490	22 (40%)	10	45	1160	20	55
Beef Melt	540	24 (40%)	10	60	1520	26	55
Taco Salad w. Salsa	850	52 (55%)	15	75	1650	32	63
Cinnamon Twists	140	6 (39%)	0	0	190	1	19
Side Items/Condiments							
Guacamole, ¾ oz	35	3 (77%)	0.5	0	140	0	2
Nacho Cheese Sauce, 2 oz	120	10 (75%)	3	5	470	2	5
Salsa, 1 pkt	30	0 (0%)	0	0	470	1	6
Sour Cream, ¾ oz	40	4 (90%)	3	10	10	1	1
Non-Fat, ¾ oz	20	0 (0%)	0	0	55	1	2
Taco Sauce, Mild/Hot, 1 pkt	0	0 (0%)	0	0	80	0	0

TACO JOHN'S

	Cal	Fat	(%Fc)	S.Fat	Chol	Sod	Pro	Carb
Burritos/Fajitas								
Bean Burrito	390	11	(25%)	4	18	870	15	57
Beef Burrito	450	20	(40%)	8	52	860	23	44
Chicken Fajita: Burrito	370	12	(29%)	5	49	1540	21	45
Salad (no dressing)	560	33	(53%)	9.5	56	1540	22	44
Combination Burrito	420	15	(32%)	7	35	865	19	50
Meat and Potato Burrito	500	25	(45%)	7	25	1340	17	53
Ranch Burrito	450	23	(46%)	8	74	805	18	44
Chicken Fajita Softshell	200	7	(31%)	3	33	905	13	20
Tacos: Crispy	180	11	(59%)	4	26	270	9	12
Softshell	230	10	(39%)	4	26	520	13	23
Bravo	345	14	(37%)	5	28	680	15	39
Burger	280	12	(39%)	5	32	580	15	28
Platters: Per Meal								
Smothered Burrito	1030	40	(35%)	16	70	2350	39	132
Chimichanga	980	38	(35%)	15	59	2340	33	127
Double Enchilada	970	43	(39%)	15	89	1920	42	106
Sampler	1410	61	(39%)	24	126	2875	61	156
Sandwiches								
Sierra Chicken Fillet	535	29	(49%)	8	68	1410	30	40
Kid's Meals: Crispy Taco	580	34	(53%)	10	35	790	13	54
Softshell Taco	620	33	(48%)	10	35	1040	15	64
Specialities: Super Nachos	920	57	(56%)	13	48	1485	26	72
Mexi Rolls w.Nacho Cheese	860	48	(50%)	11	54	1390	30	72
Taco Salad (no dressing)	585	38	(58%)	11	46	770	20	43
Sides: Beans, Refried	360	9	(23%)	2	17	1030	18	53
Chili	350	21	(54%)	10	56	865	20	19
Mexican Rice	570	18	(28%)	5	0	1295	8	40
Nachos	335	21	(56%)	2	0	610	7	27
Nacho Cheese	300	10	(30%)	0	na	600	5	0
Potato Oles:	365	23	(57%)	6	na	965	3	38
Bravo	580	38	(59%)	7	7	1550	11	47
Large	485	30	(56%)	7	na	1285	4	50
w. Nacho Cheese	485	33	(61%)	5.5	na	1565	8	38
Sour Cream, 1 oz	60	5	(75%)	na	na	15	1	1
Desserts: Apple Flauta	85	1	(10%)	0.2	0	75	1	19
Cherry Flauta	145	4	(25%)	0.5	0	110	2	27
Cream Cheese Flauta	180	8	(40%)	3	10	135	2.5	27
Choco Taco	320	17	(48%)	11	20	100	3	38
Churro	150	8	(48%)	2	4	160	2	18
Italian Ice	80	0	(0%)	0	0	5	0	19

TACO TIME

	Cal	Fat (%Fc)	S.Fat	Chol	Sod	Pro	Carb
Burritos: Bean Soft	550	21 (35%)	na	20	1030	22	68
w/o Cheese	460	14 (27%)	na	0	895	17	65
Casita, no Sour Cream/Chse	430	17 (36%)	na	25	1245	23	46
Combo, Soft	550	24 (39%)	na	48	1230	30	55
w/o Cheese	460	14 (27%)	na	0	1095	17	65
Meat Soft, w/o Cheese	470	19 (37%)	na	53	1295	32	40
Veggie	535	20 (34%)	na	20	890	21	71
w/o Sour Cream	500	17 (30%)	na	14	885	21	71
w/o Sour Cream/Cheese	480	13 (25%)	na	0	800	18	69
Cheeseburger, Taco							
no Dressing/Cheese	400	13 (29%)	na	17	1070	20	49
Refried Beans, no Cheese	295	11 (34%)	na	0	835	11	38
Rice, Brown, Mexican	160	2 (11%)	na	0	540	2	28
Taco: Chicken, Soft	390	12 (28%)	na	70	320	31	34
Chicken, Soft, no cheese	335	8 (21%)	na	56	240	29	32
Flour, Soft, no cheese	330	12 (33%)	na	26	600	19	34
Tostada: no Sour Cream/Chse	410	17 (37%)	na	25	915	22	42
Salad: Chicken Taco, no dress.	435	19 (39%)	na	70	520	31	35
Chicken Taco, no dress./chse	380	15 (35%)	na	56	435	29	33
Side Order, no dress./cheese	300	13 (39%)	na	0	715	12	36
Taco, no dressing	350	16 (41%)	na	35	720	23	22
Veggie, no dressing/cheese	300	13 (39%)	na	0	715	12	36
Sauce: Casa	40	0 (0%)	0	0	180	0	10
Enchilada	15	0 (0%)	0	0	115	0	3
Hot	10	0 (0%)	0	0	120	0	2
Ranchero	20	1 (50%)	na	0	115	1	3

TCBY TREATS

	Cal	Fat (%Fc)	S.Fat	Chol	Sod	Pro	Carb
Yogurt: Reg, all flav: Small	210	5 (21%)	3	24	95	6.5	37
Medium	285	6.5 (21%)	4.5	33	135	9	51
Large	365	8.5 (21%)	5.5	42	170	11	64
Hand-Dipped: Small	225	5 (20%)	3	8	130	5	42
Medium	310	6.5 (20%)	4.5	11	175	6.5	57
Large	390	8.5 (20%)	5.5	14	225	9	73
Non-Fat: Small	175	0 (0%)	0	72	95	6.5	37
Medium	240	0 (0%)	0	99	130	9	51
Large	310	0 (0%)	0	126	170	11	64
No Sugar Added N/F: Small	130	0 (0%)	0	5	56	6.5	32
Medium	175	0 (0%)	0	6	77	9	44
Large	225	0 (0%)	0	8	98	11	56
Ice Cream: Small	320	19 (53%)	11	56	115	6	37
Medium	440	26 (53%)	15	77	160	9	50
Large	560	34 (53%)	20	98	200	11	64
Sorbet: Small	160	0 (0%)	0	0	50	0	38
Medium	220	0 (0%)	0	0	65	0	53
Large	280	0 (0%)	0	0	85	0	67
Paradise Ice: Small	315	0 (0%)	0	0	0	0	80
Medium	430	0 (0%)	0	0	0	0	110
Large	550	0 (0%)	0	0	0	0	140

WENDY'S

	Cal	Fat	(%Fc)	S.Fat	Chol	Sod	Pro	Carb
Sandwiches								
Plain Single	360	16	(40%)	6	65	460	25	31
Single with Everything	420	20	(43%)	7	70	810	26	37
Big Bacon Classic	570	29	(46%)	12	100	1320	34	46
Jr. Hamburger	270	10	(33%)	3	30	560	15	34
Jr. Cheeseburger	320	13	(37%)	6	45	770	17	34
Deluxe	360	16	(40%)	6	45	840	18	36
Jr. Bacon Cheeseburger	380	19	(45%)	7	60	790	21	34
Kids' Meal: Hamburger	270	10	(33%)	3	30	560	15	33
Cheeseburger	320	13	(37%)	6	45	770	17	33
Grilled Chicken	310	8	(23%)	2	65	780	27	35
Breaded Chicken	440	18	(37%)	3	60	840	28	44
Chicken Club	470	20	(38%)	4	70	980	31	44
Spicy Chicken	410	15	(33%)	3	65	1280	28	43
Garden Spot Salad Bar								
Applesauce, 2 Tbsp	30	0	(0%)	0	0	0	0	7
Bacon Bits, 2 Tbsp	45	2.5	(50%)	1	10	570	6	0
B'nas & Strawb. Glaze, 1/4 cup	30	0	(0%)	0	0	0	0	8
Broccoli, 1/4 cup	5	0	(0%)	0	0	0	0	1
Cantaloupe, 1 slice	15	0	(0%)	0	0	0	0	4
Carrots, 1/4 cup	5	0	(0%)	0	0	5	0	2
Cauliflower, 1/4 cup	5	0	(0%)	0	0	0	0	1
Chse, shred. (imitation), 2 T.	50	4	(72%)	1	0	230	3	1
Chicken Salad. 2 Tbsp	70	5	(64%)	1	0	135	4	2
Chow Mein Noodles, 1/4 cup	35	2	(51%)	0	0	30	0	4
Cole Slaw, 2 Tbsp	45	3	(60%)	0	5	65	0	5
Cottage Chse, 2 Tbsp	30	1.5	(45%)	1	5	125	4	1
Croutons, 2 Tbsp	30	1	(30%)	0	0	75	0	4
Parmesan Blend, grated, 2 T.	70	4	(51%)	2	10	290	4	5
Pasta Salad, 2 Tbsp	25	0	(0%)	0	0	75	1	3
Peaches, 1 slice	15	0	(0%)	0	0	0	0	4
Pepperoni, 6 slices	30	3	(90%)	1	5	70	1	0
Pineapple, chunked, 4 pieces	20	0	(0%)	0	0	0	0	5
Potato Salad, 2 Tbsp	80	7	(79%)	3	5	180	0	5
Pudding, 1/4 cup: Choc./Vanilla	70	3	(39%)	0.5	0	60	0	10
Red Onions, 3 rings	5	0	(0%)	0	0	0	0	1
Seafood Salad, 1/4 cup	70	4	(51%)	0.5	0	300	3	5
Sesame Breadstick, 1 each	15	0	(0%)	0	0	20	0	2
Strawberries, 1 each	10	0	(0%)	0	0	0	0	2
Sunflower Seeds & Rais.,2 T.	80	5	(56%)	0.5	0	0	0	5
Tomato, wedged, 1 piece	5	0	(0%)	0	0	0	0	1
Turkey Ham, diced, 2 Tbsp	50	4	(72%)	1	25	280	3	0
Salads-To-Go: No Dressing								
Caesar Side	110	5	(41%)	2	10	660	8	8
Deluxe Garden	110	6	(49%)	1	0	320	7	10
Grilled Chicken:	200	8	(36%)	2	50	690	25	10
Caesar	260	10	(35%)	3	60	1210	28	17

WENDY'S CONT

	Cal	Fat	(%Fc)	S.Fat	Chol	Sod	Pro	Carb
Salads (Cont)								
Side Salad	60	3	(45%)	0.5	0	160	4	5
Taco Salad	590	30	(46%)	11	65	1230	29	53
Soft Breadstick	130	3	(21%)	0.5	5	250	4	24
Dressings & Sauces								
Barbeque Sauce, 1 pkt	50	0	(0%)	0	0	100	1	11
Bleu Cheese, 2 Tbsp	170	19	(100%)	3	15	190	1	0
French, 2 Tbsp	120	10	(75%)	2	0	330	0	6
French Fat Free, 2 Tbsp	30	0	(0%)	0	0	150	0	8
French Sweet Red, 2 Tbsp	130	10	(69%)	2	0	230	0	9
Hidden Valley Ranch, 2 Tbsp	90	10	(100%)	2	10	240	0	1
Reduced Fat	60	5	(75%)	1	10	240	0	2
Honey Mustard, 1 pkt	130	12	(83%)	2	10	220	0	6
Italian Caesar, 2 Tbsp	150	16	(96%)	3	20	250	1	1
Italian Red. Fat; 2 Tbsp	40	3	(67%)	0	0	340	0	2
Salad Oil, 1 Tbsp	130	14	(97%)	2	0	0	0	0
Sweet & Sour Sce, 1 pkt	50	0	(0%)	0	0	120	0	12
Thousand Island, 2 Tbsp	130	13	(90%)	2	10	170	0	3
Wine Vinegar, 1 Tbsp	0	0	(0%)	0	0	0	0	0
French Fries								
Small	260	13	(45%)	3	0	85	3	33
Medium	380	19	(45%)	4	0	120	5	47
Biggie	460	23	(45%)	5	0	150	6	58
Baked Potato: Plain	310	0	(0%)	0	0	25	7	71
Bacon & Cheese	540	18	(30%)	4	20	1430	17	78
Broccoli & Cheese	470	14	(27%)	3	5	470	9	80
Cheese	570	23	(36%)	9	30	640	14	78
Chili & Cheese	620	24	(35%)	9	40	780	20	83
Sour Cream & Chives	380	6	(14%)	4	15	40	8	74
Sour Cream, 1 pkt	60	6	(90%)	4	10	15	1	1
Whipped Marg., 1 pkt	60	7	(100%)	1	0	110	0	0
Chili: Small	210	7	(30%)	3	30	800	15	21
Large	310	10	(29%)	4	45	1190	23	32
Cheddar Chse, shred. 2 Tbsp	70	6	(77%)	3	15	110	4	1
Saltine Crackers, 2 ea.	25	0.5	(18%)	0	0	80	0	4
Chicken Nuggets & Wings								
5 Piece	210	14	(60%)	3	50	600	14	12
Spicy Buffalo Wing	25	1	(36%)	0	0	210	0	4
Desserts & Drinks								
Choc. Chip Cookie, 1 Tbsp	270	11	(45%)	8	15	150	4	38
Frosty Dairy Dessert: Small	340	10	(26%)	5	40	200	9	57
Medium	460	13	(25%)	7	55	260	12	76
Large	570	17	(27%)	9	70	330	15	95
Cola, small, 8 oz	90	0	(0%)	0	0	10	0	24
Lemon-Lime, Small	90	0	(0%)	0	0	25	0	24
Lemonade, Small	90	0	(0%)	0	0	5	0	24
Milk (2%), 8 oz	110	4	(33%)	2.5	15	115	8	11
Hot Chocolate, 6 oz	80	3	(34%)	0	0	135	1	15

WEINERSCHNITZEL

	Cal	Fat	(%Fc)	S.Fat	Chol	Sod	Pro	Carb
Breakfast Burrito	570	37	(58%)	13	530	1105	na	na
Breakfast Sando	445	27	(55%)	10	285	1040	na	na
Chicken Sandwich	540	32	(53%)	9	48	960	na	na
Chili Burger	625	40	(58%)	12	96	1350	na	na
Deluxe: Hamburger	580	37	(57%)	12	90	1145	na	na
Cheeseburger	635	42	(59%)	14	103	1350	na	na
Bacon Cheeseburger	690	46	(60%)	16	110	1520	na	na
Hickory Burger	605	37	(55%)	12	90	1215	na	na
Patty Melt	580	35	(54%)	16	108	1330	na	na
Dogs: Chili Dog	295	16	(50%)	5	28	935	na	na
Chili Cheese Dog	350	21	(54%)	8	41	1140	na	na
Corn Dog	290	23	(70%)	8	26	460	na	na
Deluxe Dog	275	14	(45%)	5	21	1620	na	na
Kraut Dog	265	14	(46%)	5	21	1150	na	na
Mustard Dog	260	14	(48%)	5	21	795	na	na
Relish Dog	280	14	(45%)	5	21	900	na	na
Western Dog	380	23	(55%)	9	43	985	na	na
Fries: Small	175	13	(67%)	8	19	345	na	na
Medium	270	21	(70%)	13	30	460	na	na
Large	380	29	(69%)	17	42	690	na	na
Chili Fries	470	36	(69%)	19	64	1000	na	na

WHATABURGER

	Cal	Fat	(%Fc)	S.Fat	Chol	Sod	Pro	Carb
Justaburger	275	11	(36%)	4	34	580	13	30
Whataburger:	600	26	(39%)	9	84	1095	30	61
Small bun, no oil	410	19	(42%)	7	84	840	25	34
Whataburger Jnr.	300	12	(36%)	4	34	580	14	35
Fajitas: Chicken	270	7	(23%)	0.5	33	690	18	35
Beef	325	12	(33%)	3	28	670	22	34
Sandwiches								
Grilled Chicken	440	14	(29%)	3	66	1100	34	48
No Dressing	385	9	(21%)	2	66	990	34	46
w.Mustard, small bun	300	3	(9%)	1	66	990	33	35
Whatachick'n	500	23	(41%)	4	40	1120	27	51
Whatacatch	470	25	(48%)	4	33	630	18	43
Sides: No Dressing								
Baked Potato: Plain	310	0	(0%)	0	0	25	7	72
w. Cheese	510	16	(28%)	8	22	865	15	80
w. Broccoli & Cheese	450	10	(20%)	0	17	635	13	79
Garden Salad	55	0	(0%)	0	0	30	3	11
Grilled Chicken Salad	150	1	(6%)	0.5	49	435	23	14
French Fries: Regular	330	18	(49%)	3	0	210	5	37
Onion Rings: Regular	330	19	(52%)	3	0	595	5	34
Shakes: Vanilla, 12 oz	325	10	(28%)	5	37	170	9	51
Strawberry; Chocolate, 12 oz	350	9	(23%)	5	35	170	9	60

WHITE CASTLE

	Cal	Fat	(%Fc)	S.Fat	Chol	Sod	Pro	Carb
Hamburgers								
Hamburger	160	8	(45%)	na	40	265	6	15
Cheeseburger	200	11	(49%)	na	50	360	8	16
Sandwiches: Chicken	185	7	(34%)	na	80	495	8	20
Fish (w/out Tartar), 1 serving	155	5	(29%)	na	80	200	6	20
Sausage	195	12	(55%)	na	80	490	7	13
Sausage & Egg	320	22	(62%)	na	280	700	13	16
French Fries: regular	300	15	(45%)	na	15	195	2	37
Onion Chips, regular	330	13	(35%)	na	10	825	4	38
Onion Rings, regular	245	16	(59%)	na	10	565	3	26

YOSHINOYA BEEF BOWL

	Cal	Fat	(%Fc)	S.Fat	Chol	Sod	Pro	Carb
Bowls								
Beef Bowl: Regular, 13 oz	720	29	(36%)	12	80	1130	31	87
Large, 18 oz	1020	40	(33%)	16	110	1640	45	127
Combo Bowl, 25 oz	1160	32	(25%)	13	110	2250	52	147
Teriyaki Chicken: Reg., 17 oz	640	11	(15%)	4	60	1440	31	105
Large, 28 oz	975	17	(15%)	6	80	2400	47	156
Teriyaki Steak: Regular, 17 oz	720	20	(25%)	11	60	1400	31	105
Large, 28 oz	1080	31	(26%)	6	80	2330	47	155
Vegetable Bowl:								
Regular, 16 1/2 oz	410	1	(2%)	0	0	880	8	93
Large, 29 oz	630	1.5	(1%)	0	0	1730	13	143
Vegetable Beef Bowl:								
Regular, 16 oz	650	21	(29%)	6	80	1250	25	91
Large, 22 oz	950	30	(28%)	12	80	2000	35	137
Extras								
Beef, 5 1/2 oz	370	26	(67%)	12	60	1200	25	6
Chicken & Vegetables, 10 oz	290	10	(31%)	4	50	140	25	24
Rice, 7 1/2 oz	350	1	(1%)	0	0	40	6	81
Steak & Vegetables, 10 oz	370	19	(45%)	11	60	1380	25	24
Vegetable, 9 oz	60	0	(0%)	0	0	840	2	12

Note: Yoshinoya Beef Bowl Restaurants are based in California.

ZANTIAGO

	Cal	Fat	(%Fc)	S.Fat	Chol	Sod	Pro	Carb
Burrito								
Hot Cheese, Chilito	329	15	(41%)	na	na	466	14	35
Mild Cheese, Chilito	330	15	(41%)	na	na	505	14	36
Enchilada: Beef	315	15	(43%)	na	na	904	18	26
Cheese	390	23	(53%)	na	na	759	20	26
Taco: Burrito	415	19	(41%)	na	na	815	21	41
Regular	198	12	(55%)	na	na	318	10	13

FATS & CHOLESTEROL GUIDE

NOTES ON CHOLESTEROL

- **Cholesterol** is a white waxy substance produced mainly by our liver. It is also found in animal food products. Plant foods have no cholesterol.

- **Cholesterol is essential to life.** It is a structural part of every body cell wall and is the building block for vitamin D, sex hormones, and bile acids which help in the digestion of dietary fats.

- **The body makes sufficient cholesterol for its needs** and does not rely on cholesterol in the diet. Dietary fats have a major influence on blood cholesterol levels - moreso than dietary cholesterol.

- **A high blood cholesterol increases the risk of atherosclerosis** - the thickening of arteries that can reduce or block blood flow to the heart muscle, brain, eyes, kidneys, sex organs and other body parts.

  This in turn increases the risk of heart attack, stroke, blindness, kidney failure, impotence and other blood circulatory problems.

- **Other risk factors** which increase the risk of atherosclerosis include high blood pressure, tobacco smoking, obesity and diabetes (uncontrolled).

BLOOD CHOLESTEROL
Check Your Risk

Cholesterol Level (mg per deciliter)	Risk of Heart Attack
240 and above	~ High Risk
200 - 239	~ Borderline/High
Below 200	~ Desirable

- Know your cholesterol level, particularly if there is a family history of heart disease or stroke. If high, see your doctor for advice.

- All adults should have their cholesterol, HDL, and triglycerides tested at least every 5 years.

HEART ATTACK WARNING SIGNALS

Many victims die before reaching hospital by ignoring warning signals and delaying medical help. Symptoms vary and commonly include:

- Chest pain, vice-like squeezing or burning sensation in centre of chest or between shoulder blades, or feeling of severe indigestion.
- Pain may spread to shoulders, neck, jaw or arms.
- Sweating, nausea, dizziness, shortness of breath, irregular pulse.

If you experience any of the above symptoms seek IMMEDIATE medical attention! Every minute counts.

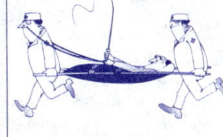

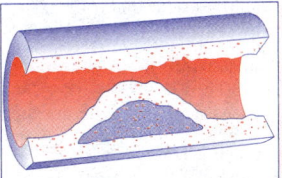

▲ *Atherosclerosis can clog arteries and impede blood flow to the heart muscle or other body organs.*

▲ *A thrombus (blood clot) can form on unstable, festering atherosclerotic plaque and rapidly block blood flow. A heart attack or stroke can result.*

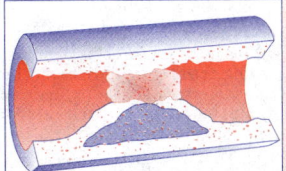

FATS & BLOOD CHOLESTEROL

The amount and type of dietary fat has the greatest influence on blood cholesterol levels.

♦ **Fats in food are a mixture of 3 basic types:** saturated, monounsaturated, and polyunsaturated. Animal fats are mainly saturated while plant oils and fish oils are mainly mono- and polyunsaturated.

♦ **Saturated fats** have subgroups known as long chain, medium chain, and short chain fats. Most of the long chain fats raise blood cholesterol; and increase the risk of blood clots and thrombosis leading to artery blockage.

Long chain saturated fats are found mainly in full cream milk, cheese, butter, cream, fatty meats and sausages, and processed foods.

♦ **Monounsaturated fats** tend to more selectively lower 'bad' LDL-cholesterol and maintain the protective 'good' HDL-cholesterol in the bloodstream - but only if they replace saturated fats in the diet.

Foods rich in monounsaturates include canola and olive oils, canola margarine, peanuts, and avocados.

♦ **Polyunsaturated fats** consist of two main classes. **Omega-6** polyunsaturates tend to lower blood cholesterol. Rich sources include safflower, sunflower and corn oils.

♦ **Omega-3** polyunsaturated fats can lower blood cholesterol, and also confer extra benefits by lowering blood triglycerides, and reducing the risk of thrombosis, heart arrhythmias, and artery spasm.

Best practical omega-3 sources include canola oil and margarine, soybean oil and fish. (See adjoining chart)

♦ **A balanced intake** of the two omega classes is important for optimal health. Increasing slightly omega-3 intake by Americans would help to attain a more ideal balance. Adequate vitamin E intake is also important.

Note: All fats are high in calories and need to be limited for weight control.

DIETARY FATS COMPARISON

- Saturated Fat
- Monounsaturated Fat
- Linoleic (Omega-6)
- Alpha-Linolenic (Omega-3)

OILS - PERCENTAGE CONTENT

Oil	Saturated	Monounsaturated	Linoleic (Omega-6)	Alpha-Linolenic (Omega-3)
CANOLA OIL	7	63	20	10
LINSEED/FLAX OIL	9	19	17	55
SAFFLOWER OIL	9	14	77	
GRAPESEED OIL	10	22	68	
SUNFLOWER OIL	11	23	66	
CORN OIL	14	32	52	2
OLIVE OIL	14	76	10	
SOYBEAN OIL	15	23	54	8
PEANUT OIL	19	45	34	2
COTTONSEED OIL	26	16	58	
PALM OIL	51	39	10	

SPREADS & FATS
Saturated Fat includes 'Trans Fats' ❏ Water Content

	Saturated	Mono	Omega-6	Omega-3	Water
LIGHT MARGARINE	14	14	21		51
CANOLA MARGARINE	18	45	12	6	19
POLYUNSATURATED MARG.	24	20	36		20
BUTTER	57	18	2		24
LARD	41	47	12		
BEEF FAT	44	37	4		15

GOOD SOURCES OF OMEGA-3 FATS

PLANT SOURCES Omega-3 Fats (Grams)

Canola Oil, 1 Tbsp, 1/2 fl oz	1.5g
Flaxseed Oil, 1 Tbsp,	8g
Soybean Oil, 1 Tbsp	1.2g
Canola Margarine, 1 Tbsp, 1/2 oz	1g
Soybeans, cooked, 1/2 cup, 4 oz	0.5g
Walnuts, 1/2 oz	0.5g

FISH - Per 4 oz Serving:

High Content: Salmon (Chinook), Tuna, Trout (Lake), Sardines, Herring, Mackerel	3g 3g
Medium Content: Salmon (Pink/Red/Coho), 4 oz	2g
Fair Content: - Per 4 oz Serving: Bass, Catfish, Cod, Grouper, Hake, Halibut, Kingfish, Perch, Pollock, Shark, Trout (rainbow), Tuna (Skipjack), Crab, Oysters, Blue Mussel, Shrimp, Squid	0.5-1g

HOW MUCH IS NEEDED?

As little as 1-2 grams daily of omega-3 fats may benefit general health. High doses of fish oil supplements should only be taken as directed by your doctor.

CHOLESTEROL IN FOOD

DIETARY CHOLESTEROL

Cholesterol in food varies in its effect on blood cholesterol level (BCL) from person to person. Much depends on the amount and type of fat, and fiber eaten at the same meal.

Any elevating effect of dietary cholesterol on BCL is more likely to occur when the diet is high in saturated fat. Little elevation, if any, generally occurs when dietary fats are balanced in favour of mono- and polyunsaturated fats (including omega-3 fats).

For example, while fish does contain cholesterol, the omega-3 fats can prevent any increase in BCL. Conversely, a meal containing no cholesterol but rich in saturated fat, may see a significant increase in BCL.

Consequently, the need to be overly concerned about dietary cholesterol is being de-emphasised in favour of a stricter approach to limiting total fats, and saturated fat in particular.

The liver usually cuts back its own cholesterol production in response to cholesterol in the diet. Perhaps 3 out of 4 people, or more, can consume normal amounts of high cholesterol foods without concern.

However, it is difficult to identify just who is at risk - the so-called 'hyper-responders' - and because over 50% of Americans have a BCL above ideal levels, the **American Heart Association** advises all Americans to be prudent and limit their cholesterol intake to less than 300mg daily.

This limitation still allows the inclusion of most foods regularly eaten - even the overly maligned egg.

Note: Eggs contain a modest 5 grams of fat per large egg of which barely 2 grams are saturated, the rest being mono- and polyunsaturated. By comparison, a cup of whole milk has almost 10g fat of which 6g are saturated.

CHOLESTEROL COUNTER

- Cholesterol is found only in foods of animal origin. Plant foods contain no cholesterol.
- AHA recommends limiting dietary cholesterol to less than 300mg/day.

Cholesterol (mg)

Food	Cholesterol (mg)
Meat - Average all types:	
Lean Meat, cooked, 4 oz	70
Fatty Meat, cooked, 4 oz	105
Fat, thick strip, 2 oz	35

(Note: While lean meat and fat have similar amounts of cholesterol, choose lean meat to limit fat intake.)

Food	Cholesterol (mg)
Chicken/Turkey, average, 4 oz	90
Organ Meats: Liver, fried, 4 oz	500
Brains, beef, pan fried, 3 oz	1700
Sausages: Frankfurter, 1.5 oz	25
Salami, 2 slices, 2 oz	40
Bacon: 3 slices, cooked, 1 oz	20
Fish: Fish fillets, average, ckd, 4 oz	70
Tuna/Salmon, canned, 3 oz	30
Scallops, 9 medium, 3 oz	30
Shrimp, 12 large, raw, 3 oz	130
Oysters, raw, 6 medium, 3 oz	45
Lobster, Crab, raw, 3 oz	80
Eggs (Chicken), 1 large	210
1 medium	180
Egg White, Egg Beaters	0
Milk/Yogurt: Whole, 1 cup, 8 fl oz	35
1% Milk, 1 cup	10
Skim/Non-fat, 1 cup	5
Soy Milk	0
Cheese: Natural/Hard/Cream 1 oz	30
Cottage, lowfat, 4 oz	5
Ricotta, part skim, 4 oz	25
Fats: Butter, 2 Tbsp, 1 oz	60
Margarine, Oils (vegetable)	0
Mayonnaise, 1 Tbsp	10
Cream: Heavy, whipping, 2 T, 1 oz	40
Half & Half/Sour, 2 Tbsp, 1 oz	10
Icecream: Regular, 1/3 cup, 4 fl oz	30
Fruit, Vegetables, Avocados	0
Nuts, Seeds, Grains	0
Coffee, Tea, Soda, Beer, Wine	0

FAST FOODS - See Fast Food Section

BLOOD CHOLESTEROL CONTROL

DIETARY HINTS TO LOWER BLOOD CHOLESTEROL

1. Maintain a healthy weight.
If overweight, lose weight with lowfat eating and daily exercise.

2. Reduce saturated fat intake by:

(a) eating less dairy fat. Choose lowfat or fat-reduced varieties of milk, yogurt, cheese, and icecream. Enjoy soy drinks.

(b) replacing saturated fats with fats and oils rich in mono- and polyunsaturated fats; and carbohydrate-rich foods. Choose margarine instead of butter; and vegetable oils such as canola, olive, sunflower, soybean. Avoid solid frying fats.

(c) eating less fat from meat and poultry. Choose lean cuts of meat and skinless chicken. Go easy on luncheon meats, salamis and fatty sausages. Enjoy fish.

(d) eating less saturated fats from baked and fried fast-foods. Avoid deep-fried foods. Go easy on donuts, cakes, pastries, cookies. Choose lower fat fast-foods. Homemade foods and recipes using healthier fats and oils are preferable.

3. Increase your 'soluble' fiber intake.

Foods rich in 'soluble' fiber include dried beans, baked beans, lentils, chick peas, hummus, nuts and seeds.

Highest in soluble fiber are psyllium seed husks, psyllium-based cereals and psyllium fiber supplements.

Oat bran, rice bran and barley are also useful, as are fruit, veges and avocados.

4. Eat more soya bean products such as: soy drinks, tofu, tempeh (cultured soya beans), soy flour, soy vegetarian foods.

Soy protein in place of animal protein can significantly decrease high blood cholesterol levels - as well as 'bad' LDL-cholesterol and blood triglycerides. 'Good' HDL-cholesterol is maintained.

At least 25g of soy protein (from 3-4 servings of soy products) per day should be consumed for best results.

5. Eat more fruit and vegetables in place of high fat foods.

Aim for 2 fruits and 5 servings of vegetables per day. They also contain valuable antioxidants.
The fat of avocados is mainly unsaturated and lowers blood cholesterol levels.

Garlic helps to lower blood cholesterol, and inhibit thrombosis.
Note: Garlic supplements (such as *Kyolic*, *Kwai*) can prevent the increase in 'bad' LDL- cholesterol resulting from fish oil supplements. Take at the same time.

6. Limit cholesterol to 300mg per day.
(Extra Notes ~ See Pevious Page)

7. Avoid brewed unfiltered coffee (espresso; plunger-style). It contains oil compounds (diterpenes) which can raise blood cholesterol. American style filtered coffee is fine.

8. Spread your food intake over the day.
Have 5-6 small meals per day rather than just 2-3 large meals. Nibbling, versus gorging, favors lower blood cholesterol.

ALCOHOL • WINE

Alcohol is a mixed bag. Moderate amounts of 2-3 drinks daily appear to reduce the risk of heart attack and ischaemic stroke.

However, larger amounts increase the risk of high blood pressure, obesity, heart failure and hemorrhagic stroke; and can aggravate hypertriglyceridemia - in addition to many other health hazards. *(See Alcohol Guide - p.128)*

The over-riding harmful effects of excess alcohol do not allow its recommendation for any aspects of health promotion.

Note: Red wine (moreso than white) contains antioxidants which may help protect cholesterol in the blood from becoming oxidized. Many fruits, vegetables and tea also contain protective antioxidants.

HOW FATS AFFECT BLOOD FLOW

Fats in the diet not only affect blood cholesterol levels. They can also strongly influence blood clot formation and thrombosis, as well as blood flow and ultimate oxygen delivery to body parts and organs.

While advanced atherosclerosis can impede blood flow to the heart and other organs, it is thrombosis (complete blockage by blood clots) or arterial spasm which commonly result in a heart attack or stroke.

Plant and fish oils rich in omega-3 fats lessen the risk of blood clots, thrombus formation and artery spasm by reducing platelet stickiness and adhesion to artery walls. This reduces the risk of atherosclerotic plaque becoming unstable and reactive.

Omega-3 fats also improve blood flow by reducing blood viscosity; and increasing the flexibility of red blood cells (**RBC**) that need to flex and twist on themselves in order to squeeze through tiny narrow capillaries often half their diameter.

A diet high in saturated fats has the opposite effect by stiffening RBC membranes and increasing blood viscosity thereby hindering blood flow. The stiffening of the RBC membrane also reduces its ability to release vital oxygen to body cells and take up carbon dioxide.

Stiff red blood cells may also form aggregates like coin stacks called rouleaux. In narrow blood vessels, this further impedes blood flow and impairs oxygen release through the much lessened surface area of red blood cell membranes exposed to blood. (Smoking, lack of exercise, and stress can have similar adverse effects on thrombosis, red blood cell flexibility and blood flow.)

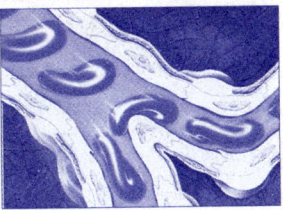

▲ *A picture of healthy blood flow.*
Flexible red blood cells twist and slide through tiny capillaries - often half the diameter of red blood cells.

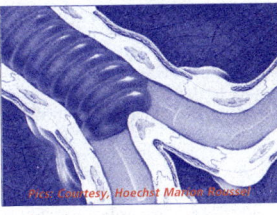

Pics: Courtesy, Hoechst Marion Roussel

▲ *A not-so-healthy picture!*
Red blood cells have lost their flexibility and ability to twist and slip through capillaries. They are stacked up thereby impeding blood flow.

A diet high in saturated fats can contribute to this picture - as can smoking, lack of exercise and stress.

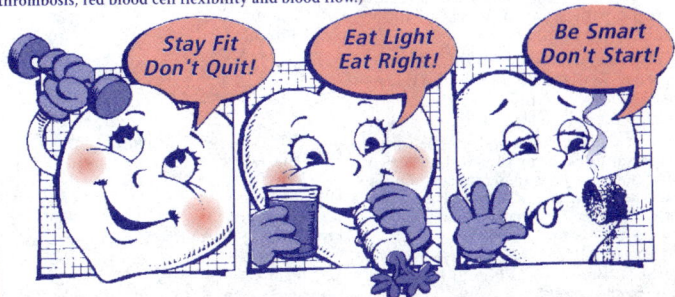

CAFFEINE GUIDE & COUNTER

- **Moderate caffeine intake** is probably not harmful to healthy adults. However, regular large amounts (over 350mg/day) may cause dependency ('caffeinism') and adversely affect health.

- **Symptoms of excessive caffeine** intake include chronic insomnia, persistent anxiety and depression, restlessness, heart palpitations, stomach upset and increased need to urinate. (It can take 4-6 hours for caffeine's effects to wear off.)

- **High caffeine intake**, combined with nicotine and alcohol may increase the risk in men of sperm damage, infertility, and birth defects in their children; and may in women, reduce their fertility.

- **Caffeine-withdrawal** headaches, fatigue and irritability are more commonly experienced on weekends when any heavy coffee drinking at work is suddenly reduced. Such headaches are relieved by drinking coffee. As little as 100-200 mg caffeine daily can produce withdrawal effects. (Withdrawal symptoms only last one week or less.) Reduce gradually.

- **Sensitivity to caffeine** may increase during pregnancy and with age. To be safe, limit caffeine to 200mg/day.

- **Persons wise to avoid caffeine** entirely include those who get irritable and jittery from just one cup of coffee, pregnant and nursing women, children under eight, people with stomach ulcers or heart arrhythmia condition.

- **Large amounts of cola drinks** (1-2 litres per day) as well as coffee may also lead to excessive caffeine intake, particularly in children. Caffeine-free colas are available.

Notes: 1. Blood cholesterol can be raised by several drinks daily of boiled unfiltered coffee (such as espresso and cafetiere/plunger pot style). American-style filtered coffee does not contain the oil compounds (diterpenes) which appear to raise blood cholesterol.

2. Coffee does not sober up an inebriated person. It simply turns him or her into a wide-awake drunk!

	Caffeine (mg)
COFFEE	
Instant Coffee:	
Weak, 1 level tsp	45
Medium, 1 rounded tsp	60
Strong, 1 heaping tsp	90
Decaffeinated, 1 rnd tsp	2
Bags(Folgers), 1 bag (6-8 fl.oz)	115
Decaffeinated, 1 bag	3
Brewed: Percolator, 8 oz cup	120
Drip Method, 8 oz cup	160
Ground, 1 Tbsp, 6g	60
Decaffeinated, 1 Tbsp	2
FLAVORED COFFEE MIXES	
Coffee with Chicory, 1 rd tsp	40
General Foods: Irish Mocha Mint	25
Orange Cappuccino	70
Other flavors, average	50
COFFEE SHOP STYLE	
Coffee: Drip-brew, average, 8 fl. oz	160
Percolated, 8 fl. oz	120
Cappuccino, 8 fl. oz	80
Decappuccino (decaffeinated)	5
Espresso: Regular/Solo	80
Double (Doppio) Espresso	160
Latte/Macchiato	80
Iced Coffee, 8 fl. oz	80
Mocha, 8 fl. oz	90
Vienna Coffee, 8 fl. oz	80
Cocoa, 8 fl. oz	10
STARBUCKS (Franchise Chain)	
Drip Coffee: Short, 8 fl. oz	140
Tall, 12 fl. oz	210
Grande, 16 fl. oz	280
Coffee Decaf: Tall	10
Cappuccino: Short or Tall	70
Grande	100
Caffe Americano: Short	75
Tall	150
Grande	220
Caffe Latte, Short or Tall	75
Grande	150
Cafe Mocha, Short or Tall	85
Grande	170
Espresso (Reg./Macchiato): Solo	75
Doppio	150
Decaf	5
Frappuccino, Reg./Mocha, Tall	75

CAFFEINE COUNTER (CONT)

COFFEE ALTERNATIVES	Caffeine (mg)
(Roasted Cereals - Caffeine-Free)	
Kaffree Roma/Postum/Teeccino Caffe	0
TEA	
Brewed or Tea Bags: Weak, 1 cup	20
Medium Strength	40
Strong	70
Instant Tea Powder: 1 tsp	30
w. lemon flavor, 1 tsp	25
+ sugar, 3 rnd tsp	30
Decaffeinated Tea (*Kaffree*)	1
Herbal Tea	0
Iced Tea, regular: 8 oz Glass	20
12 oz Glass	30
16 oz Glass	40
Flavored Teas, Ready to drink, Average, 12 fl.oz	25
COLA SOFT DRINKS: *Per 12 fl. oz*	
Coca Cola: Can/Bottle	30
Fountain/Restaurant	38
Diet Coke: Can/Bottle	40
Fountain/Restaurant	45
Pepsi: Can/Bottle	32
Fountain/Restaurant	37
Diet Pepsi: Can/Bottle	30
Fountain/Restaurant	37
Caffeine Free Coke/Pepsi	0
OTHER COLAS: *Per 12 fl. oz*	
Cherry Coke	35
Cherry Cola (Shasta)	40
Diet Rite Cola	48
Jolt Cola	55
K-Mart Amer. Fare Cola/Diet	12
Kroger Big K Cola	5
Diet Cola	30
Pepsi Kona	55
RC Cola	43
Diet RC Cola	50
Shasta Cola	42
Diet Shasta Cola	37
Slice Cola	10
Slice: Dr. Slice, Cherry Spice, Red	35
Surge	53
TAB	50
Wal-Mart Sam's Choice/Diet	12
Wild Cherry Pepsi	38
Winn-Dixie Chek Cola	8

NON-COLA SOFT DRINKS	Caffeine (mg)
Per 12 fl. oz Can/Bottle	
National: Cherry Spice; Dr Slice	35
Dr Pepper, Reg./Diet	42
Josta (Pepsi)	60
Kick	55
Mello Yellow	50
Mountain Dew, Reg./Diet	55
Mr PiBB, Reg./Diet	43
Red	35
Sunkist Orange	43
Caffeinated Water: Water Joe, 12 fl.oz	53
Average other brands, 12 fl.oz	50
Store Brands - Non- Cola Drinks	
Kroger Big K Citrus Drop, Reg./Diet	26
Kroger Dr K, Reg/Diet	17
Wal-Mart Sam's Choice:	
Southern Lightning	30
Green Lightning	50
Winn-Dixie: Dr Chek	18
Chek Kountry Mist	53
CHOCOLATE/COCOA	
Chocolate: Milk Choc., 2 oz	20
Dark Chocolate, 2 oz	35
Choc Chips, 1/4 cup., 1.5 oz	15
Bakers, semi-sweet,, 2 oz	35
Candy Bars, average, 1.5 oz	10
Cocoa, dry, unsw. 1 Tbsp, 5g	12
Cocoa/Hot Choc. Mix, 1 oz pkt	5
Chocolate Milk, 8 fl. oz	8
Chocolate. Cake, 1 pce	10
Choc Chip Cookie, 1 oz	4
Chocolate Icing, 1 serving	5
Chocolate Icecream, 1/2 cup	2
Chocolate Pudding, 1/2 cup	5
Chocolate Syrup, 2 Tbsp	6
PHARMACEUTICALS & GUARANA	
Anacin/Empirin/Midol, 2 tabs	65
Aqua-Ban (diuretic), 2 tabs	200
Dexatrim (weight control), 1 tab	200
Excedrin, 2 tablets	130
NoDoz: Regular Strength, 1 tab	100
Maximum Strength, 1 tab	200
Vivarin, 1 tablet	200
Guarana: Powder, 1 tsp, 3 g	120
Tablet/Capsules (800mg), 1	30
Drinks/Soda, average, 12 fl.oz	50

OSTEOPOROSIS GUIDE

CALCIUM'S ROLE IN THE BODY

Calcium plays a vital role in nerve and muscle function, clotting of blood, enzyme regulation, insulin secretion and overall bone strength. Bones and teeth store 99% of the body's calcium.

The calcium level in blood is kept at a steady level by the continual exchange of calcium between blood and bone. When insufficient calcium is obtained from food the body draws calcium out of the bones.

This bone loss over a period of years may lead to **osteoporosis** - thinning of the bones (*porous bones*).

The bones become weak, brittle and easy to fracture, particularly the bones of the wrist, hips and spine. Loss of height and curvature of the spine may also result, as may periodontal disease - the deterioration of the jaw bones that support the teeth.

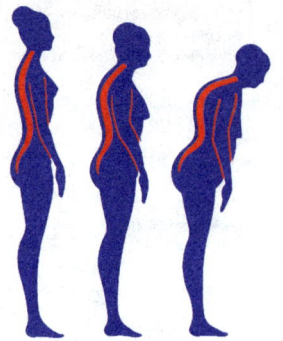

As osteoporosis progresses after menopause, vertebrae may collapse causing the spine to curve and shoulders to hunch.

COMMON IN WOMEN

While osteoporosis also occurs in men, women are particularly vulnerable (1 in 4 by age 60). They have about 30% less bone than men, and a greater bone loss at menopause when estrogen levels drop. Slender framed women are at greater risk. (A woman in her eighties can have lost up to two thirds of her skeleton.)

Insufficient dietary calcium during pregnancy and breastfeeding will see bone reserves drawn upon, increasing the risk of osteoporosis.

CAUSES OF OSTEOPOROSIS

The major factors associated with the bone loss of osteoporosis appear to be:

- Hormone changes of menopause.
- Insufficient calcium in the diet. (Absorption of dietary calcium decreases with age.)
- Insufficient exercise (weight bearing - such as walking, cycling.)
- Family history of osteoporosis.

Other contributing factors may include: excess amounts of alcohol, caffeine, protein and phosphorus (from meats and soft drinks); insufficient vitamin D (the 'sunshine' vitamin); and cigarette smoking.

RECOMMENDED DAILY INTAKE OF CALCIUM

		CALCIUM
Infants:		
	0-6 mths	360mg
	6-12 mths	540mg
Children:		
	1-10 yrs	800mg
	10-12 yrs	1200mg
Teenagers:		
	13-18 yrs	1200mg
	16-18 yrs	800mg
Adults:		
	19+ yrs	800mg
Women:		
Pre-menopausal		1000mg
Menopausal (beginning)		1200mg
Post-menopausal		1500mg
Pregnancy/breastfeeding:		
	10-18 yrs	1600mg
	19+ yrs	1200mg

OSTEOPOROSIS GUIDE

EARLY PREVENTION IMPORTANT

Gradual loss of bone begins in the thirties after maximum bone mass is reached. The stronger the bones at that time, the less trouble is likely to occur later. The earlier that prevention or treatment begins the greater the benefit. **The key to prevention** is to build strong, dense bones early in life. **By age 16**, some 80% of peak bone mass is reached.

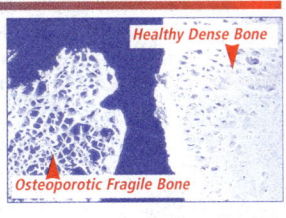

Healthy Dense Bone
Osteoporotic Fragile Bone

Young women may lessen the risk by eating high-calcium foods, not engaging in excessive dieting that results in period cessation (less estrogen), taking regular exercise and not smoking.

In menopausal women, hormone therapy as well as calcium supplements and exercise, can help retard osteoporosis. Your doctor can advise you.

Note: While dietary calcium cannot reverse age-related bone loss, it can slow down the process.

DIETARY SOURCES OF CALCIUM

Milk, yogurt, calcium-enriched soy drinks and cheese are the richest sources of calcium. (Lowfat and nonfat varieties contain similar calcium.)

Canned fish with edible bones (salmon/sardines) are high in calcium. Tofu (soybean curd), tempeh, broccoli and dried beans are also good sources.

Note: Soy drinks (calcium-enriched) may be preferable to cow's milk. Body calcium losses are much greater with animal protein. Soy protein is relatively 'bone-sparing'. Phytoestrogens in soy foods may also lessen calcium losses at menopause. Soy drinks are suitable for persons with lactose intolerance.

EXTRA NOTES ON CALCIUM

- Persons who have difficulty eating sufficient calcium-rich foods should consider a **calcium supplement**. Prescribed high doses of calcium (1.5-2g/day) may benefit persons with osteoporosis - as well as vitamin D (up to 400 IU), and magnesium (100mg).

- **Calcium in food reduces iron absorption** by up to 60% when eaten with iron-containing foods. Consume calcium-rich foods/supplements at smaller meals and mid-meal snacks. (Only the first 150-200mg calcium inhibits iron absorption.)

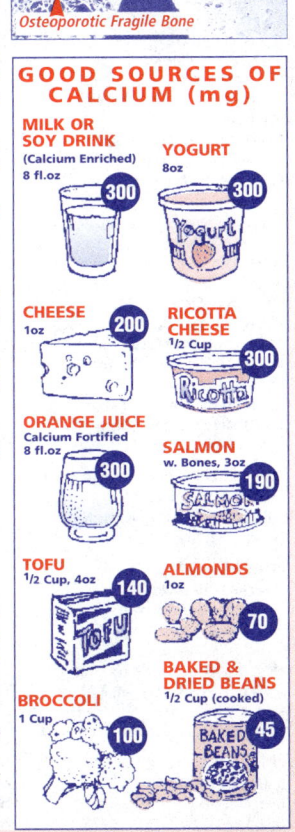

GOOD SOURCES OF CALCIUM (mg)

- MILK OR SOY DRINK (Calcium Enriched) 8 fl.oz — 300
- YOGURT 8oz — 300
- CHEESE 1oz — 200
- RICOTTA CHEESE 1/2 Cup — 300
- ORANGE JUICE Calcium Fortified 8 fl.oz — 300
- SALMON w. Bones, 3oz — 190
- TOFU 1/2 Cup, 4oz — 140
- ALMONDS 1oz — 70
- BROCCOLI 1 Cup — 100
- BAKED & DRIED BEANS 1/2 Cup (cooked) — 45

CALCIUM COUNTER

Daily Calcium Requirements - See Page 226.
Calcium Counter figures are rounded.

MILK & MILK DRINKS	Calcium (mg)
Milk Fluid:	
Whole: 1 cup, 8 fl.oz	300
1 small glass, 6 fl.oz	220
1% or 2%: 1 cup, 8 fl.oz	300
Lowfat/Skim: 1 cup, 8 fl.oz	300
Hi-Calcium (*Borden*), 1 cup	1000
Viva, w.extra Calcium, 1 cup	500
Condensed Milk, sweet, 1 fl.oz	110
Evaporated Milk, Skim, 1 fl.oz	90
Whole/Lowfat	80
Dry/Powder: Whole 1/4 cup	290
Skim/Nonfat, 1/4 cup	380
Other Milks & Drinks	
Buttermilk, average, 1 cup	300
Chocolate Milk, average, 1 cup	300
Cocoa/Chocolate w. Milk, 1 cup	300
Goats Milk, 1 cup	320
Malted Milk, 1 cup	350
Milkshakes: Small, 10 fl.oz	280
Medium, 15 fl.oz	450
Milk Drink Powders:	
Malted Milk, dry powder, 1oz	80
Chocolate, Instant, 3 Tbsp	10
Cocoa Powder: regular, 1 Tbsp	10
Cocoa Mix: *Hershey*, 1/3 cup	40
Alba High Calcium, 1 envelope	320
SOY DRINKS - Per 1 Cup, 8 fl.oz	
Regular, non-fortified	60
Calcium-fortified (*e.g. Edensoy Extra*)	300
Dry Powder, 1 oz	80
YOGURT	
Average All Brands	350
Fruit-flavored, 1 cup, 8 oz	250
Small cup, 6 oz	230
4 1/2 oz cup	350
Plain: Average, 1 cup, 8 oz	430
Dannon, Nonfat/Lowfat, 8 oz	200
Custard-style, 6 oz	100
Frozen Yogurt, average, 1/2 cup	100
FATS/OILS	
Butter, Lard, fats	Negl
Margarine, Regular/Imitation	Negl
Oils, Salad Dressings	Negl

CREAM	Calcium (mg)
Average: Unwhipped, 1 Tbsp	15
Whipped, 1 heaping Tbsp	15
Half & Half, 1 Tbsp	15
Non-dairy Creamers, 1 tsp	Negl
ICE CREAM & ICES	
Ice Cream: Regular, 1 scoop	65
1/2 cup	90
Premium, 1 serve, 4 oz	150
Soft Serve, 1/2 cup	120
Ice Milk, average, 1/2 cup	100
Sherbet, average, 1/2 cup	50
Fruit Sorbet	0
Sundae, regular, 6 fl.oz	200
Tofu Ices, average, 1/2 cup	10
CHEESE: Per 1 oz (1 1/2" cube)	
Natural, Hard: Average 1 oz	200
Processes Cheese: Average, 1 oz	150
Single-wrapped, 3/4 oz	120
Cheese Substitutes: Aveage,. 1 oz	200
Specific Cheeses: Blue, 1 oz	150
Brie	50
Camembert	110
Cheddar	200
Cottage Cheese: 1 rnd Tbsp, 1 oz	20
1/2 cup, 4 oz	80
Cream Cheese	20
Dorman's Light, average 1 oz	200
Edam, Gouda	200
Feta	140
Goat, semi-soft	85
Gruyere	290
Kraft Light Naturals, aver.	250
Light-Line (*Borden*), singles	200
Monterey Jack	210
Mozzarella, average	170
Parmesan, grated, 1 Tbsp	70
Processed, average	160
Provolone	210
Ricotta, part skim, 1/2 cup	330
Swiss	270
Cheese Dishes: Souffle, 4 oz	240
Macaroni & Cheese, 1 cup, 8 oz	150
Ham & Cheese Crepes, 8 oz	350
Quiche, 1 serve, 6 oz	200

CALCIUM COUNTER

EGGS	Calcium (mg)
1 large Egg	30
Scrambled, w. Milk	50
Omelet, w. Cheese (1/2 oz)	260

FISH & SEAFOODS
Canned Fish:

Salmon, with bones, 3 oz	190
without bones, 3 oz	10
Sardines, with bones, 3 oz	90
Tuna, canned, 3 oz	10
Fresh Fish: cooked, average, 4 oz	35
Lobster, cooked, 4 oz	60
Mussels/Oysters, (10), 4 oz	95
Crabmeat, cooked, 4 oz	50

MEATS & POULTRY
Average all types, cooked, 4 oz	20

SOUPS
Average all types:

No Milk or Cheese added, 1 serve	30
with Milk, 1/2 cup, 1 serve	180

SAUCES
Average all kinds, 1 Tbsp	10
Cheese/White Sauce, 2 Tbsp	40

SPICES & HERBS
Average all types, 1 tsp	5-20

BREAD, BAGELS
Bread: White, 1 slice	30
Wholewheat, Rye, 1 slice	30
Bagels, average	30
Buns/Rolls: Small	40
Large	90
English Muffins, 2 oz	90
Pita, 6 1/2" diameter, 2 oz	50
Tortillas, Corn, 1 oz	40

BREAKFAST CEREALS
Ready To Eat:

Average all types, 1 oz	20
with 3/4 cup Milk/Soy (enriched)	250
Hot Type, cooked	
Corn (Hominy) Grits, 1 cup	Negl
Cream of Wheat, 1 cup	50
Malt-O-Meal, 1 cup	5
Oatmeal/Rolled Oats:	
Regular, non-fortified, 1 cup	20
Instant, fortified, 1 pkt	100

Note: Breakfast cereals are a good medium for calcium-rich milk or soy drinks (150mg per 1/2 cup).

FLOURS, GRAINS, PASTA

	Calcium (mg)
Wheat Flour: All-purpose, 1 cup	20
Self-rising, 1 cup	330
Whole-wheat, 1 cup	50
Carob Flour, 1 cup, 3 1/2 oz	360
Corn meal, 1 cup, 4 oz	20
Soybean Flour, 1 cup, 3 oz	170
Grains, Barley, Rice, average:	
Cooked, 1 cup	15
Macaroni, Noodles, cookd, 1 cup	15
Macaroni & Cheese, aver., 1 cup	150
Pasta, Spaghetti, average:	
Cooked, 1 cup	15
Lasagne, average, 1 serve	300
Spaghetti w. Meat Sce, 1 serve	20
with 1 Tbsp Parmesan	90

SUGAR & SYRUPS
Sugar: White	0
Brown, 1 Tbsp	10
Syrups: Per 2 Tbsp, 1 oz	
Choc., Thin type, 2 Tbsp	5
Fudge type, 2 Tbsp	40
Molasses: Light, 2 Tbsp	70
Blackstrap, 2 Tbsp	270
Table Syrup, 2 Tbsp	0

HONEY, JAM, JELLY
Contain negligible calcium.

COOKIES & CAKES
Cookies: Average all types, 1 only	5
Crackers, average, 1 only	5
Cake: Plain, average, 2 oz	40
Carrot Cake with Icing	45
Cheesecake, 1 piece	80
Fruitcake, 1 piece	40
Croissants, average, 2 oz	20
Danish pastry, average, 2 oz	60
Donuts, average, 2 oz	20
Muffins: Regular, aver. 1 1/2 oz	40
English Muffins, 2 oz	90
Pancakes, 4" diam. aver., 1 oz	40
Pies:	
Apple/Fruit, average, 5 oz	20
Custard Pie, average, 5 oz	140
Pecan Pie, 1 piece, 5 oz	70
Pumpkin Pie, 1 piece, 5 oz	80
Waffles, 7" diam. average	160

CALCIUM COUNTER

DESSERTS	Calcium (mg)
Custard, average, 1/2 cup	150
Gelatin, plain w. water, 1/2 cup	2
Puddings: Canned, aver., 5 oz	80
Dry Mix, made w. milk, 1/2 cup	150
Rice Pudding: 1/2 cup	120
Snack Can, 5 oz	60
Pancakes, 4" diam., 2	120

CANDY, CHOCOLATE

Chocolate: Milk	50
Plain/Fruit, 1 oz	65
with Almonds, 1 oz	80
Kit Kat Wafer, 1 1/2 oz	80
Mars Bar	80
Milky Way Bar, 2 oz	60
Carob Bar, average, 2 oz	220
Plain candy, uncoated, 1 oz	Negl
Jelly Beans, M'shmallow, 1 oz	Negl

SNACKS & BARS

Breakfast Bars (*Carnation*)	20
Corn Chips; Tortilla Chips, 1 oz	40
Granola Bars, average	30
Popcorn, 1 cup	Negl
Potato Chips, 1 oz	10
Sandoz Nutritional Bars	400
Power Bar 300	
Tiger's Milk/Sport	350

NUTS & SEEDS (Shelled)

Almonds, 12-15 nuts, 1/2 oz	40
Brazil Nuts, 4 medium, 1/2 oz	30
Cashews, 6-8 nuts, 1/2 oz	5
Coconut, fresh, 1/2 oz	5
Filberts (Hazelnuts), 1/2 oz	40
Macadamias, 6 medium, 1/2 oz	10
Peanuts, raw, 1 oz	25
Walnuts, 1 oz	20
Seeds: Pumpkin, 1 oz	15
Sesame, 1 Tbsp	10
Sunflower, 1 oz	30
Tahini, 1 Tbsp, 1/2 oz	20

BEVERAGES - ALCOHOL, SODA

Beer, Cider, Wine, 1 glass	8
Spirits, 1 fl.oz	0
Coffee, Tea, Soda, Fruit Drinks	Negl
Water: Tap, average, 1 cup	5
Perrier, 1 glass, 6 oz	20

FRUIT	Calcium (mg)
Fresh Fruit: Average all types, 1 serve	20
Apple, 1 medium	10
Avocado, 1 medium	20
Banana, 1 medium	10
Orange, 1 medium	50
Pear, 1 medium	20
Rhubarb, cooked, 1/2 cup	170
(calcium largely not available to body)	
Dried Fruit: Average, 1 oz	20
Figs, 3 medium, 2 oz	80
Fruit Juice: Average, 1 cup	25
Orange Juice, calcium fortified:	
Citrus Hill Plus Calcium,	
Minute Maid (Premium Calcium Rich)	300

VEGETABLES

Average all types, 1/2 cup	20
1 cup	40
Higher Calcium Content:	
Beans, dried:cooked, 1/2 cup	50
Baked/Refried Beans, 1/2 cup	60
Broccoli, chopped, 1 cup	100
Chickpeas, boiled, 1/2 cup	40
Collards, cooked, 1 cup	150
Dandelion Greens, cooked, 1 cup	150
Kale, 1 cup	130
Mustard Greens, 1 cup	100
Potato: Plain, 1 large	20
Au Gratin, 1 cup	200
Mashed w.Milk, 1 cup	60
Spinach, cooked, 1/2 cup	120
Soybeans, cooked, 1/2 cup, 3 oz	90

TOFU, MISO, TEMPEH

Tofu: Hinoichi, regular, 4 oz	140
Nasoya, firm, 4 oz	100
Soft (*Hinoichi/Nasoya*), 4 oz	190
Silken (*Mori Nu*) 4 oz	90

CALCIUM SUPPLEMENTS

Caltrate 600, 1 tablet	600
Cal-Sup, 1 tablet	300
Citracal, 1 tablet	200
Mature Essentials, 1 tablet	600
Os-cal, 1 tablet	500
Ostal, 1 tablet	500
Posture Calcium, 1 tablet	600
Shaklee (Non-chewable), 1 tablet	400
Tums, 1 tablet	200

CALCIUM COUNTER

FROZEN ENTREES/MEALS	Calcium (mg)
Budget Gourmet Light	
Chicken Parmigiana; Ziti Parmesano	160
Three Cheese Lasagne	360
Cheese Manicotti w. Meat Sauce	200
Healthy Choice: Chick.Parmigiana	100
Chicken & Pasta Divan	150
Fettucini Alfredo; Lasagne	100
Le Menu: Beef Sirloin/Strogan.	100
Manicotti, Cheese (Entree)	400
Chicken Florentine/Parmagiana	150
Light Style: Turkey Dinner	100
Chicken Cacciatore	100
3-Cheese Stuffed Shells	150
Lean Cuisine	
Cheese Ravioli	160
Cheddar Bake w. Pasta	200
Classic Cheese Lasagna	360
Chicken Fettucine w. Broccoli	160
Mandarin Chicken	30
Turkey Pie	120
French Bread Pizza: Cheese Deluxe;	360
Pepperoni	200
Nasoya: Vegetable Lasagne	150
Stuffed Shells (2); Manicotti (2)	160
Mexican Enchil; Shells Provenc.	200
Stouffer's: Cheese Manicotti	320
Chicken Enchilada; Fettucini Alfredo	200
Double Cheese Pizza	280
Four Cheese/Vegetable Lasagna	400
Turkey Pie/Tetrazzini	80
Swanson: Beef Enchiladas	150
Entrees: Lasag., Macaroni & Ch.	450
Salisbury Steak	250
Scalloped Potatoes & Ham	300
Weight Watchers	
Bowtie Pasta & Mushroom	160
Broccoli & Cheese Baked Potato	200
Chicken Fettucini	80
Chicken Enchiladas Suiza	200
Cheese Manicotti; Garden Lasagna	320
Fettucini Alfredo; Lasagna Florentine	200
Italian Cheese Lasagna	400
Tuna Noodle Casserole	160
Pizza: Deluxe Combo; Pepperoni	400
Extra Cheese	560

FAST FOODS, RESTAURANTS	Calcium(mg)
Chicken: Grilled/BBQ, 1/4 chicken	20
Battered & Fried, 2 pieces	80
Nuggets, 6 pack	20
Crispy Chicken Deluxe S'wich	50
Croissant Sandwich: Plain	40
with Cheese, 1 oz	240
Fish Sandwich: no Cheese	60
with Cheese	140
Fish Filet Deluxe	70
Fish, fried, 2 pieces	20
French Fries: Small Serving	10
Hamburgers: Average all outlets	
Regular, no Cheese	120
Cheeseburger: Regular	120
McDonald's: Big Mac	160
Arch Deluxe w. Bacon	70
Quarter Pounder w. Cheese	120
Egg McMuffin	120
Hot Dog: Plain	60
with Cheese	150
Mexican: Burrito	120
Enchilada	300
Nachos, regular	200
Taco, regular	140
Taco (Bell) Salad	400
Pizza: Average all types	
Medium (12"), 2 slices	250
Double Cheese, 2 slices	350
Large (16"), 2 slices	350
Double Cheese, 2 slices	500
Pizza Hut, Medium:	
Cheese, 2 slices	290
Pepperoni, 2 slices	300
Potato: Plain, baked, 8oz	20
Stuffed w. Cheese Topping	100
with Cheese Filling	300
Sandwiches: Average	
no Cheese	60
with 1 oz Cheese	200
with 2 oz Cheese	460
Subway: 6" S/wich average	100
Tuna, 6"; Tuna Salad (sm.)	100
Salads, small, average	100
Salads: Chef, regular	300
Coleslaw, small	20
Milkshakes, average	330

FIBER GUIDE

INTRODUCTION

- **Fiber** is the general term for those parts of **plant** food that we cannot digest (although bacteria in the large bowel partly digests fiber through fermentation). It is **not** found in foods of animal origin (meats, dairy products).

- **Fiber promotes intestinal health**, bowel regularity, can benefit diabetes and blood cholesterol levels, and may help prevent colon cancer. High fiber foods also assist weight control.

- **Most Americans** don't eat enough fiber - less than 20 grams/day - instead of a **healthier 25 to 35 grams/day**.

TYPES OF FIBER

Plant foods contain a mixture of different fibers in varying proportions. Insoluble and soluble fiber categories are based on their solubility in water. All types of fiber are beneficial to the body.

(a) **Insoluble fibers** (cellulose, hemi-celluloses, lignin) make up the structural parts of plant cell walls. The **best sources** are wheat bran, corn bran, rice bran, wholegrain cereals and breads, dried beans and peas, nuts, seeds and the skins of fruits and vegetables.

These fibers absorb many times their own weight in water. They create a soft bulk and hasten the passage of waste products through the intestines.

They promote bowel regularity, and aid in the prevention and treatment of uncomplicated forms of **constipation, diverticulosis and haemorrhoids**.

The risk of colon cancer may also be reduced by fiber's diluting effect of potentially harmful substances.

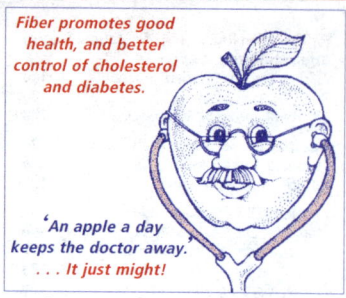

Fiber promotes good health, and better control of cholesterol and diabetes.

'An apple a day keeps the doctor away.'
... It just might!

TYPES OF FIBER (CONT)

(b) **Soluble fibers** (pectin, gums, mucilages) are found mainly within plant cells, soy milk (whole bean) and products.

Best Sources: Fruits and vegetables, oat bran, barley, dried beans and peas, psyllium and flax seed.

These fibers form a gel which slows both stomach emptying and the absorption of sugars from the intestines. This helps to control **blood sugar** levels.

Weight control is also aided by the slower emptying of the stomach and the feeling of fullness provided by soluble fiber.

Some soluble fibers can lower **blood cholesterol** by binding bile acids and excreting them. More body cholesterol must then be broken down to supply bile acids for emulsification of dietary fats. Rice bran, while not high in soluble fiber can also lower blood cholesterol.

(c) **Resistant starch** is that part of starchy foods (approx. 10%) which is tightly bound by fiber and resists normal digestion. Friendly bacteria in the large bowel ferment and change the resistant starch into short-chain fatty acids which are important to bowel health and may protect against colon cancer.

Starchy foods include bread, cereals, rice, pasta, potatoes and legumes.

FIBER GUIDE

FIBER & WEIGHT CONTROL

Fiber can assist weight control in several ways. Fiber-rich foods such as fresh fruit and vegetables, potatoes and whole-grain bread contain few calories for their large volume (due to their lowfat, high water content).

Their bulk fills the stomach and satisfies appetite much earlier than fiber-depleted foods. The extra chewing time also contributes to satiety, and gives the stomach time to register a feeling of fullness. Excessive calories are less likely to be consumed.

Fiber-depleted foods and drinks are more concentrated in calories; e.g. fats, sugar, candy, soft drinks, fruit juices, alcohol. They require little or no chewing. Large amounts with excessive calories can be consumed before appetite is satisfied.

Example: Whereas one fresh apple might satisfy our appetite, an apple juice drink with the equivalent sugars and calories of 2-3 apples does little to satisfy appetite. (See illustration below.)

LOW FIBER FOODS are more concentrated in calories. More food must be eaten to fill the stomach.

HIGH FIBER FOODS fill the stomach. Fewer calories are consumed.

EFFECTS OF REMOVING FIBER FROM FOOD
2-3 pieces of fresh fruit produces 1 glass of fruit juice.
The removal of fiber concentrates the sugar and calories.

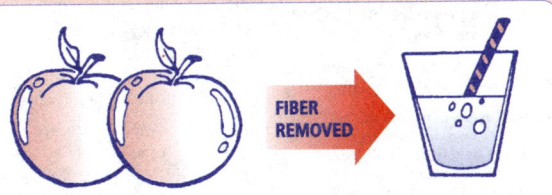

FRESH FRUIT
- High Fiber
- Low Calorie Density
- Long Eating Time
- Satisfies Hunger
- Sugar Slowly Absorbed
- Less Insulin Required

FRUIT JUICE
- Negligible Fiber
- High Calorie Density
- No Eating Time (Drink)
- Does Not Satisfy Hunger
- Sugar More Quickly Absorbed
- More Insulin Required

FIBER GUIDE - CONSTIPATION

CONSTIPATION

Constipation can reasonably be defined as a failure to have a bowel movement at least every second day - and just as importantly, without straining or pain.

Typically, stools are too hard, too narrow, and too small... *sinkers* rather than *floaters*.

The **main cause** is simply a lack of dietary fiber. Other contributing factors include insufficient fluids, too little exercise, emotional stress, gastro-intestinal disease, lack of proper dentition to chew high-fiber foods, and some medications (e.g. some antacids, antidepressants, tranquilizers).

Note: Check with your doctor to rule out any underlying medical problem - especially if you have a change in bowel habits in middle-age or later years.

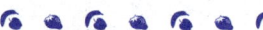

DESIRABLE FIBER INTAKE

Adults: 25-35 Grams Per Day
Children/Adolescents, 3-18 Years:
(Age + 5) grams/day
Example: A 6-year old would require 11g (6 + 5) per day.

SAMPLE FOOD QUANTITIES TO OBTAIN 35g FIBER

	Fiber
Breakfast Cereal (higher-fiber)	5g
plus 4 slices whole wheat Bread	6g
plus 3 servings fresh Fruit	9g
plus 1 medium Potato (w. skin)	
or 1 cup Brown Rice	4g
or 1/2 cup whole-wheat Pasta	
plus 3-4 servings Veges/Salad	6g
plus 1 cup Bean Soup	
or 1/4 cup Baked Beans/Soy Beans	
or 1/2 cup Corn/Peas/Lentils	5g
or 1 1/4 oz Almonds (natural)	

HINTS TO INCREASE FIBER & AVOID CONSTIPATION

1. **Breakfast is an important contributor** to daily fiber intake. Eat high-fiber breakfast cereals (bran-based cereals, oatmeal etc.). Add 1-2 tablespoons of unprocessed bran (wheat/barley/rice) and wheat germ if required.

   Dried fruits, chopped nuts, soy grits, and seeds are also excellent additions to cereals.

   Note: A gradual increase in fiber will prevent bloating, gas or pain. Persons intolerant to bran may benefit from psyllium-based fiber supplements and cereals.

2. **Drink 6-8 glasses of water or fluid daily.** Fiber works by absorbing many times its own weight of water.

3. **Eat wholegrain breads, or fiber-enriched breads.** One slice of whole-wheat bread has over double the fiber of regular white bread.

4. **Enjoy fruit as fresh fruit** with skins rather than as fruit juice. Enjoy whole-wheat pasta, barley, brown rice, nuts and seeds.

5. **Eat more vegetables, salads and legumes** - especially dried beans, baked beans, lentils, potatoes with skins, avocado, broccoli, brussel sprouts, cabbage, carrots, celery, and peas.

6. **Add bran** (barley/rice/wheat) or soy grits to soups, casseroles, yogurt, desserts, biscuits, cakes. Also use wholemeal flour or soy flour in place of white flour. Use nuts and seeds.

7. **Snack** on fresh or dried fruits, carrot or celery sticks, popcorn, nuts or seeds, wholegrain crackers, high-fiber bars (low-fat). Limit amounts if overweight.

8. **Exercise regularly** to strengthen abdominal muscles and stimulate the gut. Keep up fluids, especially in warm weather.

9. **Avoid indiscriminate and regular use of harsh laxatives.** They can overstimulate the intestinal muscles and may make normal bowel activity impossible. It may take several weeks to restore normal bowel function.

FIBER COUNTER

BREAKFAST CEREALS	FIBER (g)
Breadshop:	
Oat Bran, 1/3 cup, 1 oz	4
Triple Bran, 1 oz	6.5
Nectar-Sweet Granolas, 1 oz	3
Health Valley: *Per Serving*	
Amaranth Flakes, 3/4 cup	4
Bran w. Apple & Cinnamon, 3/4 cup	7
Bran w. Raisins, 3/4 cup	6
Corn Bran Flakes, 3/4 cup	4
Fiber 7 Flakes	4
Golden Flax, 1/4 cup	6
Granola (Fat Free), 2/3 cup	6
Healthy Crunches & Flakes, 3/4 cup	4
Healthy Fiber Flakes, 3/4 cup	4
Oat Bran O's, 3/4 cup	5
Oat Bran Flakes, all types, , 3/4 cup	4
Real Oat Bran 1/2 cup	5
10 Bran O's, 3/4 cup	4
General Mills:	
Cheerios, 1 cup, 1 oz	3
Basic 4, 1 cup, 2 oz	3
Crispy Wheaties 'N Raisins, 1 cup, 2 oz	4
Fiber One, 1/2 cup, 1 oz	13
Raisin Nut Bran, 3/4 cup, 2 oz	5
Oatmeal Crisp, 1 cup, 2 oz	4
Kellogg's: (Per 1 oz):	
All-Bran, 1/2 cup	10
All-Bran w. Extra Fiber, 1/2 cup	13
Bran Buds, 3/4 cup	12
Bran Flakes (3/4 c.) Raisin Bran, (1 c.)	6
Common Sense Oat Bran, 3/4 cup	4
Corn Flakes, Frt.Loops, Smacks, 1 cup	1
Special K, 1 cup	1
Cocoa/Rice Krispies, 3/4 cup	0
Healthy Choice, all types, 1 cup	5
Nutri-Grain (Almond Raisin), 1 1/4 cup	4
Mueslix, Apple Almond, 3/4 cup	5
Nabisco:	
100% Bran, 1/2 cup, 1 oz	10
Shreaded Wheat, 2 biscuits	6
Nature Valley: Average, 3/4 cup, 1 oz	1
Quaker (& Brands): Per 1 oz	
Cap'n Crunch (3/4 c.) Cr.Nut Oh's (1 c)	1
Crunchy Bran, 2/3 cup, 1 oz	5
Life Cereal (2/3 cup), Oat Squares (1/2 c.)	2.5
Oat Bran (Quaker & Mothers), 1/3 cup	4.2
Oatmeal, average, 1 packet	2.7
100% natural cereals, aver., 1/4 cup	0.2
Puffed Rice, 1 cup	1
Puffed Wheat, Popeye Crunch, 1 cup	1.8

BREAKFAST CEREALS (Cont)	FIBER (g)
Post: Alpha Bits, Corn Flakes, 1 oz	0
Bran Flakes (Natural), 3/4 cup, 1 oz	5
Fruit & Fiber, 1 1/4 oz	5
Granola (Hearty), Fruity Pebbles	0
Grape-Nuts Brand/Flakes, 1 oz	3
Honey Bunches of Oats, 1 oz	1
Oat Flakes, 1 cup, 1 oz	2
Smurf Magic, Super Golden, 1 oz	0
Ralston: Fruit Muesli, 1/2 cup, 1 1/2 oz	3
Multi-Bran Chex, 2/3 cup, 1 oz	4
Wheat Chex, 2/3 cup, 1 oz	2
BRANS & SUPPLEMENTS	
Oat Bran: 1 Tbsp (level)	0.8
1/3 cup, (5 1/3 Tbsp) 1 oz	4.2
Rice Bran: 1/3 cup, 1 oz	6
Wheat Bran: unprocessed: 1 Tbsp	1.6
2 Tbsp (level), 1/4 cup	3.2
1/4 cup, (4 Tbsp), 1/2 oz	6.4
1/2 cup, 1 oz	13
Corn Germ: 1/4 cup, 1 oz	5
Wheat Germ: 1/4 cup, 1 oz	3
Psyllium Seed Husks, 2 Tbsp	8
LiFiber (Enrich), 1 serving	5.6
Metamucil, 1 dose	3.4
HOT CEREALS, OATMEAL	
Bulgur (cracked Wheat), ckd, 1 cup	8
Cream of Wheat, ckd, 2/3 cup	1
Hominy Grits, dry, 3 Tbsp, 1 oz	1.2
Kashi (Breakfast Pilaf), 5 oz	5
5 Bran Kashi, 1/2 envelope	16
Oatmeal, uncooked, 1/3 cup, 1 oz	2.7
cooked, 2/3 cup	2.7

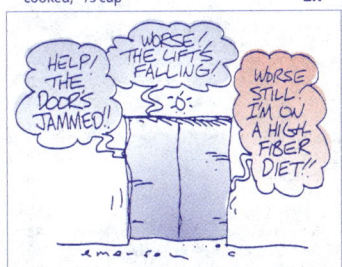

FIBER COUNTER

FOODS WITH ZERO FIBER
- Dairy Products (Milk, Cheese, etc)
- Meats, Poultry, Fish, Eggs
- Fats/Oils, Sugar/Syrups

(Only foods of plant origin contain fiber.)

BREADS & CRACKERS

Item	FIBER (g)
Bread: White, 1 slice, 1 oz	0.7
Whole-wheat, 1 slice, 1 oz	1.5
Whole-grain, 1 slice, 1 oz	2
Rye, Pumpernickel, 1 oz	1.5
Bagel/Roll/Bun, 1 medium, 2 oz	1.5
Pita, whole wheat, 5" pocket	4.5
Crackers: Graham, average, 2	1.4
Saltine, 4 crackers	0.3
Crispbreads (Rye), average, 2	4
Matzo 1 board, 1 oz	1
Rice Cakes Average, 1 cake	0.3
Tortilla: Regular, 6"	0.5
Whole-wheat, 6"	1.3

BARLEY, PASTA, RICE & FLOURS

Item	FIBER (g)
Barley, pearled, raw, 1/4 cup, 1.7 oz	5
Rice: White, cooked, 1 cup 7 oz	1.6
Brown, cooked, 1 cup	3.2
Rice-A-Roni, average, 1 cup	1.5
Spaghetti/Noodles: cooked, 1 cup	2
Whole-wheat, cooked, 1 cup	7
Amaranth (Health Valley), 1 cup	9
Flour: All-purpose, 1 cup, 4 oz	<1
Whole-wheat, 1 cup	10
Cornmeal, stone ground, 1 cup	8
Carob Flour, 1 cup, 3 1/2 oz	11
Soymeal, defatted, 1 cup	14

FROZEN ENTREES & DINNERS
Average All Brands - Per Serving

Item	FIBER (g)
Potato/Pasta base, average	4-6
Vegetable base, average	3
Meat/Chicken base, average	2-3
Pizzas, 1/4 large, average	3

SOUPS

Item	FIBER (g)
Chicken Noodle, 1 cup	<0.5
Tomato Soup, average, 1 cup	<1
Vegetable Soup, average, 1 cup	3
Health Valley - Per 1 Cup Serving:	
Black Bean Soup	10
Tomato	4
Organic Split Pea Soup	8
5-Bean Vegetable	13
Minestrone Soup	10
Mushroom & Barley; Vegetable	7
Lentil & Carrots	14

FAST FOODS & RESTAURANTS

Item	FIBER (g)
Hamburgers: Small, average	1.5
Large/Whopper, average	2.5
Hot Dog, Regular	1.5
French Fries: Small serving, 2 1/2 oz	2.5
Regular/Medium, 3 1/2 oz	3.5
Chicken Nuggets, 6 pack	<0.5
Chicken Sandwich, average	2
Taco, average	4
Sundaes, Shakes, Soft Drinks	0
Arby's: Baked Potato w.Broccoli	9
Roast Beef Sandwich, regular	3
Denny's: Oriental Chicken Salad	7
Dennyburger w. fries	3
Club Sandwich	3
Grilled Chicken Sandwich	1
Domino's (Pizza): Veggie, 2 sl. (12")	4
Pepperoni, 2 slices (12")	2.5
Cheese., Saus/Mushr., 2 slices, (12")	3
McDonald's: Arch Deluxe; Crispy Chicken	4
Big Mac	3
Egg McMuffin	1
Salads: Garden; Grilled Chicken	2
Pizza Hut: (Per 2 slices, Medium)	
Pan Pizza: Cheese, Pepperoni	2
Supreme	4
Thin 'n Crispy: Supreme	4
Hand-Tossed, average	3
Personal Pan Pizza, 1 whole	5
Subway: Sandwich, white roll	2.5
w.honey Wheat Roll	3.2
Footlong, w.Wheat Roll	6.4
Salads, average	3

CAKES, COOKIES, SNACK BARS

Item	FIBER (g)
Apple/Fruit Pie, 1 serving	2
Cake, w. plain flour, 1 serving	1
w. whole-wheat flour, 1 serving	3
Carrot Cake, 1 serving	2
Cookies, oatmeal, (3 small/1 large)	3
Donuts	0
Fruit Cake, 1 serving	3
Fi-Bar (Natural Nectar), 1 bar	4
Fig Bars, 2	1.3
Granola Bars, average	1
Health Valley: Fat-Free Fruit Bars	3.7
Oat Bran Jumbo Fruit Bars	7
Fat-Free Cookies, 2	2
Fat-Free Fruit Muffins, 1	5
Muffins, Oat Bran (2 small, 1 large)	5
Break Bar (IDN)	6
Meal On The Go (Omnitrition), 1 1/2 oz	4

FIBER COUNTER

CHOCOLATE, CHIPS, POPCORN	FIBER (g)
Chocolate, Hard Candy, Cheese Balls	0
Chocolate with nuts/fruit, 2oz bar	1
Mars Bar	1
Cheese Balls/Curls/Twists	0
Potato Chips, corn chips, 1 oz	1
Popcorn, 3 cups	2
Pretzels, Twists, 6	1

NUTS, SEEDS

Almonds: Natural, 25 kernels, 1 oz	4
Blanched (skins removed), 1 oz	3
Cashews, Filberts, Pecans, 1 oz	1.7
Peanuts, Mixed Nuts, Coconut, 1 oz	2.5
Peanut Butter, 2 Tbsp, 1 oz	1.8
Pistachio Nuts, dried, shelled, 1 oz	3
Walnuts, Black/English, dried, 1 oz	1.5
Seeds: Amaranth, 2½ Tbsp, 1oz	3.5
Flax Seeds, 3 Tbsp, 1 oz	6
Quinoa Seeds, 3 Tbsp, 1 oz	2.7
Psyllium Seed Husks, 5 Tbsp, 1 oz	20
Sesame Seeds, whole, 1 oz	3
Sesame Butter/Tahini, 2 tbsp, 1.1 oz	3
Sunflower kernels, ¼ cup, 1 oz	4.4
Teff Seeds, 1 oz	3.8

FRUIT - FRESH

Apples: Early season, 1 medium, 6oz (whole)	
with skin + core	5.5
with skin, no core	4.5
without skin, no core	3.7
Late season, 1 med. 6 oz, w.skin, no core	3
Apricots, 2 medium, 4 oz	2
Avocado, average, ½ medium	3
Banana, 1 medium, 6 oz (w.skin)	2
Blueberries, raw, ½ cup, 5 oz	4.4
Cherries, sweet, raw, 10 fruits, 2½ oz	1.5
Grapefruit, average, ½ fruit, 8½ oz	1
Grapes, 1 med.bunch, seedless, 7 oz	3
Kiwifruit, 1 medium, 3 oz	3
Mango, 1 medium, 11 oz (whole)	1.6
Melons, cantaloup, 4 oz (edible)	1
Nectarine, 1 medium, 4 oz	1.8
Olives, average all types, 7 jumbo, 2 oz	1.5
Oranges, 1 medium (7-8 oz w.skin)	
5½ oz (peeled)	3.8
Passionfruit, 2 medium, 2½ oz	2
Peaches, 1 large, 6 oz	2
Pears, raw, 1 medium, 6 oz	4.5
Pineapple, 1 slice, 3 oz	1.8
Plums, 2 medium, 6 oz	2.8
Strawberries, 6 medium/3 large, 2 oz	1.5
Watermelon, 4 oz (edible)	0.5

FRUIT - DRIED, JUICE	FIBER (g)
Dried Fruit: Apricots, 8 halves, 1 oz	2.2
Dates (3 med); Raisins (2 Tbsp), 1 oz	1.5
Figs, 2 medium, 1.4 oz	3.5
Prunes, 4 medium, 1 oz	2
Fruit Juice: Orange/Apple etc, 1 glass	<0.5
Prune Juice, 5 oz	1.4
Carrot Juice, 8 oz	1.8

VEGETABLES

Asparagus, 4 spears	2
Bean Sprouts, ½ cup, 2¼ oz	1.5
Beans: Snap/Green, ½ cup, 2½ oz	2
Baked Beans in Tom Sce, ½ c, 4½ oz	10
Dried BEans, ckd, average, ½ cup	7
Beets, ckd, slices, ½ cup, 3 oz	1.5
Broccoli, cooked, ½ cup, 3 oz	2.2
Brussels Sprouts, ckd, ½ cup, 3 oz	3.5
Cabbage: White, ckd, ½ cup, 2½ oz	1
Red, ckd, ½ cup, 2½ oz	2
Carrots, 1 medium (7½"), ½ cup, 3 oz	2.7
Cauliflower, cooked, ½ cup, 3 oz	2.8
Celery, raw, diced, ½ cup, 2½ oz	1
Chick Peas (Garbanzos), ckd, ½ c., 3½ oz	6
Corn, kernels, ckd, ½ cup, 2½ oz	2.5
Cream-style, ½ cup, 4½ oz	1.5
Cucumber/Lettuce/Mushrooms, 2 oz	0.5
Eggplant, raw, sliced, ½ cup	2.5
Lentils, cooked, ½ cup, 3½ oz	4
Lettuce	
Onions, 1 medium, 4 oz	2
Spring Onions, chop., ¼ cup, 1oz	1.5
Peas: Green, ½ cup, 3 oz	3
Cowpeas (Black-eyed), ckd, ½ cup	10
Split Peas, ckd, ½ cup, 2½ oz	6.5
Peppers, sweet, raw, 1 large, 3½ oz	1.5
Potatoes: 1 medium, with skin, 5 oz	4
without skin	2
½ cup mashed, 3½ oz	1.5
French Fries, 3 oz serving	3
Spinach, cooked, ½ cup, 3 oz	2
Squash: Summer, cookd, 3 oz	1.2
Winter, cooked, 3 oz	2.4
Tomatoes: 1 medium, 5 oz	2
Tomato Sauce, 1 cup	0.3
Frozen: Mixed Vegetables, ckd, ½ cup	3
Soybean Products: Miso, ½ c., 5 oz	7.7
Tempeh, 1 piece, 3 oz	2
Tofu, 4 oz	1.4
SALADS: Side Salad, average	1
Bean Salad, ½ cup	5
Coleslaw, ½ cup	1
Potato Salad, ½ cup	2

PROTEIN GUIDE

GENERAL NOTES

- **Protein has many important body functions.** It builds and repairs muscle, and is the basis of our body's organs, hormones, enzymes and antibodies.

- **Protein is also an emergency fuel** in the absence of sufficient carbohydrate and fats. For this reason, weight loss should be gradual so as to preserve protein levels in muscle, the heart and other body organs.

- **It is easy to obtain sufficient protein,** even if vegetarian. **Plant proteins are not inferior to animal proteins.** In fact, eating more soy and other plant proteins, and less animal protein, may help to build stronger bones and prevent osteoporosis; and may help to control blood cholesterol levels.

- **When changing to a vegetarian diet,** include soybeans, and other dried beans, soy milk drinks (calcium-enriched), lentils, tofu, nuts, and wholegrain breads and cereals. Milk, yogurt, cheese and eggs may enhance nutrient intake.

PROTEIN & MUSCLE

- Although muscles are built of protein, protein is not a special fuel for working muscle cells - carbohydrates and fats are.

  In fact, a diet high in protein (and fat) and low in carbohydrate, can significantly reduce the performance of endurance sports athletes. **Carbohydrate** is the best fuel for muscles exercised for long periods.

- Any **extra protein** required by athletes and bodybuilders, can easily be obtained from the extra food eaten to satisfy hunger and energy needs - even allowing an excessive 120g protein daily for a 170 lb athlete (0.7g/lb body wt; twice the RDI).

- Remember, **excess protein** in food will not build bigger muscles. It is converted and stored as fat. Excess protein can also strain the kidneys which excrete the waste products of protein metabolism.

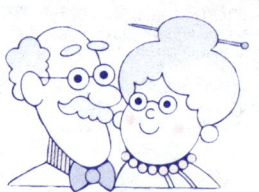

Elderly people (and dieters) must eat sufficient food to ensure adequate protein intake.

Inadequate protein leads to a drop in immune response with greater susceptibility to illness and infections. Muscle strength and muscle mass also drop.

Protein needs are easily met with sensible eating. Athletes who eat enough food for their energy needs, can obtain sufficient protein.

RECOMMENDED DAILY PROTEIN INTAKE (Grams)

(Figure in brackets - Recommended amount of protein per lb of ideal body weight.)

Infants:	0-6 mths	**13g**	(1g/lb)
	6-12 mths	**14g**	(0.7g/lb)
Children:	1-3 yrs	**16g**	(0.6g/lb)
	4-6 yrs	**24g**	(0.5g/lb)
	7-10	**28g**	(0.5g/lb)
Males:	11-14 yrs	**45g**	(0.45g/lb)
	15-18	**59g**	(0.4g/lb)
	19-24	**58g**	(0.36g/lb)
	25+	**50g**	(0.4g/lb)
Females:	11-14 yrs	**46g**	(0.45g/lb)
	15-18	**44g**	(0.37g/lb)
	19-24	**46g**	(0.36g/lb)
	25+	**50g**	(0.36g/lb)
Pregnancy:		**60g**	
Breastfeeding:		**65g**	

Note: Above figures allow for a large safety margin for most persons.

IRON GUIDE

IRON & ANEMIA GUIDE

- **Iron deficiency** is one of the most common nutritional deficiencies in women. The risk is increased in dieters who do not eat well-balanced meals. Chronic shortage of iron leads to **anemia**.

- **Women** between 11 and 50 years of age are at greater risk because of the monthly loss of menstrual blood. Pregnancy, growth, and endurance sports also demand extra iron.

- **In** red blood cells, iron combines with protein to form **hemoglobin** - the red pigment which carries oxygen in the blood. A lack of iron limits the production of hemoglobin and hence the amount of vital oxygen delivered to body cells.

Note: A blood test will tell you whether your Hb and iron stores (ferritin) are adequate. (Iron stores can be low even when Hb is normal.)

- **Vitamin C** (in fruits/veges/salads) enhances absorption of 'non-heme' iron in bread, cereals, milk, vegetables, nuts, eggs and iron supplements. Small amounts of meat, fish or poultry also help. (They contain 'heme' iron).

- **Iron absorption is lessened** by up to 60% when high calcium foods are consumed with iron-rich main meals. Tea, coffee, phytates (in bran) and oxalates lessen absorption of non-heme iron.

- **For infants to 1 year**, use iron-fortified milk/soy formula if not breast-feeding. Introduce iron-fortified baby cereals at 4-6 mths.

Note: Iron deficiency in children (even without anemia), can result in lethargy, irritability, repeated infections, and development problems.

IRON SUPPLEMENTS

- **Most people** can obtain adequate iron from their diet. A **wide variety** of animal and plant foods contain iron. *(See Iron Counter)*

- **Iron supplements** are only recommended for women with heavy menstrual blood losses, during pregnancy (if tests show a low-iron status), endurance athletes with low blood ferritin (iron stores) and for persons with diagnosed anemia.

- While the 5 mg of iron in multi-vitamin/mineral supplements is safe for most people, large amounts can be toxic, (especially in persons with hemochromatosis iron overload condition).

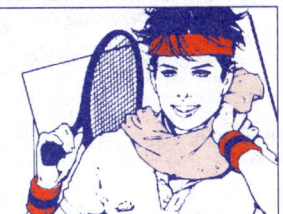

A nutritious diet with adequate iron is important - particularly for women and athletes.

ANEMIA SYMPTOMS

Anemia reduces the amount of oxygen carried in the blood. The body tissues become starved of oxygen. Symptoms include:

- Pale skin; brittle finger nails (may turn up into spoon shape).
- Excessive tiredness or fatigue
- Breathlessness
- General feeling of malaise and irritability.
- Always feel cold.
- Decrease in attention span.

Note: Other medical conditions may also cause similar symptoms. Check with your doctor.

RECOMMENDED DAILY INTAKE OF IRON (mg)

Infants:	0-6 mths	
	Breastfed	0.5mg
	Bottlefed	3mg
	6-12 mths	9mg
Children:	1-11 yrs	6-8mg
Males:	12-18 yrs	10-13mg
	19+ yrs	7mg
Females:	12-50yrs	12-16mg
	51+ yrs	5-7mg
	Pregnancy:	22-36mg
	Breastfeeding:	12-16mg

PROTEIN & IRON COUNTER

P ~ PROTEIN (Grams) **I** ~ IRON (mg)

MEAT	P	I
Steak: Average all cuts, lean (no fat)		
Small (4 oz raw/3 oz ckd)	23	2.3
Medium (6 oz raw/ $4^{1}/_{4}$ oz ckd)	34	3.4
Large (10 oz raw/ $7^{1}/_{4}$ oz ckd)	57	5.7
Roast Beef: lean, 2 slices, 3 oz	24	2.5
Ground Beef patty, lean, ckd, 3oz	21	2
Lamb chop, broiled, 3 oz	22	1.5
Liver, Cooked, 3 oz	23	5.5
Veal cutlet, 1 medium	23	1
Pork, cooked, lean, 3 oz	24	1
Bacon, 3 medium slices	6	0.3
Ham, roasted, 2 pieces, 3 oz	18	1
Ham, luncheon, 2 slices, $1^{1}/_{2}$ oz	7	0.3
Pastrami (*Oscar Mayer*), 3 sl., $1^{3}/_{4}$ oz	10	1.3
Sausages: Bologna, 2 sl., 2 oz	7	1
Braunschweiger, 2 sl., 2 oz	8	5.3
Pork link, thick, 2 oz	6	0.4
Frankfurter, $1^{1}/_{3}$ oz	5	0.5
Salami, hard, 3 slices, 1 oz	7	0.5
CHICKEN/TURKEY		
Chicken, ckd; Brst. portion 3 oz	27	1
Leg/Thigh, lean, 3 oz	24	1
$1/2$ Whole Chicken	60	2.5
Drumstick, 1 medium, 3 oz	12	0.6
Turkey, cooked: Light meat, 3 oz	24	2
Dark meat, lean, 3 oz	24	2
FISH		
Finfish - Per 4 oz, cooked		
Cod, Flounder/Sole, Pollock	28	0.5
Catfish, Haddock, Halibut, M/Mahi	28	1.3
Ocean Perch, Swordf., Orange Roughy	28	1.3
Canned Fish: Tuna, Light, 3 oz	25	1.5
White, 3 oz	23	0.5
Salmon, pink, 3 oz	17	0.7
Salmon, red, 3 oz	17	1
Sardines, 3 whole (3"), $1^{1}/_{4}$ oz	9	1
Anchovies, 1 can, $1^{1}/_{2}$ oz	13	2
Shellfish: Crabmeat, 3 oz	17.5	0.7
Clams, raw, 4 lge/9sml, 3 oz	11	12
Crayfish, cooked, 3 oz	20	2.7
Lobster, cooked, 3 oz	17	0.5
Oysters, raw, 6 medium, 3 oz	7	5
Scallops, 2 lge/5 small, 1 oz	5	0.1
Shrimp, raw, 6 large, $1^{1}/_{2}$ oz	8.5	1
Fish Products: Fish Sticks, 4 sticks	10	0.5
Fish Portions, in batter, 4 oz	13	0.6
Gefilte Fish, 1 med. ball, 2 oz	8	1

EGGS	P	I
1 Large Egg, whole	6	0.7
Egg Yolk	3	0.7
Egg White	3	0
Omelet: Plain, 2 eggs	13	1.4
Ham & Cheese	17	3
Egg Substitutes (liquid):		
Eggbeaters, 1 egg equiv.	4.5	1
Scramblers, $1/4$ cup, 2oz	6	0.7
MILK & DAIRY PRODUCTS		
Milk, Whole/Lowfat/Skim, 8 fl.oz cup	8	0.1
Protein Enriched, 1 cup	10	0.1
Chocolate Milk, 1 cup	8	0.6
Thick Shake, Chocolate, 10 oz	9	1
Vanilla, 10 oz	11	0.3
Soymilk (fortified), aver., 1 cup	7	1
Yogurt: Plain, 6 oz	10	0.1
Fruit flavors, 6 oz	8	0.3
8 oz	11	0.5
Ice Cream: Rich, $1/2$ cup	2	0
Regular, vanilla, $1/2$ cup	2.5	0
Sherbet, $1/2$ cup	1	0
Custard, baked, $1/2$ cup	7	0.5
CHEESE		
Hard Cheeses, average, 1 oz	7	0.2
4 oz	28	0.8
Cottage Cheese, $1/2$ cup	13	0.3
Ricotta, part skim	14	1
BREAD, BAGELS, BISCUITS		
Bread (w/enriched flour): 1 slice, 1 oz	2	1
4 slices, 4 oz	8	4
4 thick slices, 6 oz	1.2	6
Bagel, plain 2 oz	6	1.5
Biscuits, 1 oz	2	0.7
Pita Bread, 1 pita, $1^{1}/_{2}$ oz	4	1
Pumperknickel, 1 slice, 1 oz	3	1

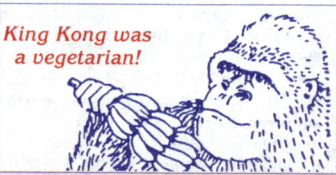

King Kong was a vegetarian!

PROTEIN & IRON COUNTER

BREAKFAST CEREALS	P	I
Hot Type, cooked		
Bulgur, cooked, 1 cup, 5 oz	9	2
Oatmeal: Reg., non-fortified., 1 cup	6	1.5
Instant, fortified, aver., 1 pkt	4	6
Quaker, reg. w.Cin.Spice	4	8
Quaker Extra, all flavors	4	18
Total, all types, 1 pkt	4	18
Corn/Hominy Grits: Reg., 1 cup	3	1.5
Quaker: Reg., 3 Tbsp, 1 oz	2	0.8
Instant White, 1 packet	2	8
Cream of Wheat, 1 cup	4	10
Ready-To-Eat (Per 1 oz serving)		
Arrowhead, Average, all varieties	3	1
General Mills: Basic 4, 1 cup, 2 oz	4	3.8
Cheerios, regular, 1 cup, 1 oz	3	6.8
Cocoa Puffs, 1 cup, 1 oz	1	3.8
Corn Flakes, 1 cup	2	6.8
Fiber One, 1/2 cup	2	3.8
Kix, 1 1/3 cups; Kaboom, 1 1/4 cup	2	6.8
Total, Raisin Bran, 1 cup, 2 oz	4	15
Wheaties, 1 cup	3	6.8
Health Valley: 10 Bran O's, 3/4 cup	3	0.9
Amaranth Flakes, 3/4 cup	3	0.6
Bran Cereal w. Raisins, 3/4 cup	5	1.5
98% Fat Free Granola, 2/3 cup	5	1.2
Real Oat Bran, 1/2 cup	6	0.6
Golden Flax, 1/4 cup	6	1.2
Kellogg's: All Bran, 1/2 cup	4	4.5
Bran Flakes, 3/4 cup	3	8.5
Cocoa Krispies, 3/4 cup	2	1.8
Corn Flakes, 1 cup	2	8.4
Just Right, 1 cup	4	16
Nutrigrain Almond Raisin, 1 1/4 cup	4	1.4
Product 19, 1 cup, 2 oz	2	18
Raisin Bran, 1 cup, 2 oz	6	4.5
Raisin Squares, 3/4 cup	4	16
Rice Krispies, 1 1/4 cup	2	1.8
Special K, 1 cup	6	8.7
Nature Valley: All varieties, 1/3 cup	2	0.7
Post: Raisin Bran, 1 oz	3	4.5
Grape Nuts, 1 oz	3	1
Quaker: Crunchy Bran, 2/3 cup	2	8
Oat Squares, 1/2 cup	4	6
100% natural cereal, 1/4 cup	3	1
Puffed Rice/Wheat, 1 c., 1/2 oz	1	0.5
Shreaded Wheat, 2 biscuits	4	1

BRANS & WHEATGERM	P	I
Oat Bran, raw, 1 Tbsp	2	0.5
Rice Bran, raw, 2 Tbsp	1	1
Wheat Bran, unproc., 2 Tbsp	1	1
Wheat Germ, 2 Tbsp, 1/2 oz	4	1.3
GRAINS & FLOURS		
Amaranth, 1 cup, 1/2 oz	10	3
Barley, 1/2 cup, 3 1/2 oz	8	2
Buckwheat Flour, dark, 1 cup	11.5	2.7
light, 1 cup	6	1
Carob Flour, 1 cup	5	3
Corn Flour, 1 cup, 4 oz	9	2
Corn Meal, enriched, 1 cup	11	3.5
Flour: White, enriched, 1 cup, 4 1/2 oz	13	6
Wholegrain, 1 cup, 4 1/4 oz	16	5
Millet, wholegrain, 1 cup, 3 1/2 oz	10	7
Rye Flour, dark, 1 cup, 4 1/2 oz	21	6
light, 1 cup, 3 1/2 oz	10	1
Soy Flour, full fat, 1 cup, 3 oz	32	5.5
NUTRITION & HI PROTEIN DRINKS		
Bariatrix Shakes, dry, 1 oz	15	3.6
Fruit Drinks, mix, 2/3 oz	15	0
Proti-Max Meal Replacement, 67g	35	6.3
Boost Nutrition Energy Drink, 8 oz	10	3.6
Ensure, all flavors, 8 oz	9	2.3
Ensure Plus, 8 oz	13	3
Carnation Instant Breakfast, 10 oz	12	4.5
Kindercal, 8 fl. oz	8	2.5
Met-Rx, Drink Mix, 72g	38	9
Nature's Best, Protein Shake, 11 oz	20	3.6
Nutra Start, 11 oz	10	3.6
Resource Nutritional Food, 8 fl. oz	9	2.7
Sweet Success Shake (Nestle), 10 oz	10	4.5
Sustacal/Plus, 8 oz	15	4
Ultra Slim Fast, powder, 3 Tbsp, 33g	5	6.3
Weider: Muscle Builder, 2 scoops	18	9
90% Plus Protein, 3 Tbsp	24	2.7
YEAST: Brewer's, dry, 1 Tbsp	3	1.5

INFANT/BABY FOODS	P	I
Infant Formula Milk:		
Enfamil/Gerber/Similac, 5 fl. oz		
Regular/Low Iron	2.2	0.2
With Iron	2.2	1.8
Isomil/Nursoy/ProSobee	3	1.8
Baby Cereals, average all brands		
Dry, 4 Tbsp, 1/2 oz	1	7
Jars (w.fruit), 4 1/2 oz	1	7

241

PROTEIN & IRON COUNTER

RICE, SPAGHETTI
	P	I
Rice, brown/white, average 1 cup cooked, 6 1/2 oz	5	1
Spaghetti/Macaroni/Noodles (enriched) cooked, 1 cup, 4 1/2 oz	7	2
Canned: in Tomato Sce, 1/2 cup	2	0.5
w. Meatballs, 1 cup, 8oz	9	2

SOUPS
With Noodles/Vegetables, 1 cup	3	0.5
With Meat/Beans/Peas, 1 cup	8	1.5

FRUIT
Fresh/Canned: Average, all types, 1 serving 1 medium/2 small fruit	1	0.5
Avocado, 1/2 medium	2	1
Dried Fruit: Apricots, 8 halves, 1 oz	1	1.3
Dates, 6 dates, 2 oz	1.5	0.7
Figs, 3 medium figs, 2 oz	1	1.3
Prunes, 5 medium, 1 1/2 oz	1	1
Raisins, 1 oz	1	0.7
Fruit Juice: Average, 1 cup	0.5	0.5
Prune Juice, 6 fl.oz	1	2.5
Tomato Juice, 6 fl.oz	0.5	1

VEGETABLES
Beans: Snap/green, 1/2 cup	1	0.8
Dried: Average all types, cooked, 1/2 cup	7	2.5
Baked Beans, 1/2 cup 4 1/2 oz	5	2
Bean Sprouts, mung, 1 cup	3	1
Broccoli, 3/4 cup pieces, 4 oz	4	1.4
Cabbage; Cauliflower, 1 cup	1	0.6
Corn, 1/2 cup kernels, 3 oz	2.5	0.3
1 ear trimmed to 3 1/2"	2	0.4
Lentils, cooked, 1/2 cup, 3 1/2 oz	9	3.3
Mushrooms, raw, 1/2 cup, sliced	0.5	0.5
Peas: green, 1/2 cup, 3 oz	4	1.2
Split Peas, cooked, 1 cup	16	2.5
Potatoes, cooked:		
1 medium, with skin, 5 oz	3.3	2
without skin, 4 oz	2.3	1
French Fries, 3 oz	3	1
Potato Salad, 1/2 cup	3.5	2
Pumpkin, 1/2 cup mashed	1	2.5
Seaweed, kelp, 1 oz	<1	2.5
Spinach, cooked, 1/2 cup, 3 oz	2.7	2.5
Squash, ckd, all types, 1/2 cup	1	0.3
Tomatoes, 1 medium, 4 1/2 oz	1	0.6
Vegetables, mixed, ckd, 1 cup	2.5	0.7
Soybeans, cooked, 1/2 cup, 3 oz	14	4.4

TOFU, TEMPEH, MISO
	P	I
Tofu, raw, firm, 1/2 cup, 4 1/2 oz	10	1.5
Tempeh, 1/2 cup, 3 oz	16	2
Miso, 1/2 cup, 4 3/4 oz	16	4
Soybean Protein (TVP), 1 oz	18	3

CAKES, PASTRIES, PIES
(Made with enriched flour)
Carrot w.cream cheese frosting, 4 oz	4	1.3
Cheesecake, 1 piece, 3 1/2 oz	5	0.5
Chocolate, 1 piece, 2 oz	2	2
Fruitcake, 1 piece, 1 1/2 oz	2	1.2
Plain, 1 piece, 3 oz	4	1.2
Croissant, plain, 2 oz	5	2
Danish Pastry, 1 pastry, 2 1/4 oz	4	1.3
Donuts, average, 2 oz	4	1.2
Muffins, aver., 1 medium, 1 1/2 oz	3	1
Pancakes, 4" diam., two, 2 oz	4	1
Pies: Fruit, 1 piece, 5 1/2 oz	4	1.5
Pecan, 1 piece, 5 oz	7	4.5
Puddings, aver., 1/2 cup, 4 1/2 oz	4	0.3
Waffles, 1 large, 2 1/2 oz	7	1.5

COOKIES, CRACKERS, CHIPS
Cookies, average 4 cookies	2	1
Crackers: Graham, 2 1/2" sq., two	1	0
Rice Cakes, average, one	1	0
Corn/Potato Chips, 1 oz	2	0.3

SUGAR, HONEY, JAM
Sugar: White	0	0
Brown, 1 Tbsp	0	0.3
Molasses: Light/Medium, 1 Tbsp	0	1
Blackstrap, 1 Tbsp, 3/4 oz	0	3
Corn Syrup, 1 Tbsp, 3/4 oz	0	1
Honey, Jams, Jelly	0	0.2

CANDY, CHOCOLATE, CAROB
Candy, sugar-based	0	0
Chocolate: Plain, 2 oz bar	4	0.8
with nuts, 2 oz bar	6	0.8
Carob, plain, 2 oz	6	0.7

GRANOLA & FOOD/PROTEIN BARS
Granola Bar, average	2	0.5
Peanut Bar (Planters), 1 1/2 oz	7	0.7
Bariatrix: Nutra Bars, 1	11	3.6
Proti Bars, 1	15	1.5
MetaForm Bar	30	7.2
Met-Rx Bar, 100g	26	7.2
Power Bar, 1 bar	10	6.3
Slim-Fast Bar, 34g	6	4.5
Tiger Sport, 65g	11	4.5
Sandoz Nutritional Bar, 1	8	4.5

PROTEIN & IRON COUNTER

NUTS & SEEDS- Per 1 oz | P | I
Item	P	I
Almonds, shelled, 20-25 nuts	6	1
Brazil Nuts, 7-8 medium nuts	4	1
Cashews, 12-16 nuts	5	1.5
Coconut, raw, $1^{1}/_{2}$ oz pce (2" x $2^{1}/_{2}$")	1	1
Filberts, 1oz	4	1
Macadamias, 1 oz	2	0.5
Mixed Nuts, 1 oz	5	1
Peanuts, dry roasted, 40 nuts, 1 oz	6	0.6
Peanut Butter, 1 Tbsp	1	0.5
Pecans, 24 halves, 1 oz	2	0.5
Pumpkin Kernels, dry, hulled, 1 oz	7	4.2
Sesame Seeds, dry, 1 Tbsp	2	0.6
Sunflower Seeds, dried, hulled, 1 oz	6	2
Tahini, 1 Tbsp, $^{1}/_{2}$ oz	2.5	1.4
Walnuts, 15 halves, 1 oz	4	0.7

COFFEE, TEA, SODA
Item	P	I
Coffee, Coffee Substitutes, 1 cup	0	0.1
Tea (all types); Soft Drinks/Soda	0	0
Hot Chocolate, 6 fl.oz	2	2.2

BEER, WINE, SPIRITS
Item	P	I
Beer, 12 fl.oz	1	0
Wines, red/white, 1 glass	0	0.4
Spirits/Liquor	0	0

FAST FOODS/BURGERS

Note: See Fast Foods Section for comprehensive protein counts.

Item	P	I
Arby's: Roast Beef S/wich, reg.	23	4
Giant Roast Beef S/wich	35	6
Italian Sub	30	2
Roast Turkey Deluxe	20	3
Burger King: Whopper S/wich	27	2.5
Hamburger	20	1.5
Double Bacon Cheeseburger	44	2.5
Chicken Sandwich; Big Fish Sandwich	26	2
Carl's Jr: Famous Star H/burger	26	2
Super Star Hamburger	43	3
Chicken Club Sandwich	35	2
Hot & Crispy Sandwich	14	1
Domino's Pizza: Deep Dish (12"), 2 sl.		
Cheese, 2 slices	18	4
Pepperoni, Sausage/Pepperoni	21	4
X-tra Cheese & Pepperoni	24	4.5
French Fries: Medium, $3^{1}/_{2}$ oz	4.5	0.7
Hardees: Frisco Burger	33	5
Cravin' Bacon Cheeseburger	30	2.5
Roast Beef, regular	17	4
Fisherman's Fillet	26	4

KFC | P | I
Item	P	I
Original, Wing & Breast	38	0.4
3-Pce. Dinner, Original	51	0.4
Kentucky Nuggets, 6	16	0.4
Colonel's Chicken Sandwich	29	1.5
Long John Silver's		
Flavorbaked Fish, 1 pce	20	1
Flavorbaked Chicken, 1 pce	26	1.5
Ultimate Fish	18	na
McDonald's: Arch Deluxe	29	2.5
Big Mac	25	2.5
Cheeseburger	15	1.5
Chicken McNuggets(6)	18	0.6
Fish Filet Deluxe	24	1.5
Grilled Crispy Chicken Deluxe	27	1.5
Hamburger	12	1.5
Quarter Pounder	23	2.5
French Fries: Small, $2^{1}/_{2}$ oz	3	0.2
Large, 5 oz	6	0.6
Breakfast: Egg McMuffin	17	1.5
Hotcakes w. Marg/Syrup	9	1.5
Sausage McMuffin w. Egg	19	1.5
Grilled Chicken Salad Deluxe	21	1
Muffin, Lowfat, Apple Bran	6	1
Shake, Chocolate	12	0.4
Pancakes: 3 Pancakes	8	2
Pizza Hut: Medium, 2 slices		
Pan Pizzas, average	26	4
Thin 'n Crispy: Supreme	28	2
Hand Tossed: Pepperoni	24	3
Supreme; Personal Pan Pizza	32	4.5
Subway: 6" Subs, average	22	2
Del Style S/wiches, average	12	1
Subway Club Salad, reg.	16	2
Sundaes: Average	7	0.3
Taco Bell: Bean Burrito	13	3.5
Beef Burrito	22	3.7
Tostado	10	1.5
Enchirito; Nachos Bellgrande	20	3
Taco Bellgrande	18	2
Taco Light	19	2.5
Taco Salad w. Shell	35	7
Wendy's: Single w. Everything	26	3
Big Bacon Classic	34	3
Hamburger Kid's Meal	15	2
Grilled Chicken Sandwich	27	1.5
Stuffed Potatoes: Broc. & Cheese	9	2.5
Bacon & Cheese	17	2.5
Taco Salad	29	2.5

243

HIGH BLOOD PRESSURE GUIDE

HIGH BLOOD PRESSURE

Many American adults have hypertension (high blood pressure), and are unaware of it. It is generally symptomless, so **have your blood pressure checked annually** - particularly if there is a family history of hypertension.

♦ **Untreated hypertension** overworks the heart, damages arteries and promotes atherosclerosis. This in turn greatly increases the risk of heart disease, stroke, blindness, kidney disease and impotence. The earlier hypertension is detected, the sooner it can be brought under control.

TREATING HYPERTENSION

If your blood pressure is high, consult your doctor about diet and medication. You may be referred to a dietitian for more detailed dietary advice and meal planning.

♦ **High-Normal and Stage 1 hypertension** can often be treated by reducing sodium intake, losing weight if overweight, limiting alcohol to 2 drinks or less daily, exercising regularly, and dealing with stress.

♦ **Stages 2, 3 and 4 hypertension** usually require drug therapy. However, salt restriction, abstaining from alcohol and the above lifestyle changes will improve the success of drug therapy, and enable smaller drug doses to be prescribed.

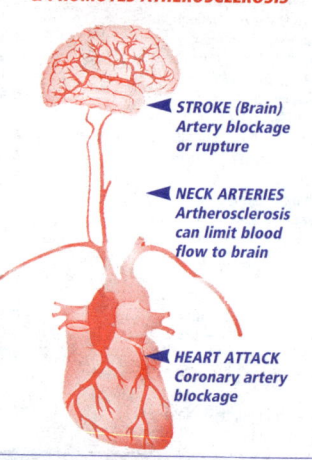

HYPERTENSION DAMAGES ARTERIES & PROMOTES ATHEROSCLEROSIS

◄ **STROKE (Brain)** Artery blockage or rupture

◄ **NECK ARTERIES** Artherosclerosis can limit blood flow to brain

◄ **HEART ATTACK** Coronary artery blockage

BLOOD PRESSURE CLASSIFICATIONS
National High Blood Pressure Educ. Prog. (1993)

	DIASTOLIC	SYSTOLIC
Normal	80-84	120-129
High-Normal	85-89	130-139
Stage 1	90-99	140-159
Stage 2	100-109	160-179
Stage 3	110-119	180-209
Stage 4	120 or over	210 or over

STROKE
KNOW THE WARNING SIGNS

If you notice one or more of these signs, **call your doctor immediately**. They may be signalling a possible stroke or transient ischemic attack:

♦ **Sudden weakness** or numbness in your face, arm or leg on one side of your body.

♦ **Sudden dimness**, blurring or loss of vision, particularly in one eye.

♦ **Loss of speech**, or trouble talking or understanding speech.

♦ **Sudden severe headache** - 'a bolt out of the blue' - with no apparent cause.

♦ **Unexplained dizziness**, unsteadiness or a sudden fall, especially if accompanied by any of the other symptoms.

SALT · SODIUM GUIDE

SALT & SODIUM

- **Sodium is a mineral element** most commonly found in salt (sodium chloride). It also occurs naturally in much smaller amounts in animal and plant foods, and water - normally sufficient for our needs without having to add salt.

- **Sodium is required** for nerve and muscle function as well as to balance the amount of fluid in our tissues and blood.

  Sodium acts like a sponge to attract and hold fluids in body tissues.

- **Excess sodium** can cause water retention, and increase the risk of developing hypertension. Very high salt intake may also increase the risk of stomach cancer.

- **Too little sodium** may cause low blood pressure (hypotension), and decrease blood flow to the heart, brain and kidneys - especially during exercise. (A certain blood volume is required to sustain the blood pressure needed for adequate blood flow in the capillaries).

SALT-SENSITIVE PERSONS

- Normally, our **kidneys** excrete excess dietary sodium. The thirst we feel after a salty meal is the body calling for water to dilute the sodium, and enable the kidneys to flush out excess sodium.

- However, 'salt sensitive' persons (perhaps 1 in 2-3 adults) tend to retain excess sodium (above approximately 3000mg daily) instead of excreting it. Such persons are more likely to develop hypertension and would most benefit from sodium restriction. Assume you are susceptible if there is a family history of hypertension.

- Although not everyone will benefit, all Americans are being asked to **moderate their salt and sodium intake** as a public health measure - particularly that so many do not know whether or not they have hypertension; and also because we do not know just who is salt-sensitive.

SAFE SODIUM LEVELS

The American Heart Association recommends a maximum sodium intake of 2400mg per day for adults with normal blood pressure. Many Americans have double this amount.

Persons with hypertension and kidney ailments are usually restricted to as little as **1000mg sodium per day**. Your doctor will discuss the correct sodium level for you.

Persons engaged in prolonged strenuous work or exercise may lose sodium through heavy sweating - especially in hot, humid weather. Adequate salt (and fluids) is necessary to avoid dehydration. A little extra salt at mealtimes is usually sufficient to satisfy any extra need. Do not take salt tablets.

FINDING HIDDEN SODIUM

On average, only one third of our sodium intake comes from the salt shaker. The rest is hidden in processed foods that have salt added during manufacture.

Additionally, sodium compounds added to food or medicinals can contribute significant sodium.

Sodium bicarbonate in particular is widely used in antacid tablets and powders, and saline drink powders (such as *Alka Seltzer*). Sodium bicarbonate contains 27% sodium by weight. Each gram contributes 270mg sodium. Large amounts of sodium can be unwittingly consumed.

Other sodium compounds include monosodium glutamate (MSG), sodium ascorbate, sodium nitrite, and sodium citrate.

ALCOHOL

Alcohol causes up to 20% of hypertension in America.
Susceptible persons should abstain to normalize their blood pressure.

SALT · SODIUM GUIDE

Sodium accounts for only 40% of the weight of salt (sodium chloride). Examples:
1 gram (1000mg) Salt has 400mg Sodium
1 teasp. (5g) Salt has 2000mg Sodium

HINTS TO REDUCE SODIUM

♦ **Watch the salt shaker.** Start with an easy 50% cut in sodium by using Lite Salt (*Morton*). Then gradually cut back until you can leave the salt shaker off the table.

♦ **Taste your food before salting.** Use the pepper shaker (small holes) for more controlled sprinkling of salt.

♦ **Choose low sodium**, sodium free, and reduced sodium products in place of regular salted products.

♦ **Check labels for sodium levels.** The following sodium descriptors may appear on labels:

Reduced Sodium: At least 75% less sodium than the original product.
Low Sodium: 140 mg or less/serving.
Very Low Sodium: 35mg or less/serving.
Sodium Free: Less than 5mg per serving.

♦ Use reduced sodium breads, butter and margarine. Regular varieties contain up to 2% salt. This is considered high in view of their significant contribution to our diet.

♦ **Go easy on condiments and sauces** such as tomato sauce, mustard, soy sauce and spaghetti sauces, as well as salad dressings. Use low sodium varieties.

♦ **Limit pizzas and salty fast foods.** Check the *Fast Food Restaurant* Section.

♦ **Avoid salty snack foods** such as potato chips, corn chips, salted nuts, pretzels and cheesy-flavoured snacks. **Choose unsalted** popcorn, nuts or seeds. Eat more fruit.

♦ **Don't salt children's food** to your taste.

♦ **Limit or avoid antacids and saline powders** with sodium bicarbonate (such as *Alka-Seltzer*). They are high in sodium.

FOODS HIGH IN SODIUM
- Cheese, Butter, Margarine
- Pickles, Sauerkraut, Olives
- Condiments, Sauces
- Salad Dressings
- Canned vegetables/salads/beans
- Deli Salads (with dressing)
- Frozen/Packaged Meals/Entrees
- Soups: Canned/dry; bouillon cubes
- Meats: Ham, bacon, sausage, luncheon meats, smoked meats
- Canned Fish (in brine)
- Seasoning Salts (e.g. garlic, celery)
- Snack Foods (potato chips, pretzels)
- Tomato Jce (Canned), V8 Vegetable Jce
- Fast Foods: Pizza, Burgers, Chicken
- *Alka-Seltzer* Antacid

MODERATE SODIUM
- Bread (Reduced Salt)
- Meat, Fish, Poultry - Unprocessed
- Milk, Yogurt, Soy Drinks, Eggs
- Peanut Butter
- Breakfast Cereals (<200mg/serving)
- Chocolate Candy, Fruit/Nut Bars
- *Reduced & Low-Sodium* Products

FOODS LOW IN SODIUM
- Products labelled *Very Low Sodium*, or *Sodium Free*
- Fresh fruits and vegetables
- Canned and Dried Fruits
- Potatoes, Rice, Pasta
- Dried Beans & Lentils, Tofu
- Nuts & Seeds (unsalted)
- Corn & Popcorn (unsalted)
- Pepper, Spices, Herbs
- Jam, Honey, Syrup
- Candy, Gum
- Hard & Jelly Candy
- Coffee, Tea, Alcohol
- Fresh Fruit Juices, Water

SODIUM COUNTER

> The American Heart Association recommends a sodium intake of LESS THAN 2400mg/day

Sod ~ SODIUM (mg)

MILK & DAIRY PRODUCTS (Sod)

Milk: Whole/lowfat/skim, aver. 1 cup, 8 fl.oz	120
Whole, low sodium, 1 cup	6
Choc Milk (*Hershey's*), 1 cup	130
Human Milk, 8 fl.oz	40
Soy Milk, 8 fl.oz	30
Buttermilk, cultured, 8 fl.oz	250
Dry/Powder, skim, 1/4 cup, 1 oz	110
Yogurt: with fruit aver., 8 oz	130
Cheese, *Kraft:* Cheddar, 1 oz	180
Swiss, 1 oz	40
Parmesan, 1 oz	450
Blue, 1 oz	330
Philadelphia Brand Cream	85
Process Cheese., aver.,1 oz	430
Cottage Cheese, 1/2 cup, 4 oz	450
Ricotta Cheese, 1/2 cup, 4 oz	150

ICECREAM, FROZEN YOGURT

Icecream, average, 1/2 cup	50
Frozen Yogurt, 1/2 cup	50

FATS/OILS

Butter/Margarine, reg., 2 Tbsp,1 oz	230
Unsalted, reg., 2 Tbsp,1 oz	<5
Mayonnaise, aver., 2 Tbsp.,1 oz	160
Molly McButter, 1 tsp	120
Oils/Lard/Dripping	0
Cream, average, 1 Tbsp	6
Coffee-Mate: Powdered, 1 tsp	2
Liquid, 1 Tbsp	5

EGGS: Whole, 1 large

EGGS: Whole, 1 large	70
Egg White, 1 large	50
Omelette, 2 egg, plain	220
w.cheese	400
Egg Beaters (*Fleischmann's*), 1/4 cup	80

MEATS

Meat, average all types, cooked (Beef/Lamb/Veal/Pork), 4 oz	80
Corned Beef, cooked, 3 oz	800
Bacon, cooked, 2 slices, 1/2 oz	270
Ham, 3 oz	1100

CHICKEN & TURKEY

Chicken, cooked, unsalted, 4 oz	80

SAUSAGES & MEATS (Sod)

Bologna, 1 oz	280
Frankfurter, 2 oz	640
Ham, chopped, 3/4 oz slice	290
Liverwurst (Braunschweiger), 1 oz	320
Pepperoni, 5 slices, 1 oz	570
Salami, cooked, 1 oz	350
dry/hard, 1 oz	600
Sausage, 1 oz link	220
Pork, 2 oz patty	260
Turkey Roll, 1 oz	160

FISH: Fresh Fish, average, plain

Cooked, 4 oz (no bone)	60
Broiled w. butter, 4 oz	150
Breaded & fried, 4 oz	320
Fish fillets, bat.-dipped 3 oz	350
Fish sticks, 1 oz stick	160
Gefilte Fish (w.broth), 1 pce, 1 1/2 oz	220
Herring, pickled, 2 pces., 1 oz	260
Lobster, meat only, 4 oz	180
Oysters, fresh, 6 med., 3 oz	95
Salmon, canned, 3 oz	460
No Salt Added, 3 oz	65
Smoked fish, average, 3 oz	650
Tuna, canned, 3 oz	330
No Added Salt, 3 oz	40

ENTREES & MEALS

Frozen Meals, average	600-900
Lean Cuisine, average	900
Stouffer's, average	580
Dinners, average	900-1200
Side Dishes, average	400-600
Pizza, frozen, 1/4 large, 6 oz	800-1200
Microwave Cup Meals	900-1200
Cup O'Noodles, average	1500

FAST FOODS & RESTAURANTS

(Comprehensive listings see **Fast-Foods Section**)

Cheeseburger	750
Hamburger: Regular	500
Large with cheese	1100
Fish/Chicken Sandwich	1000
French Fries, medium, 2 1/4 oz	150
Chicken Dinner (3 piece)	2200
Chicken Nuggets w. Sauce	800
Hot Dog (Frankfurter)	800
Pizza, 2 medium slices	1200
Taco	400
Shake, chocolate	250

SODIUM COUNTER

Sod ~ SODIUM (mg)

SOUPS: Condensed, 1 cup, 8 oz — 800-1000
   Low Sodium — 70
Chicken Noodle, 1 cup — 900
Bouillon Cube, average — 950
Cup-A-Soup, average — 850
   Lite, average — 450
Soup Mixes, aver. 1 cup — 900

CONDIMENTS, SAUCES, DRESSINGS

A-1 Sauce, 1 Tbsp — 270
Barbecue Sauce, 1 Tbsp — 130
Chili Sauce, 1 Tbsp — 230
Ketchup, tomato, 1 Tbsp — 180
   Low Sodium, 1 Tbsp — 20
Mayonnaise, 1 Tbsp — 80
Mustard, 1 tsp — 70
Pizza Sauce, 1/2 cup — 700
Salad Dressings, 2Tbsp., 1 oz — 160-400
Spaghetti Sauce, 1/2 cup — 500
Soy Sauce, 1 Tbsp — 1000
Sweet & Sour, 1/2 cup — 250
Tabasco, 1 tsp — 25
Vinegar, Lemon Juice, 1/2 cup — 1
Worcestershire, 1 Tbsp — 200
Tomato: Sauce, 1 cup — 1200
   Paste/Puree (salted), 1/2 cup — 1000
   No Salt Added, 1/2 cup — 25

SALT & SALT SUBSTITUTES

Table Salt: 1 tsp, 6g — 2400
   Single Serve packet, 1 g — 400
Lite Salt (*Morton*), 1 tsp, 6g — 1200
Salt Substitute (Potassium), 1 tsp — <1
Garlic Salt, 1 tsp, 6g — 1800
Seasoned or Sea Salt, 1 tsp, 5g — 1600

SEASONINGS, HERBS & SPICES

Baking Powder, 1 tsp, 3g — 340
Baking Soda (Sod.bicarb), 1 tsp, 3g — 810
Accent (Flavor Enhancer), 1 tsp — 600
Chili Powder, 1 tsp, 3g — 25
Herbs/Spices: Curry Powder — <1
Lemon Pepper (*Lawry's*), 1 tsp — 340
Meat Tenderizer, 1 tsp, 5g — 1750
MSG (Monosodium glutamate), 5g — 500
Mrs Dash (Herb/Spice Blend), 1 tsp — 0
Pepper, Mustard (dry), 1 tsp — 1
Vegit, 1 tsp — 3
Yeast, Nutritional, 1 Tbsp — 10
Stuffing Mixes, average., 1/2 cup — 500

BREAKFAST CEREALS

Kellogg's:
   All-Bran, 1/3 cup, 1 oz — 260
   Bran Flakes, 2/3 cup, 1 oz — 220
   Corn Flakes, 1 cup, 1 oz — 290
   Just Right, 2/3 cup, 1 oz — 200
   Shredded Wheat Squares,
      1/2 cup, 1 oz — 5
Health Valley Cereals, 1 serving — 5
Quaker: Crunchy Bran, 1 oz — 320
   100% Natural, 1 oz — 15
   Puffed Rice/Wheat, 1 oz — 1
Cap'n Crunch, average, 1 oz — 250
Total, 1 cup, 1 oz — 140
Nature Valley: Average, 1 oz — 90
Oatmeal: Regular, 3/4 cup — 1
   Instant (*Quaker*), 2/3 cup (1pkt) — 270

BREADS, BAGELS, CRACKERS

Bread: Average all types, 1 oz — 140
   Low Sodium, 1 oz — 10
Bagels, plain, 2 oz — 200
   Sara Lee, 3 oz — 500
Biscuits, average, 1 oz — 180
Bun/Roll, 1 medium, 1 1/2 oz — 200
Crackers: Saltine, 2 — 70
   Low Salt (Premium), 2 — 45
   Graham, 2 — 50
Croissant, average, 2 oz — 280
Rice Cakes, average — 25
RyKrisp Crispbread, Sesame, 2 — 100

COOKIES, CAKES, DESSERTS

Cookies, average, 1 cookie — 30
Baked Custard, 1/2 cup — 100
Brownie, 1/4 oz piece — 75
Cake, average, 3 oz piece — 250
Cinnamon Sweet Roll, 2 oz — 250
Danish, Apple — 250
Donut, average — 150
Muffins, 1 medium, 2 oz — 150
   Sara Lee, average, 2 1/2 oz — 300
Pancakes, 3 x 4" — 360
Pie, average 1/6 of 9" pie — 300
Pudding, average, 1/2 cup — 160
   Jell-O (Mix), Instant, 1/2 cup — 400
Waffles: Home-made, 7", 2 1/2 oz — 350
   Frozen, average, 1 1/4 oz — 260
   Aunt Jemima, aver., 2 1/2 oz — 630

SODIUM COUNTER

(< = less than)

FRUIT & JUICES | Sod
Item	Sod
Fresh Fruit, aver., 1 serving	1
Dried/Canned Fruit, 1/2 cup	<5
Fruit Juice: Fresh, sqz'd, 6 fl.oz	<5
Commercial, aver., 6 fl.oz	20
Carrot Juice (*Ferraro's*), 8 fl.oz	230
Tomato Juice (*Campbell's*), 6 fl.oz	570
Low Sodium (No Salt Added)	20
V8 Vegetable (*Campbell's*), 6 fl.oz	600
(No Salt Added), 6 fl.oz	45

VEGETABLES
Fresh/Frozen (No Salt Added), 1/2 cup

Item	Sod
Asparagus, Bean Sprouts, Corn	3
Cucumber, Green Beans, Mushroom, Okra	3
Onions, Potato, Pumpkin, Squash	3
Broccoli, Cabbage, Cauliflower	10
Peppers, Hot Chili, raw 1	3
Tomato, 1 medium, 5 oz	10
Beets, Carrots, Celery, 1/2 cup	40
Spinach, Turnips, 1/2 cup, ckd.	40
Canned: Asparagus, 4 spears	300
Beans, baked in tom.sce	450
Beets, 1/2 cup, 3 oz	240
Corn Kernels, 1/2 cup, 3 oz	190
Creamed, 1/2 cup, 4 1/2 oz	330
Mushrooms w. butter sce, 2 oz	550
Peas, 1/2 cup, 3 oz	250
Sauerkraut, 1/2 cup, 4 oz	750

PICKLES, OLIVES
Item	Sod
Olives, pickled: Green, 1 large	90
Ripe/black, 1 large	40
Pickles: Bread & Butter, 4 sl., 1 oz	200
Dill, 1 pickle, 2 1/2 oz	900
Sweet, 1 gherkin, 1/2 oz	130

SOYBEAN PRODUCTS
Item	Sod
Miso (Soy Paste), 1/4 c., 2 1/2 oz	2500
Soybean Protein Isolate, 1 oz	280
Tempeh, 1/2 cup, 3 oz	5
Tofu, average, 1/2 cup, 4 oz	5

JAM, HONEY, SYRUPS
Item	Sod
Jam/Jelly, 1 Tbsp	2
Honey/Maple Syrup, 1 Tbsp	1
Log Cabin Syrup, 1 fl.oz	35
Lite, 1 fl.oz	90

PEANUT BUTTER
Item	Sod
Peanut Butter, regular, 1 Tbsp	70
Unsalted, 1 Tbsp	1

SNACKS, NUTS | Sod
Item	Sod
Cheese Balls/Curls, 1 oz	280
Corn/Tortilla Chips, aver., 1 oz	220
Granola bars, aver., 1 bar	80
Nuts: Plain, unsalted, 1 oz	1
Lightly salted, 1 oz	80
Salted or Honey Roasted, 1 oz	160
Popcorn: Plain (unsalted), 1 cup	1
Flavored, average, 1 cup	60
Salt added, 1 cup	180
Potato Chips, plain, 1 oz	160
Flavored, average, 1 oz	250
Pretzels, regular, 3, 1 oz	450

CANDY, CHOCOLATE
Item	Sod
Chocolate, milk, 1 oz	30
Carob Milk Bar, 1 oz portion	55
Fudge, chocolate, 1 oz	55
Candy Bars, average, 1 1/2 oz	60
Hard Candy, Jelly Beans, 1 oz	10
Licorice, 1 oz	30

BEVERAGES, ALCOHOL
Item	Sod
Coffee (& Substitutes), Tea, 1 cup	1
Cocoa, dry, plain, 1 Tbsp	0
Mix, average, 1 envelope	120
Quik (*Nestle*), 2 tsp	35
Soft Drinks, average, 8 fl.oz	20
Mineral Water, Perrier, 8 fl.oz	5
Gatorade Thirst Quencher, 8 fl.oz	110
Water, average, 1 cup, 8 fl.oz	5
Drier regions, 1 cup	20+
Alcohol: Beer, average, 12 fl.oz	15
Wines, average, 4 fl.oz	10
Spirits (distilled), 1 1/2 fl.oz	1

ANTACIDS ~ ALKA-SELTZER
Item	Sod
Alka-Seltzer (Per Tablet):	
Original (Light Blue Box)	570
Extra Strength (Dark Blue Box)	590
Flavored Lemon/Lime	500
Antacid (yellow Box)	310
Gelatine Capsule, 1	0
Alka-Mints, chewable	0
Bromo Seltzer, 3/4 capful	760
Rolaids: Original, 1 tablet	50
Sodium-Free; Extra Strength	0
Tums: Regular/Extra Strength	<5
Sodium Bicarb. (27% sodium), 1 g	270

INDEX (A-C)

Aero Bar, 100
Alcohol, 128-132
Ale, 129
Alfalfa, 118
All Bran, 79
Almonds: 108
   Butter, 109
   Joy, 100
   Paste, 95
   Roca, 100
Aloe Vera, 109
Amaranth, 81
Anchovy, 46
Angel Food Cake, 90
Angostura Bitters, 132
Antipasto Salad, 122
Apple: 110
   Caramel, 110
   Juice, 114
   Pie, 92
   Sauce, 68
Apricot, 110
Arby's, 140-141
Artichokes, 118, 121
Asparagus, 118
Aunt Jemima, 97, 99
Avocado, 29, 110

Baba Ghannouj, 137
Baby Ruth, 100
Babybel Cheese, 31
Baci, 100
Bacon, 40
   Bits, 122
   Chips, 67
Bagel: 83, 133, 136
   Chips, 83
Baked Beans, 57
Baking Ingredients, 95
Baking Powder, 95
Baklava, 135
Bamboo Shoots, 118
Banana, 110
Banana Chips, 112
Banquet Meals, 49
Barley, 81
Barley Sugar, 100
Baskin Robbins, 142
BBQ Sauce, 68
Beans, 118
Beanut Butter, 109
Bee Pollen, 77
Beechies, 102
Beef, 37
   Fat, 29
   rky, 42, 105

Beers, 129
Beerwurst, 42
Bernaise Sauce, 68
Best Foods, 72
Betty Crocker:
   Cakes, 94
   Cereals, 78
   Frostings, 95
   Meals, 57
   Muffins, 90
   Pancakes, 97
Biscuits, 89
Bisquick, 92, 97
Black Forest Cake, 90, 134
Blancmange, 96
Blintzes, 136
Bloody Mary, 132
Blue Thunder, 125
Boar, 40
Bok Choy, 118
Bologna, 42
Borscht, 64, 136
Boston Market, 150
Bouillabaisse, 134
Bouillon Cubes, 63
Brains, 40
Bran, 77, 79
Bratwurst, 42
Brazil Nuts, 108
Bread: 83
   & Butter Pickles, 71
   Crumbs, 84
   Dough, 84
   Pudding, 96
Breadsticks, 84
Breakfast Cereals, 77
Brie, 31
Brioche, 134
Brisket, 38
Broadbeans, 118
Broccoli, 118
Buckwheat, 77, 81
Budget Gourmet, 49
Buffalo, 40
Bugles, 105
Bulgar, 77, 81, 122
Buns, 83
Burger King, 151
Burgundy, 131
Burritos, 137
Butermilk, 20
Butter, 29, 109
Butter Buds, 29, 67
Butterbeans, 118
Butterscotch, 100
   Topping, 99

Cabbage Rolls, 137
Caesar Salad, 122
Cajun Meals, 134
Cakes: 90-95
   Frostings, 95
Calamari, 46, 135
Camembert, 31
Canada Dry, 126
Candied Fruit, 112
Candy, 100
Canned Meals, 57
Canned Veges, 121
Cannelloni, 82, 135
Capon, 44
Cappuccino, 123
Caramel Apples, 110
Caramello, 101
Caramels, 101
Caraway, 109
Carefree, 102
Carob Candy, 104
Carob Flour, 81, 95
Carrot Juice, 114
Cashew Butter, 109
Cashews, 108
Cassava, 110
Catsup, 68
Cauliflower, 118
   Pickles, 71
Caviar, 46, 138
Celeriac, 118
Cereal, 77
Certs, 101
Challah, 83
Champagne, 131
Chapati, 135
Cheese: 31-34
   Balls, 31
   Crackers, 105
   Dips, 34
   Spreads, 34
Cheesecake, 90, 93
Cheez Balls, 105
Chef Salad, 122
Cherries, 113
Chevre, 31
Chianti, 131
Chick Pea, 81, 118
Chicken, 44
   Broth, 136
   Cacciatore, 135
   Fat, 29
   Liver Pate, 43
   Pilaf, 135
   Spread, 42
Chicory, 118, 123

Chili, 119
Chili con Carne, 137
Chili Powder, 67
Chinese: Chard, 118
   Egg Noodles, 82
   Meals, 134
Chips Ahoy, 87
Chitterlings, 40
Chocolate: 100
   Baking Bars, 95
   Baking Chips, 95
   Chip Cookie, 85
   Cake, 90
   Pie, 92
Cholent, 136
Chop Suey, 134
Chopped Liver, 136
Choux Pastry, 92
Chow Mein Noodles, 122
Chuck Steak, 38
Churros, 105
Chutney, 71
Cider, 130
Cinnamon, 67
Clams, 46
Clams Marinara, 138
Claret, 131
Clarified Butter, 29
Club Sandwich, 133
Coating Mixes, 84
Coca Cola, 126
Cochifrito, 138
Cocktail Sauce, 68
Cocktails, 131-132
Cocoa: Drinks, 21, 123
   Krispies, 79
   Powder, 95
   Puffs, 78
Coconut, 108, 110
   Cream Pie, 92
   Cream, 30
   Dried, 95
   Milk, 30
   Water, 30
Cod Liver Oil, 109
Coffee: 123
   Cakes, 93
   Creamers, 30
   Essence, 123
   Whiteners, 123
Coffee-Mate, 30
Cointreau, 132
Cold Meat, 42
Coleslaw Salad, 122
Colombo, 22, 23
Condensed Milk, 20

INDEX (C-H)

Condiments, 68
Cookies, 85
Cooking Choc, 100
Cool Whip, 30
Coolers, Wine 131
Coq au Vin, 134
Cordials, 132
Corn: 81
   Bran, 81
   Bread, 83
   Chips, 105
   Dogs, 41
   Flakes, 77-79
   Flake Crumbs, 84
   Flour, 81
   Grits, 77, 81
Cornbread, 137
Corned Beef, 42
Cornmeal, 81
Cornstarch, 81, 95
Cottage Cheese, 31
Cough Drops, 104
Cough Syrups, 109
Cous Cous, 81, 137
Crab, 46
Crackers, 85
Cranberry, 68, 110
Cranberry Juice, 114
Cranberry Sauce, 68
Crawfish, 134
Crayfish, 46
Cream: 30
   Cheese, 34
   of Rice, 77
   of Wheat, 77
   Toppings, 30
Creamers, 30
Creme Caramel, 134
Cremora, 30
Creole Meals, 134
Crepe Suzette, 134
Crispbread, 84
Croissants, 84, 133
Croutons, 84, 122
Crunch, 101
Cup-A-Ramen, 66
Cup-a-Soup, 65
Cupcake, 90
Currants, 110
Custard, 96
   Pie, 92

Dal, 135
Danish Pastry, 90
Dates, 112
Deer, 40

Deli Meats, 42
Denny's, 161
Desserts: 90-95
Deviled Eggs, 35
Dextrose, 98
Diet Coke, 126
Diet Pepsi, 126
Dill Pickle, 71
Dim Sum, 134
Dipping Sauces, 136
Dole: Bars, 27
   Salads, 122
Domino's, 165
Donuts, 91
Doritos, 106
Dove: 134
   Bars, 27
   Candy, 101
Drambuie, 132
Dried Fruit, 112
Dripping, 29
Drumstick, 27
Duck, 45
Duck Eggs, 35
Duck Fat, 29
Duncan Hines Cakes, 94
Dunkeroos, 105
Dunkin Donuts, 167

Eclair, 90
Edensoy, 20
Eel, 46
Eggs: 35
   Dishes, 36
   Nogs, 35
   Noodles, 82
   Rolls, 36, 134
   Salad, 122
   Substitutes, 35
Eggplant, 118
Empanada, 137
Enchilada, 137
Enchirito, 137
Endive, 118
Energy Bars, 106
English Muffins, 84
Ensure, 125
Entrees, 49-54
Equal, 98
Escargot, 134
Eskimo Pie, 27
Espresso, 123
Ethnic Meals, 134
Evaporated Milk, 20

Fajitas, 137
Famous Amos, 85
Fanta, 126
Farfel, 136
Farina, 77, 81
Fats, 29
Featherweight: Candy, 101
   Cookies, 85
   Sauce, 69
Felafel, 136
Fennel, 109, 118
Fenugreek, 67
Ferrero Rocher, 101
Fig Bars, 90
Figs, 110
Filberts, 108
Filet Mignon, 37
Filo Pastry, 92
Fish: 46
   Oil, 29, 109
   Sticks, 48
Flaky Pastry, 92
Flavor Extracts, 95
Flavorings, 67
Flax Seeds, 81
Flour, 81
Foie Gras, 43
Fortune Cookie, 134
Frankfurter, 41
Frappucino, 123
French Fries, 119
French Toast, 83
Fresh Fruit, 110
Frito Lay: Dips, 34
   Snacks, 105
Frogs Legs, 134, 138
Froot Loops, 79
Frostings, 95
Frozen Meals, 49-54
Fructose, 98
Fruit: 110-117
   Butters, 98
   Cake, 90
   Canned, 113
   Cocktail, 113
   Juices, 114
   Leather, 101, 112
   Nectar, 114
   Pectin, 95
   Rolls, 112
   Salad, 113
   Snacks, 113
   Spreads, 98
Fruitopia, 115
Frusen Gladje, 24
Fudge, 101

Galactobureko, 135
Game Meats, 40
Garbanzo, 81
Garlic: 118
   Bread, 83
   Powder, 67
   Tablets, 109
Gatorade, 125
Gazpacho, 135
Gefilte Fish, 136
Gelatin, 95
General Mills, 78
German Meals, 135
Ghee, 29
Gherkins, 71
Giblets, 44
Gin, 131
Ginger Ale, 126
Ginger, 112, 118
Gingerbread, 90
Glace Fruit, 112
Glucose: 98
   Tablets, 109
Gnocchi, 135
Goats Milk: 20
   Cheese, 31
Goldfish, 105
Goose: 45
   Eggs, 35
   Fat, 29
Gooseberries, 113
Gourmet Food, 138
Graham, 85, 88
   Cracker Crumbs, 84
Grains, 81
Granola, 77
Granola Bars, 106
Grapes, 110
Gravy, 38, 71
Greek Food, 135
Green Chilies, 71
Grenadine, 132
Grits, 80
Ground Beef, 38
Guacamole, 34, 137
Guiltless Indulgence, 89
Gum, 102
Guylian Candy, 103

Haagen-Daaz, 25, 27
Haggis, 138
Hain Dressing, 73
Hallah, 136
Halvah, 102
Ham Hock, 137
Ham, 40, 42

INDEX (H-N)

Hamburger Helper, 57
Hamburger Roll, 83
Hardees, 174
Haricot Beans, 118
Hash Browns, 119
Hazelnut Butter, 109
Hazelnuts, 108
Head Cheese, 42
Health Valley: Bars, 106
    Cereals, 79
    Cookies, 85
    Meals, 50
    Pizza, 55
Heart, 40
Hearts of Palm, 121
Herb-Ox, 63
Herbal Tea, 124
Herbs, 67
Herring, 46
Hershey's, 21, 102
Hi-C, 115
Hickory, 108
Hidden Valley, 73
Hoagie, 83
Hogshead Cheese, 134
Hominy Grits, 77
Hominy, 137
Honey, 98
Honeycomb, 102
Horseradish, 68, 118
Hot Dog, 41
Hot Fudge, 99
Hubba Bubba, 102
Hummus, 34, 136
Hush Puppies, 137

Ice Milk, 23
Icecream: 23
    Bars, 27
    Cones, 25
    Toppings, 99
Iced Tea, 124
Ices, 23
Inari Zushi, 136
Indian Food, 135
Instant Grits, 80
Instant Pudding, 96
Irish Coffee, 123
Italian: Bread, 83
    Dressing, 72
    Meals, 135
    Seasoning, 67

Jack In The Box, 178
Jalapeno Relish, 71
Jam, 98

Jambalaya, 134
Japanese Food, 135
Japanese Soba, 82
Jell-O: 96
    Icecream Bars, 28
    Yogurt, 22
Jellies, 98
Jelly Beans, 102
Jelly, 98
Jewish Foods, 136
Jolt Cola, 126
Jujube, 110

Kaffree, 123
Karo, 99
Kasha, 136
Keebler, 86
Kelloggs, 79
KFC, 181
Kid Cuisine, 51
Kidney Beans, 118
Kidneys, 40
Kielbasa, 137
Kipfel, 136
Kisses, 102
Kit Kat, 102
Knackwurst, 42
Knaidlach, 136
Knish, 136
Knorr, 58, 71
Kool-Aid, 127
Kraft: Butter Spread, 29
    Cheese, 33
    Cream Topping, 30
    Dips, 34
    Dressing, 74
    Sauce, 69
Kreplach, 136
Kugel, 136

La Loma, 60, 79
Lactaid, 20, 21
Lamb, 39
Land 'O Lakes, 21
Lard, 29
Latke, 136
Lean Cuisine: Meals, 51
    Pizza, 55
Lecithin, 77, 109
Leeks, 118
Lemon: 110
    Meringue, 92
    Peel, 95
Lentil Puree, 135
Lentils, 118
Lettuce, 118

Licorice, 102
Lifesavers, 102
Lightlife, 60
Lima Beans, 118
Lime Juice, 114, 132
Lime, 110
Linzer Torte, 135
Lipton, 65
Liqueur Coffee, 123
Liqueurs, 132
Liver Pate, 42
Liver, 40
Liverwurst, 42
Lobster, 47
Lochshen, 136
Loma Linda, 60
Lox, 136
Lozenges, 104
Lucozade, 126
Lunch 'n Munch, 43
Lunch Packs, 43
Lunchables, 43
Luncheon Meats, 42
Lychees, 110

M & M's, 103
Macadamia Nuts, 108
Macaroni, 82
Mackerel, 47
Madeira, 131
Malt Liquor, 129
Mandarin, 111
Mandelbrot, 136
Mango, 111, 112
Manicotti, 82, 135
Margarine, 29
Margarita, 137
Marie Callender's, 52, 93
Marinara Sauce, 69
Marmalade, 98
Mars Bar, 103
Marsala, 131
Marshmallow, 99, 103
Martini, 132
Marzipan, 95
Mascarpone, 32
Matzo: 84
    Balls, 136
    Meal, 81
Mayonnaise, 29, 72
Mazola, 29
McCormick, 71
Meals, 49-54
Meat: 37-45
    Spreads, 42
    Tenderizer, 67

Meringue, 96
Met-Rx, 107, 125
MetaForm, 107
Metamucil, 109
Mexican Foods, 137
Milk, 20
    Chocolate, 21
    Condensed, 20
    Evaporated, 20
    Flavored, 21
Milky Way: 103
    Icecream Bar, 28
Millet, 77, 81
Mince Pie, 92
Mineral Water, 126
Minestrone, 64
Mints, 103
Miracle, 29
Miso: 62
    Soup, 136
Mixed Fruit, 112
Mocha, 123
Mochaccino, 123
Molasses, 99
Molly McButter, 29
Morningstar Farms, 60
Moussaka, 135
Mozzarella, 32
Mrs Fields: Cookies, 86
    Icecream Bars, 28
Muffins, 90
Mulberries, 111
Mung Beans, 118
Muscatel, 131
Mushrooms, 118
Mussels, 47
Mustard, 67, 71

Nabisco, 80, 87
Nasoya, 75
Natto, 62
Nestea, 124
Nestle: Choc Milk, 21
    Cocoa Mix, 21
    Icecream Bars, 28
    Sweet Success, 125
Neufchatel, 32
Noodles, 82
Nori-Maki Zushi, 136
Nougat, 100
Nut Butters, 109
Nuteena, 60
Nutmeg, 67
NutraSweet, 98
Nutri-Grain, 79
Nuts, 108

INDEX (O-S)

Oatbran, 77
Oatmeal, 77
Oats, 81
Octopus, 47
Oh Henry!, 103
Oils, 29
Okra, 118
Old El Paso: 34
   Meals, 58
   Sauce, 69
   Seasonings, 67
   Soup, 66
Olives, 111
Omelet, 35, 134
Onion Powder, 67
Onions, 119
Opossum, 137, 138
Orange: 111
   Juice, 114
   Peel, 95
Oreo: Cookies, 88
   Icecream Bars, 28
Osso Buco, 135
Ouzo, 132
Ovaltine, 21
Oxtail, 137
Oyster Tablets, 109
Oysters, 47

Paella, 138
Pakistan Meals, 135
Pancakes, 97
Pancreas, 40
Pappadom, 135
Parmesan, 32
Parsley, 67
Pasta: 82
   Sauce, 70
Pastrami, 42
Pastries, 90-95
Pastry, 92
Pate, 43
Peach Melba, 90
Peanut, 108
Peanut Butter, 29, 109
Pear, 111
Peas, 119
Pecan Pie, 92
Pecans, 108
Pepper, 67
Pepperidge Farm:
   Bread, 83
   Cakes, 93
   Cookies, 88
   Muffins, 90
   Pizza, 55

Peppermints, 103
Pepperoni, 42
Peppers, 71, 119
Pepsi, 127
Perrier, 127
Philadelphia Cheese, 34
Pickled Onions, 121
Pickles, 71
Pies: 49-62, 92
   Crust, 92
   Filling, 92
Pierogi, 136
Pillbury: Cakes, 94
   Cookies, 89
   Gravy, 71
   Pizza, 55
Pina Colada, 132
Pineapple, 111
Pinenuts, 108
Pinto Beans, 118
Pistachios, 108
Pita Bread, 83
Pizza: Frozen, 55
   Crust, 92
   Pizza Hut, 191
   Sauce, 70
Planters Bars, 107
Plum: 111
   Pudding, 96
Pocket Bread, 83
Poi, 119
Polenta, 81
Pollen Granules, 77
Pollen Meal, 109
Pomegranate, 111
Pop Tarts, 79
Popcorn, 105
Poppyseed, 67
Popsicles, 28
Pork, 39
   Crackling, 137
   Ears, Feet 40
   Goulash, 137
   Skin/Rind, 105
Port, 131
Potato: 119
   au Gratin, 119
   Chips, 105
   Flour, 81
   Latke, 136
   Pancakes, 119
   Salad, 122
Poultry, 44, 45
Pound Cake, 90
Preserves, 98
Pretzels, 106

Prosciutto, 42
Protein Powders, 109
Prunes, 112
Psyllium, 81
Puddings, 96
Puff Pastry, 92
Puffed Rice, 77
Pumpernickel, 83
Pumpkin: 119
   Seeds, 109
   Pie, 92

Quail: 45
Quail Eggs, 35
Quaker: 80
   Bars, 107
Quark Cheese, 32
Quik, 21
Quinoa, 81

Rabbit, 40
Raisins: 112
   Bran, 77
   Bread, 83
Ramen Noodle, 66
Ravioli, 135
Reddi-Wip, 30
Reece's: Candy, 103
   Icecream Bars, 28
Refried Beans, 137
Relishes, 71
Rennin, 95
Reuben Sandwich, 133
Rhubarb, 111
Rice: 82
   Bran, 77
   Cakes, 84
   Chips, 106
   Crisps, 77
   Dream, 20, 26
   Drinks, 20
   Polish, 82
   Pudding, 96
Rice-A-Roni, 58
Ricotta Cheese, 32
Risotto, 135
Roast Beef, 38
Rogan Josh, 135
Rolaids, 104
Root Beer, 126
Roti, 135
Rum, 131
Russian Dressing, 72
Rye, 81
Rye Bread, 83
Ryvita, 84

Safflower Seeds, 109
Saffron, 67
Sake, 131, 136
Salads: 122
   Dressings, 72
Salami, 42
Salmon, 47
Salsa, 70
Salt, 67
Sandwiches, 133
Sara Lee: Bagel, 83
   Muffins, 90
Sardines, 47
Sashimi, 136
Sauces, 68
Sauerkraut, 71, 119
Sausages, 41
Schmaltz, 136
Schnapps, 132
Scotch, 131
Scramblers, 35
Seasonings, 67
Seaweed, 109, 119
Seeds, 109
Seltzers, 126
Semolina, 81
Sesame Seeds, 109
Sesame Sticks, 106
Shakes, 21, 125
Shawourma, 137
Sherbet, 23
Shish Kabob, 137
Shooters, 132
Shrimps. 47
Silkworms, 138
Simple Pleasures, 26
Simply Lite Candy, 103
Slim-Fast, 125
Smoked Sausages, 41
Smucker's: Honey, 109
   Fruit Syrup, 99
Snacks, 105
Snack Cups, 96, 113
Snackers, 43
Snackwell's: Bars, 107
   Cakes, 95
   Muffins, 90
   Cookies, 88
Snapple, 117, 124
Snickers: 103
   Icecream Bar, 28
Soda, 126
Soft Drinks, 126
Somen, 82
Sorbet, 23
Sorbitol, 98

253

INDEX (S-Z)

Sorghum 81
Soup: 63-67
   Oyster Crackers, 63
Souplantation, 205
Sour Cream, 30
Sourdough, 83
Soursop, 112
Sousemeat, 138
Soy: Cheese, 33
   Flour, 81
   Milk, 20
   Sauce, 68
Soyagen, 20
Soybeans: 57-62, 118
   Flakes, 81
   Nuts, 108
   Products, 62
Spaghetti: 82, 135
   Sauce, 70
Spam, 42
Spices, 67
Spinach: 120
   Pie, 137
Spirits, 131
Spirulina, 109
Spleen, 40
Split Peas, 119
Sponge, 90
Sports Bars, 106
Sports Drinks, 125
Spreads, 29, 42, 109
Spring Roll, 134
Sprinklin's, 22
Squab, 134
Squid, 46
Ssips, 124
Starbucks, 26
Steak, 37
Strawberry, 112
Strudel, 90
Stuffing, 84
Succotash, 120, 138
Sugar, 98
Sukiyaki, 136
Sunflower Seeds, 109
Surimi, 47
Sushi, 135
Sustacal, 125
Sweet Rewards, 107
   Cakes, 95
   Muffins, 90
Syrups, 99

T-Bone Steak, 37
TAB, 127
Tabasco Sauce, 68

Tabouli, 122, 137
Taco: 84
   Bell, 211
   Shells, 84
Tahini: 109, 137
   Sauce, 137
Tail, 40
Tallow, 29
Tamales, 137
Tamarillo, 112
Tandoori Chicken, 135
Tang, 117, 127
Tapioca, 81, 96
Taramosalata, 135
Tartar Sauce, 68
Tarts, 92
Tea, 124
Tempeh, 61, 62
Temptations, 79
Tempura, 136
Teppan Yaki, 136
Tequila, 131, 137
Teriyaki Beef, 136
Teriyaki Sauce, 68
Three Bean Salad, 122
Tic Tac, 104
Tiger's Milk: 125
   Bars, 107
Toaster Pastry, 90
Toffees, 104
Tofu, 62
   Desserts, 26
Tom Collins, 132
Tomato, 112, 121
   Ketchup, 68
   Paste, 68
   Products, 69
   Puree, 68
   Sauce, 68
   Sundried, 121
Tongue, 40
Tonic Water, 126
Top Ramen, 58
Toppings, 99
Torte, 135
Tortellini, 135
Tortilla, 84
   Chips, 106
   Chips, 122
Tostada Shells, 84
Tostitos, 106
Totino's Pizza, 56
Trident, 102
Trifle, 96
Tripe, 40, 138
Triticale, 81

Tropicana, 124
Trout, 47
Tumeric, 67
Tuna: 47
   Helper, 58
   Spread, 42
Turkey: 42, 45
   Eggs, 35
   Fat, 29
   Franks, 41
   Jerky, 106
   Pastrami, 42
Turkish Coffee, 123
Turnovers, 90
Turtle: 138
   Eggs, 35
TVP, 62
Twix, 104
Tylenol, 109
Tyson, 45
Tzatziki, 34, 135

Ultra Slim Fast:
   Dressing, 76
   Icecream, 28

Veal: 39
   Cordon Bleu, 134
   Marsala, 135
Vegetables: 118-121
   Juice, 114
   Shortening, 29
   Snacks, 106
Vegetarian: Burgers, 59-64
   Meals, 59
   Products, 59
   Sausages, 41
Velveeta, 33
Venison, 40
Vermouth, 131
Vichyssoise, 134
Vienna Sausages, 41
Vietnamese Food, 138
Vine Leaves, 135
Vinegar, 68, 95
Vitamins, 109
Vitamite, 20
Vitari, 28
Vitasoy, 20, 61
Vodka, 131

Waffles, 97
Walnuts, 108
Wasa, 84
Water, 125

Watercress, 120
Watermelon: 112
   Seeds, 109
Weetabix, 81
Weider, 125
Weight Watchers:
   Cheese, 33
   Cookies, 89
   Desserts, 94
   Dressing, 76
   Icecream, 26, 28
   Meals, 54
   Muffins, 90
   Pizza, 56
   Salads, 122
   Snacks, 106
   Soup, 67
   Spreads, 29
   Yogurt, 22
Weiner Schnitzel, 135
Werther's Candy, 104
Westsoy, 20
Wheat: 81
   Bran, 77
   Flakes, 77
   Flour, 81
   Germ, 77
   Hearts, 77
Whey: 95
   Cheese, 32
Whipped Butter, 97
Whiskey, 131
Wild Rice, 82
Wine: 131
   Coolers, 131
Witloof, 118
Wonton, 134
Worcestershire, 68
Worthington, 62
Wraps, 133

Yam 120
Yeast: 95
   Cake, 134
   Tablets, 109
Yogurt: 22
   Candy, 104
   Raisins, 106

Ziti, 82
Zoglo's, 62
Zucchini, 120
Zushi, 136

Notes

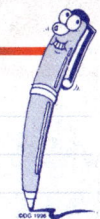

Feedback Welcome

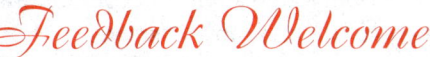

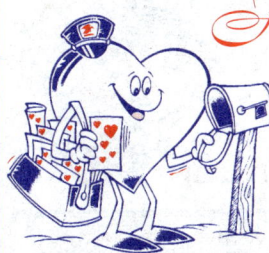

Your comments and suggestions for popular food products to be included in future editions are welcome.

Please write to:
Family Health Publications
PO Box 1616,
Costa Mesa, CA 92628
or Fax (714) 642 8900.

NO MORE EXCUSES!!

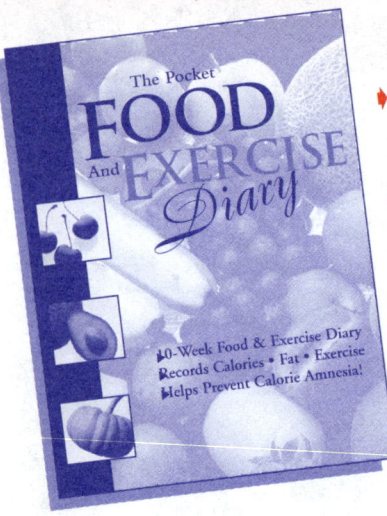

♦ Use this diary to record your food and exercise.

♦ You'll lose more weight and keep it off too!

♦ Records Calories, Fat & Exercise Calories

♦ Helps prevent 'Calorie Amnesia'!

10 Weeks (One Day Per Page)
Weekly Summary Pages

University studies show that persons who use a food diary not only lose more weight - they also keep it off!

The Pocket Food & Exercise Diary records both food and exercise. At day's end, you simply deduct exercise calories from food calories. Record fat grams too!

It's easy to use and most effective!

So get serious and start your diary today.
No more excuses!

A MUST!
For Serious Weight Control

FREE SAMPLE BOOK FOR DOCTORS CLINICS & HEALTH PROFESSIONALS
PUBLISHER: FAMILY HEALTH PUBLICATIONS ▪ PO BOX 1616 COSTA MESA, CA 92628
PHONE (714) 642 8500 ▪ FAX (714) 642 8900